The 50 Healthiest Habits and Lifestyle Changes

The 50 Healthiest Habits and Lifestyle Changes

Myrna Chandler Goldstein and
Mark Allan Goldstein, MD

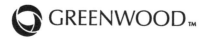 GREENWOOD™

An Imprint of ABC-CLIO, LLC
Santa Barbara, California • Denver, Colorado

Library of Congress Cataloging-in-Publication Data

Names: Goldstein, Myrna Chandler, 1948- author. | Goldstein, Mark A.
    (Mark Allan), 1947- author.
Title: The 50 healthiest habits and lifestyle changes / Myrna Chandler Goldstein
    and Mark Allan Goldstein, MD.
Other titles: Fifty healthiest habits and lifestyle changes
Description: Santa Barbara, California : Greenwood, an Imprint
    of ABC-CLIO, LLC, [2016] | Includes index.
Identifiers: LCCN 2016010070| ISBN 9781440834714 (alk. paper) |
    ISBN 9781440834721 (EISBN)
Subjects: LCSH: Health promotion. | Nutrition. | Health behavior.
Classification: LCC RA427.8 .G654 2016 | DDC 613—dc23
    LC record available at https://lccn.loc.gov/2016010070

ISBN: 978-1-4408-3471-4
EISBN: 978-1-4408-3472-1

20 19 18 17   2 3 4 5

This book is also available as an eBook.

Greenwood
An Imprint of ABC-CLIO, LLC

ABC-CLIO, LLC
130 Cremona Drive, P.O. Box 1911
Santa Barbara, California 93116-1911
www.abc-clio.com

This book is printed on acid-free paper ∞
Manufactured in the United States of America

Contents

Introduction ix

Forming and Reforming Habits xiii

Food and Healthy Eating 1

Avoid Unhealthy Diets and Weight-Loss Methods 1

Don't Skip Breakfast 6

Drink Sufficient Water 11

Eat Meals as a Family as Often as Possible 16

Eat More Local Foods 21

Eat Organically Grown Foods When Possible, Especially for Certain Foods 27

Eat the Recommended Amount of Fruits and Vegetables 32

Eliminate or Greatly Reduce the Trans Fats in Your Diet 38

Incorporate Healthier Snacks into Your Diet 43

Limit Fast Food Intake 48

Limit the Intake of Caffeine and Energy Drinks 53

Limit Processed Food 59

Limit Sodium and Salt Intake 64

Read Food Labels 69

Reduce Your Intake of Refined Sugar 76

Exercise and Physical Activity 85

Make Time for Frequent Exercise 85

Participate in Group Sports 91

Walk or Bike Instead of Driving Whenever Possible 97

Medical Care and Avoiding Medical Issues   **103**
Don't Use Antibiotics Unless Necessary   103
Get Vaccinated for Conditions That Affect Teens   109
Maintain Good Bone Density   114
Practice Excellent Home Dental Care   119
Prevent Vitamin D Deficiency   125
Protect Your Hearing   131
Take Care of Your Feet   137

Safety   **143**
Don't Text While Driving   143
Learn Ways to Prevent Violence   148
Prevent Sports Injuries   153
Use Protective Gear   158
Use Seatbelts   166

Mental, Emotional, and Social Health   **173**
Build Social Connections and Friendships with Peers   173
Build Your Resilience   178
Don't Become a Bully   183
Improve Self-Esteem   188
Maintain a Healthy Body Image   194
Practice Mindfulness   199

Sex and Dating   **205**
Get Screened for STIs   205
Get Vaccinated for HPV (Human Papillomavirus)   210
Cultivate Healthy Dating Relationships   216
Practice Safer Sex   221
Use Emergency Contraception When Necessary   227

Other Lifestyle Choices   **233**
Avoid Electronic Cigarettes   233
Avoid Indoor Tanning Beds   238
Get Enough Sleep   242
Improve Health Literacy Skills   249
Learn More About Internet Addiction   254
Limit Exposure to Electromagnetic Fields   260
Limit Screen Time   265
Reduce Stress   270
Use Sunscreen   276

Glossary   283

Index   289

About the Authors   305

Introduction

As a physician who completed special training in adolescent and young adult medicine and who founded and directs a division at Massachusetts General Hospital that meets the medical needs of this group of people, Mark A. Goldstein, MD, is always interested in ways to improve the lifestyle habits of his patients. That is why when he and his wife, Myrna Chandler Goldstein, were first approached to research and write a book on 50 healthy habits, they instantly replied in the affirmative. People who begin to follow healthier habits at younger ages are more likely to adhere to healthier lifestyles as they grow into their young adult years, their middle years, and eventually into their senior years.

Of course, teenagers are not the only people who have habits or regular and recurring patterns of behavior. People of all ages acquire habits. Even young children demonstrate them. What happens when a parent tries to read one bedtime story instead of three? The child will immediately plead for the other two. The child and parent have created the habit of three bedtime stories, and that is what the child wants and expects.

According to a study published in 2014 in the journal *Nursing and Midwifery Studies*, "the best time for establishing healthy lifestyle habits is during adolescence." In this cross-sectional descriptive study, researchers from Iran investigated the health-promoting behaviors of 424 high school students in Rasht, Iran, during the first semester of 2012. Students from both private and public schools were included in the cohort; all the students completed questionnaires. The researchers found that although the students tended to engage in health-promoting habits, there was room for improvement. Moreover, the male students participated in more health-promoting behaviors than the female students. On the other hand, the older students, who were working hard to gain admission into the competitive university system, tended to be too busy to adhere to healthy habits. The researchers emphasized that health instructors, teachers, and families need to pay more attention to these students to ensure that they follow healthy habits. "As most of lifelong healthy and unhealthy lifestyle habits are established during adolescence, developing effective health promotion and disease prevention strategies for adolescents seems crucial."[1]

These results are not uncommon. Large numbers of teens and young adults fail to follow healthy habits. A study published in 2015 in the journal *Collegium Antropologicum* investigated the nutritional knowledge and dietary habits of Croatian adolescents, but it could easily have described teens in many other locations throughout the world. The cohort consisted of 117 teens between the ages of 17 and 19 years; all the teens completed self-administered questionnaires. The researchers learned that less than one-third of the adolescents demonstrated adequate knowledge about nutrition and dietary habits. The males as well as teens from rural locations and teens who were overweight had even less knowledge than the others. Teens frequently skipped meals, especially breakfast, and males consumed high amounts of meat and meat products. Females and overweight females practiced fad dieting. The males consumed high amounts of soft drinks while the females ate too many sweets. Most of their nutrition and dietary information was obtained from television. Evidently, these teens, as well as countless numbers of teens throughout the world, need to make a number of changes in their everyday habits. These changes included eating more meals per day, eating breakfast, higher intakes of fish, and lower intakes of meat and sweetened food and drinks. The researchers noted that "the final outcome would result in long-term positive impact on dietary habits."[2]

And, intervention programs may improve habits. That is what Spanish researchers found in a study conducted during the 2013 to 2014 academic year and published in 2015 in the journal *Nutrición Hospitalaria*. A total of 158 students between the ages of 10 and 12 years were divided into an intervention group and a control group. For eight months, the researchers administered a Healthy Habits Program (HHP), a specially designed twice-weekly curriculum, to students in the intervention group. The students in the control group continued with their usual daily habits and did not participate in the program. In addition to the students, HHP included the parents and teachers of four schools. At the beginning of the study, there were no differences in eating habits between the two groups. By the end of the study, the intervention group had improved eating habits, and the eating habits of the members of the control group had worsened. The researchers commented that their findings demonstrated "that healthy lifestyle habits in adolescents are controllable and improvable, even in a relatively short period of time, despite this being a stage of life that is characterized by major changes, progressive independence and increased risk-taking."[3]

This book discusses 50 healthy habits that are useful for teens and young adults. But it also addresses barriers and problems associated with these habits. It is hoped that these entries serve as the foundation for interesting explorations and discussions.

NOTES

1. Azra Sadat Musavian, Afsaneh Pasha, Seyyedeh-Marzeyeh et al., "Health Promoting Behaviors Among Adolescents: A Cross-Sectional Study," *Nursing and Midwifery Studies* 3, no. 1 (April 2014): e14560.

2. Dragana Milosavljević, Milena L. Mandić, and Ines Banjari, "Nutritional Knowledge and Dietary Habits Survey in High School Population," *Collegium Antropologicum* 39, no. 1 (2015): 101–7.

3. Vicente Nebot Paradells, Ana Pablos Monzó, Laura Elvira Macagno et al., "Effects of An Intervention Program (HHP) on the Promotion of Healthy Habits in Early Adolescence," *Nutrición Hospitalaria* 32, no. 6 (2015): 2640–49.

Forming and Reforming Habits

Habit formation is the process by which new behaviors become automatic. People who awaken in the morning and quickly dress and go out for a run have developed a positive, life-supporting, healthy habit. On the other hand, people who begin their day with a hot drink filled with saturated fats and lots of chemicals have created an unhealthy habit, which may eventually have negative health consequences.

The formation of both good and not-so-good habits appears to have three essential steps. In the first step, there is a reminder or trigger that initiates that habit; in the second step, the behavior itself becomes routine; and, in the final step, there is a reward or benefit gained from doing the behavior. So, for example, if one wishes to remember to exercise, it might be a good idea to put sneakers or exercise clothing in a prominent place that cannot be ignored. Going out to exercise should serve as the second step. And, the reward comes with feeling so much better from the exercise itself and the knowledge that one had made regular exercise a true habit. During the process of habit formation, neural pathways are created in the brain. As the habits are repeated, the pathways become increasingly more secure. All brains are able to build new pathways, even those who have sustained an injury. So, everyone may build new positive habits and stop habits that negatively impact their lives.

When beginning a new habit, it is best to start small. Do not decide that you will be running two hours a day, every day. In the beginning, it is better to run every other day for 15 minutes. Then, over time, the running may be increased.

And, do not believe the notion that it may take weeks or months to create a true habit. Habit formation timing varies from person to person. In some, it may be quite quick; others may require longer periods of time. Motivation plays a key role. People who are truly motivated to implement a new positive habit into their life probably accomplish their goal without much delay.

There are a few theories about how habits are created. In a study published in 2016 in the *Journal of Health Economics*, researchers from Pennsylvania and Utah examined the role of short-term incentives in promoting healthy eating habits in children. Focusing on fruits and vegetables, the researchers implemented an incentive program at 40 elementary schools in Utah. The cohort included 8,000 students. Over a three- or five-week period of time, students received a small incentive—a special token—for eating at least one serving of fruits or vegetables during lunch. During the incentive period, these tokens produced a dramatic increase in fruit and vegetable consumption, and this behavior continued for at least two months after the incentive period ended. Once the rewards ended, the five-week incentive period appeared to produce a more sustained response than the three-week incentive period. The researchers noted that "there are many other positive health behaviors for which sustaining a period of active involvement can result in behavioral change persisting even after the incentive is removed and where an approach similar to the intervention described here could be effective."[1]

The role that incentives may play in habit formation was also addressed in a study published in 2016 in *Preventive Medicine*. Researchers from Minneapolis, Minnesota, wanted to estimate the effect of an incentive-based wellness program on self-reported exercise. They noted that since 2008, the University of Minnesota's Fitness Rewards Program has offered a $20-per-month incentive to encourage employees to use the fitness center. Employees who use the fitness center at least eight times a month received the $20 credit. Was this incentive making a difference? In a retrospective study that included 2,972 employees, the researchers determined that the incentive program led to an increase of 0.59 vigorous exercise days per week. While the employees who exercised the least before the program were less likely to participate, when they did, they had the largest increases in exercise compared to nonparticipants. The researchers concluded that incentives encouraged higher levels of exercise. "Participants of an incentivized, fit-based wellness program maintained higher levels of exercise than non-participants over a 3-year period."[2] And, when people exercised more, there was an increased potential that the exercise would develop into a habit.

Another study, which was conducted in the United Kingdom and published in 2013 in the *British Journal of Health Psychology*, examined the psychological determinants of habit formation from the perspective of dental flossing. The cohort consisted of 50 participants. All of the participants received a motivational intervention that was designed to trigger flossing behavior and flossing habit formation. The intervention focused on the benefits of flossing. Half of the participants were told to floss before brushing and half were instructed to floss after brushing. Participants self-reported their flossing behavior during the study, four weeks later, and at an eight-month follow-up. The researchers found that the participants with stronger prospective memory ability, with higher levels of past behavior, and with a more positive attitude flossed more frequently during the study. Those who flossed after brushing, rather than before brushing, tended to form stronger flossing habits. The researchers noted that their findings "suggested that factors additional to repetition, including the location of a new behaviour within existing routines, may aid the process of making behaviour automatic. In fact, successfully integrating a new action into a pre-existing everyday behavior pattern, or 'routine,' will increase the likelihood of consistent repetition and so lead to habit formation."[3]

In an article published in 2012 in the *British Journal of General Practice*, researchers from London outlined a role that medical practitioners may play in the development of positive habits. The researchers noted that patients often seek lifestyle advice from their healthcare providers. Still, such advice is not always provided. The researchers suggested that medical professionals give habit formation advice, and they offered the following format:

Make a New Healthy Habit

1. Decide on a goal that you would like to achieve for your health.
2. Choose a simple action that will get you toward your goal, which you can do on a daily basis.
3. Plan when and where you do your chosen action. Be consistent: choose a time and place that you encounter every day of the week.
4. Every time you encounter that time and place, do the action.
5. It will get easier with time, and within 10 weeks you should find you are doing it automatically without even having to think about it.
6. Congratulations, you've made a healthy habit![4]

NOTES

1. G. Loewenstein, J. Price, and K. Volpp, "Habit Formation in Children: Evidence from Incentives for Healthy Eating," *Journal of Health Economics* 45 (2016): 47–54.

2. Daniel J. Crespin, Jean M. Abraham, and Alexander J. Rothman, "The Effects of Participation in an Incentive-Based Wellness Program on Self-Reported Exercise," *Preventive Medicine* 82 (2016): 92–98.

3. Gaby Judah, Benjamin Gardner, and Robert Aunger, "Forming a Flossing Habit: An Exploratory Study of the Psychological Determinants of Habit Formation," *British Journal of Health Psychology* 18, no. 2 (May 2013): 338–53.

4. Benjamin Gardner, Phillippa Lally, and Jane Wardle, "Making Health Habitual: The Psychology of 'Habit-Formation' and General Practice," *British Journal of General Practice* 62, no. 605 (December 2012): 664–66.

REFERENCES AND RESOURCES

Magazines, Journals, and Newspapers

Crespin, Daniel J., Jean M. Abraham, and Alexander J. Rothman. "The Effects of Participation in an Incentive-Based Wellness Program on Self-Reported Exercise." *Preventive Medicine* 82 (2016): 92–98.

Gardner, Benjamin, Phillippa Lally, and Jane Wardle. "Making Health Habitual: The Psychology of 'Habit-Formation' and General Practice." *British Journal of General Practice* 62, no. 605 (2012): 664–66.

Judah, Gaby, Benjamin Gardner, and Robert Aunger. "Forming a Flossing Habit: An Exploratory Study of the Psychological Determinants of Habit Formation." *British Journal of Health Psychology* 18, no. 2 (2013): 338–53.

Loewenstein, G., J. Price, and K. Volpp. "Habit Formation in Children: Evidence from Incentives for Healthy Eating." *Journal of Health Economics* 45 (2016): 47–54.

Food and Healthy Eating

Avoid Unhealthy Diets and Weight-Loss Methods

OVERVIEW

During the teen years, when the body is rapidly changing, it is very common to be concerned about your weight and the shape of your body. For decades, the various media outlets have portrayed the ideal woman as pencil thin, a goal that most females can never attain. The media have also described scores of different diets. While the list of diets is too long to mention, it includes the South Beach diet, the blood-type diet, Weight Watchers, the Subway diet, Nutrisystem, Jenny Craig, the paleo diet, and the low-fat diet. They entice teens, and a host of other people, into different ways to drop the pounds. And, people on diets do lose weight. However, when they stop the diet, they tend to regain the weight, often adding even more pounds.

And, there are many teens who need to lose weight. According to the American Heart Association, about one in three teens is overweight or obese. In the United States, childhood obesity is now the top health concern of parents. Today, teens are being diagnosed with high blood pressure, type 2 diabetes, and elevated levels of cholesterol. The extra pounds also take a psychological toll. Severely overweight teens are at increased risk for low self-esteem, negative body image, and depression.[1]

In a study published in 2013 in the journal *Circulation*, researchers from several locations in the United States examined elements of cardiovascular health in 4,673 teens between the ages of 12 and 19 years from the 2005 to 2010 National Health and Nutrition Examination Surveys. The majority of the respondents were non-Hispanic white, non-Hispanic black, or Mexican American. The researchers found that high numbers of the teens had excellent blood pressure readings and did not smoke. They also did fairly well on blood glucose levels. However, females had fewer "ideal" total cholesterol levels than males and fewer "ideal" levels of physical activity than males. Only a small percentage of both males and females had an "ideal" diet. About two-thirds of all the teens had an "ideal" body mass index (BMI). The researchers noted that the "low prevalence of ideal cardiovascular health behaviors" in teens in the United States, especially physical activity and dietary intake, will contribute to a number of future health problems.[2]

So, there is obviously a need for large numbers of teens to lose some weight. But, there are healthier ways to lose weight and not-so-healthy ways to lose weight. Healthier ways to lose weight include increasing the intake of fruits, vegetables, and whole grains; reductions in the intake of fat; and moderate increases in exercise. Unhealthy weight loss methods include fasting, skipping meals, self-induced vomiting, diet pills, smoking cigarettes, and excess exercising. These behaviors are associated with a host of different medical and psychological problems such as nutritional deficiencies, particularly iron and calcium; menstrual irregularity; osteopenia; anorexia; and bulimia nervosa.

WHAT THE EXPERTS SAY

Teens Who Diet and Have Unhealthy Weight Control Behaviors Tend to Gain Weight

In a study published in 2012 in the *Journal of Adolescent Health*, researchers from Minneapolis and New York City examined the long-term effect on BMI of unhealthy dieting and weight control. The cohort consisted of 1,902 middle- and high-school adolescents who participated in Project EAT (Eating and Activity in Teens and Young Adults). This study followed students from Minneapolis and St. Paul for 10 years. Among the females, 37.8 percent reported persistent dieting and 43.7 percent noted continuous use of unhealthy weight control behaviors, such as eating little and skipping meals. These figures were, respectively, 10.3 percent and 18.7 percent in males. Still, when compared with the women who did not diet or practice unhealthy weight control behaviors, the women who engaged in these behaviors had higher BMI values when the study ended. So, the teens who practiced unhealthy dieting were heavier than the teens who did not. In fact, the researchers noted that "the large magnitude of the BMI increases associated with the use of these behaviors was a matter of concern."[3]

Family Meals May Help Prevent Unhealthy Dieting and Other Types of Disordered Eating in Teens

In a study published in 2015 in the *International Journal of Eating Disorders*, researchers from several locations in the United States wanted to learn more about the association between family meals and unhealthy dieting and disordered eating in teens. Surveys were completed by 2,382 middle and high school students with a mean age of 14.4 years and by 2,792 parents or guardians. Thirty-eight percent of the males and 50 percent of the females reported that they engaged in unhealthy weight control behaviors. The researchers found that the students who had more frequent family meals had a decreased risk of engaging in unhealthy weight control behaviors, such as unhealthy dieting. The researchers advised healthcare providers to make patients and their parents "aware that participating in regular family meals offers some protection for their teen against engaging in disordered eating behaviors."[4]

Unhealthy Diets Are Linked to Depression

In a study published in 2012 in the journal *Eating Behaviors*, researchers from Pennsylvania and New Jersey wanted to determine if there was an association between unhealthy dieting behaviors and depression. The cohort consisted of 198 young adults with a mean age of 24.8 years. Forty percent of the men were overweight; 25 percent were obese. Among the women, 22 percent were overweight and 8 percent were obese. All the participants completed questionnaires on health behaviors and attitudes. The researchers found that men and women with high BMIs were more likely to engage in both healthy and unhealthy dieting than the men and women with lower BMIs. In addition, women with symptoms of depression engaged in more unhealthy dieting practices and fewer healthy dietary practices. No such link between diets and depression was found in men. The researchers commented that "the association between depression and dieting behaviors among women, but not men, highlights the psychological nature of dieting for women."

BARRIERS AND PROBLEMS

Parents Have the Potential to Trigger Teens' Unhealthy Dieting

In a study published in 2013 in *JAMA Pediatrics*, researchers from Minneapolis, Minnesota, wanted to learn more about the effect parents have when they discuss healthful eating and weight with their adolescents. The cohort consisted of a socioeconomically and racially diverse sample of 2,793 teens with a mean age of 14.4 years and 3,709 parents or caregivers with a mean age of 42.3 years. The researchers learned that about 34 percent of the mothers and 38 percent of the fathers of adolescents who were not overweight did not have eating or weight talks with their teens. At the same time, 20 percent of the mothers and 23 percent of the fathers of overweight teens did not have these conversations. Meanwhile, about 28 percent of mothers and 23 percent of fathers of non-overweight teens and 15 percent of mothers and 14 percent of fathers of overweight teens had conversations that focused on healthful eating. And, about 33 percent of mothers and 32 percent of fathers of non-overweight teens and 60 percent of mothers and 59 percent of father of overweight teens had talks about weight or the need to lose weight. The researchers found that parental conversations about healthful eating were associated with the lowest levels of disordered eating behaviors, while parental conversations about weight were associated with the highest prevalence of disordered eating behaviors. According to the researchers, their findings "suggest that parents should avoid conversations that focus on weight or losing weight and instead engage in conversations that focus on healthful eating, without reference to weight issues." Moreover, "this approach may be particularly important for parents of overweight or obese adolescents."[5]

Adolescents Are Influenced by the Dieting and Disordered Eating Behaviors of Their Friends

In a cross-sectional study published in 2010 in the *Journal of Adolescent Health*, researchers from Minneapolis used the previously mentioned Project EAT survey to learn more about how friends of teens influenced their dieting and disordered eating behavior practices. A total of 2,516 teens provided data in 1998–1999 and at follow-up in 2003–2004. They provided information on their own chronic dieting, unhealthy weight control, extreme weight control, and binge eating; they also gave input on their friends' experiences with these behaviors. At baseline, one-third of the participants reported that their friends were "not at all" involved in dieting; 8.8 percent reported that their friends were "very involved." Females who reported more friends involved with dieting were more likely to report their own chronic dieting, extreme weight control behaviors, and binge eating five years later. Among the males, similar associations were seen in extreme weight control behaviors. In fact, the males who had friends who used extreme weight control behaviors at baseline were almost four times as likely to practice these behaviors five years later. The researchers noted that their work "is among the first longitudinal studies to demonstrate the influence of friends on disordered eating behaviors in a large and diverse sample of male and female adolescents." The researchers concluded that parents need to heighten their awareness about the dieting practices of the friends of their children. Schools need to conduct interventions within peer groups. And, healthcare providers need to ask more questions about the eating patterns of their patients' friends. "Ideas for dealing with peer behaviors—such as ignoring them, realizing they are not behaviors to adopt, or even raising one's concerns with a friend—can be discussed and explored with the adolescent."[6]

NOTES

1. American Heart Association, www.heart.org.
2. Christina M. Shay, Hongyan Ning, Stephen R. Daniels et al., "Status of Cardiovascular Health in US Adolescents: Prevalence Estimates from the National Health and Nutrition Examination Surveys (NHANES) 2005–2010," *Circulation* 127, no. 13 (2013): 1369–76.
3. Dianne Neumark-Sztainer, Melanie Wall, Mary Story, and Amber R. Standish, "Dieting and Unhealthy Weight Control Behaviors During Adolescence: Associations with 10-Year Changes in Body Mass Index," *Journal of Adolescent Health* 50 (2012): 80–86.

4. Katie Loth, Melanie Wall, Chien-Wen Choi et al., "Family Meals and Disordered Eating in Adolescents: Are the Benefits the Same for Everyone?" *International Journal of Eating Disorders* 48, no. 1 (2015): 100–110.

5. Jerica M. Berge, Rich MacLehose, Katie A. Loth et al., "Parents' Conversations About Healthful Eating and Weight," *JAMA Pediatrics* 167, no. 8 (2013): 746–53.

6. Marla E. Eisenberg and D. Neumark-Sztainer, "Friends' Dieting and Disordered Eating Behaviors Among Adolescents Five Years Later: Findings from Project EAT," *Journal of Adolescent Health* 47 (2010): 67–73.

REFERENCES AND RESOURCES

Magazines, Journals, and Newspapers

Amrock, Stephen M. and Michael Weitzman. "Adolescent Indoor Tanning Use and Unhealthy Weight Control Behaviors." *Journal of Development & Behavioral Pediatrics* 35, no. 3 (2014): 165–71.

Berge, Jerica M., Rich MacLehose, Katie A. Loth et al. "Parents' Conversations About Healthful Eating and Weight." *JAMA Pediatrics* 167, no. 8 (2013): 746–53.

Eisenberg, Marla E., and Dianne Neumark-Sztainer. "Friends' Dieting and Disordered Eating Behaviors Among Adolescents Five Years Later: Findings From Project EAT." *Journal of Adolescent Health* 47 (2010): 67–73.

Gillen, Meghan M., Charlotte N. Markey, and Patrick M. Markey. "An Examination of Dieting Behaviors Among Adults: Links with Depression." *Eating Behaviors* 13 (2012): 88–93.

Hirth, Jacqueline M., Mahbubur Rahman, and Abbey B. Berenson. "The Association of Posttraumatic Stress Disorder with Fast Food and Soda Consumption and Unhealthy Weight Loss Behaviors Among Young Women." *Journal of Women's Health* 20, no. 8 (2011): 1141–49.

Loth, Katie, Melanie Wall, Chien-Wen Choi et al. "Family Meals and Disordered Eating in Adolescents: Are the Benefits the Same for Everyone?" *International Journal of Eating Disorders* 48, no. 1 (2015): 100–110.

Mooney, E., H. Farley, and C. Strugnell. "A Qualitative Investigation into the Opinions of Adolescent Females Regarding Their Body Image Concerns and Dieting Practices in the Republic of Ireland." *Appetite* 52 (2009): 485–91.

Neumark-Sztainer, Dianne, Melanie Wall, Mary Story, and Amber R. Standish. "Dieting and Unhealthy Weight Control Behaviors During Adolescence: Associations with 10-Year Changes in Body Mass Index." *Journal of Adolescent Health* 50 (2012): 80–86.

Shay, Christina M., Hongyan Ning, Stephen R. Daniels et al. "Status of Cardiovascular Health in US Adolescents: Prevalence Estimates from the National Health and Nutrition Examination Surveys (NHANES) 2005–2010." *Circulation* 127, no. 13 (2013): 1369–76.

Web Site

American Heart Association. www.heart.org.

Don't Skip Breakfast

OVERVIEW

We all know that we should eat three meals each day. But, sometimes the day is filled with classes and work and household responsibilities, such as laundry and running errands. There is just too much to do. When time becomes so pressed, it is often easier to skip a meal, especially breakfast. Sure, one may be hungry, but skipping breakfast doesn't impact health. Or does it?

According to an article published in 2012 in the *British Journal of Nutrition*, researchers from Australia reported that it is not at all uncommon for teens, especially middle and late teens, to skip meals. However, this practice may have a "detrimental effect on multiple aspects of adolescent health." While breakfast provides the energy to begin the day, it is the meal that is most often missed. And, females are more likely than males to skip meals. The researchers underscored the fact that adolescent behaviors are "strongly influenced" by family, friends, and peers. Teens who have two parents who eat breakfast will tend to eat breakfast. But, as the teens grow older, friends and peers play a greater role in whether they skip meals. In fact, after 3,001 male and female teens from Victoria, Australia, completed a Web-based survey, these researchers found that teens who thought their best friend skipped meals were at increased risk for skipping breakfast and dinner. Male and female teens who thought that their mothers frequently didn't eat meals were at increased risk for skipping breakfast and lunch. The researchers maintained that their findings are important, "since little is known about the social influences of meal-skipping patterns of adolescents."[1]

WHAT THE EXPERTS SAY

Eating Breakfast May Reduce the Incidence of Obesity

In a study published in 2014 in the *Indian Journal of Endocrinology and Metabolism*, researchers from India examined the association between skipping breakfast and the prevalence of obesity. The cohort consisted of 186 subjects who visited a metabolic clinic. They were asked to complete a questionnaire on the food that they consumed during the previous 24 hours. The researchers found that 132 patients (71 percent) reported that they do not regularly consume breakfast. Of these, 84 (63.65 percent) were obese and 48 (36.3 percent) had a normal weight. Frequent breakfast eaters were more likely than non–breakfast eaters to have a normal body weight. When compared to males, more females were overweight; the difference between the males and females was statistically significant. "The skipping of breakfast impacted overweight positively."[2]

Consuming Breakfast May Reduce Behavioral Problems in Teens

In a 2012 study published in *Food & Nutrition Research*, researchers from Norway examined the association between dietary factors and behavioral problems in teens in Norway. The cohort consisted of 236 male and 239 female students who were in the ninth and tenth grades. The students completed questionnaires about their dietary intake and how they behaved in school. The researchers found that teens who frequently ate breakfast and a moderate amount of fruit and fish had a lower incidence of behavior problems at school. "Having an optimal diet and not skipping meals are associated with decreased odds of behavioral problems at school in Norwegian adolescents."[3]

Consuming a Protein-Rich Breakfast Is Associated with Increased Satiety

In a study published in 2010 in the *International Journal of Obesity*, researchers from Kansas City, Kansas, compared the impact of a normal protein breakfast to a protein-rich breakfast on appetite and food intake in adolescents who frequently skipped breakfast. The cohort consisted of 13 adolescents between the age of 13 and 17 years. During three separate five-hour testing periods completed on three different days, the teens had varied breakfast experiences. On one day, they ate a normal protein breakfast; on another day, they ate a protein-rich breakfast; and, on another day, they skipped breakfast. Blood samples were collected and questionnaires were completed. The researchers found that the participants who ate both types of breakfast had "increased satiety." When they ate the meal with extra protein, there were additional reductions in appetite and subsequent meal intake. The researchers noted that their findings support the consumption of a breakfast rich in protein. Perhaps, they noted, additional research on this topic will help "to identify whether acute changes lead to long-term alterations in daily appetite control, food intake and energy regulation when breakfast is consumed on a daily basis."[4]

Skipping Breakfast May Be Associated with Lower Bone Mineral Density

In a cross-sectional study published in 2013 in the *Asian Pacific Journal of Clinical Nutrition*, researchers from Japan investigated the association between consumption of breakfast and bone mineral density, the amount of calcium and other minerals that are in the body's bones. The cohort consisted of 275 Japanese female students between the ages of 19 and 25 years. The students completed questionnaires on their dietary habits and had medical tests, such as the Dexa scan, which measures bone density. The researchers found that the women were more likely to skip breakfast than they were to skip lunch or dinner. Moreover, the women who skipped breakfast were at increased risk for lower bone mineral density. "The frequency of skipping breakfast was an independent risk factor for lower hip BMD [bone mineral density], and the threshold for the effect was over 3 meals/week." The researchers concluded that "managing the frequency of skipping breakfast and reducing it to < 3 times per week may be beneficial for maintenance of bone health in younger women."[5]

BARRIERS AND PROBLEMS

Making Breakfast More Readily Available at School May Increase Consumption

In an article published in 2013 in the *Journal of School Nursing*, a school nurse from South Elgin, Illinois, noted that although there is good evidence that eating breakfast has a number of positive effects on students' academic achievement and psychosocial health, significant numbers of students do not eat breakfast. In general, students maintained that they missed breakfast because of a lack of time or an inability to eat early in the morning. Students also indicated that they did not want to participate in a breakfast program created for low-income students or to arrive earlier than the school starting time in order to eat breakfast. As a result, the author of the article described a breakfast program developed in her suburban high school "designed to provide students with opportunities to obtain a complete breakfast after the beginning of the school day." The goal was to "reduce barriers and provide healthy options." The school extended the breakfast cafeteria hours and offered a mobile cart filled with breakfast foods that students could purchase and consume during morning study hall classes. Though challenging to create, the breakfast program has been incredibly successful. "By the end of the school year, average daily school breakfast participation increased by more than 400 percent."[6]

Some People Have Limited Access to Food

In a qualitative study focused on in-depth discussion published in 2014 in *BMC Pediatrics*, researchers from South Africa explored some of the barriers to healthier eating among adolescent girls in rural South Africa. The cohort consisted of 11 pairs of female friends between the ages of 16 and 19 years. More than half of the participants commented that breakfast was the most important meal of the day. At the same time, "many did not eat breakfast at home owing to limited choices or lack of food." The researchers also observed that some participants noted that if they ate breakfast they would feel hungrier sooner and would not be able to concentrate in class. Moreover, few of the participants who ate breakfast had more than one option available. Participants who actually had lunch money commented that they had too little to purchase healthier options. So, they purchased "cheaper" snacks, such as deep-fried potato chips and sugar-sweetened beverages. Because of a lack of access to healthier foods, the researchers suggested that the participants would benefit from a free school-based breakfast program, which is not a common practice in the government-supported high schools. "School meal programmes should be expanded and improved as a contribution to healthy eating among adolescents who do not have sufficient access to healthy options at home."[7]

Cyberbullying and School Bullying Victimization May Be Associated with Skipping Breakfast

In a study published in 2014 in *Appetite*, researchers from Canada and the United Kingdom investigated the association between bullying and cyberbullying and breakfast skipping. Data were obtained from the Eastern Ontario 2011 Youth Risk Behavior Survey, a survey of middle and high school students between the ages of 11 and 20 years. The data included self-reported information from 3,035 students on breakfast eating habits and instances of bullying victimization. Slightly more than half of the students reported that they regularly did not eat breakfast. Interestingly, victims of both cyberbullying and school bullying were more likely to skip breakfast.

The researchers commented that their study is the first "to provide evidence of (a) troubling relationship between cyberbullying, school bullying, and breakfast skipping." The researchers advised parents who observe that their children are skipping breakfast to determine if their children are victims of cyberbullying and school bullying.[8]

NOTES

1. Natalie Pearson, Lauren Williams, David Crawford, and Kylie Ball, "Maternal and Best Friends' Influences on Meal-Skipping Behaviours," *British Journal of Nutrition* 108 (2012): 932–38.

2. Raksha Goyal and Sandeep Julka, "Impact of Breakfast Skipping on the Health Status of the Population," *Indian Journal of Endocrinology and Metabolism* 18, no. 5 (2014): 683–87.

3. Nina Øverby and Rune Høigaard, "Diet and Behavioral Problems at School in Norwegian Adolescents," *Food & Nutrition Research* 56 (2012): 17231+.

4. H. J. Leidy and E. M. Racki, "The Addition of a Protein-Rich Breakfast and Its Effects on Acute Appetite Control and Food Intake in 'Breakfast-Skipping' Adolescents," *International Journal of Obesity* 34 (2010): 1125–33.

5. T. Kuroda, Y. Onoe, R. Yoshikata, and H. Ohta, "Relationship Between Skipping Breakfast and Bone Mineral Density in Young Japanese Women," *Asian Pacific Journal of Clinical Nutrition* 22, no. 4 (2013): 583–89.

6. Julia Olsta, "Bringing Breakfast to Our Students: A Program to Increase School Breakfast Participation," *Journal of School Nursing* 29, no. 4 (2013): 263–70.

7. H. M. Sedibe, K. Kahn, K. Edin et al. "Qualitative Study Exploring Healthy Eating Practices and Physical Activity Among Adolescent Girls in Rural South Africa," *BMC Pediatrics* 14 (2014): 211+.

8. Hugues Sampasa-Kanyinga, Paul Roumeliotis, Claire V. Farrow, and Yuanfeng F. Shi, "Breakfast Skipping Is Associated with Cyberbullying and School Bullying Victimization. A School-Based Cross-Sectional Study," *Appetite* 79 (2014): 76–82.

REFERENCES AND RESOURCES

Magazines, Journals, and Newspapers

Cahill, Leah E., Stephanie E. Chiuve, Rania A. Mekary et al. "Prospective Study of Breakfast Eating and Incident Coronary Heart Disease in a Cohort of Male US Health Professionals." *Circulation* 128 (2013): 337–43.

Fujiwara, Tomoko, and Rieko Nakata. "Skipping Breakfast Is Associated with Reproductive Dysfunction in Post-Adolescent Female College Students." *Appetite* 55 (2010): 714–17.

Goyal, Raksha, and Sandeep Julka. "Impact of Breakfast Skipping on the Health Status of the Population." *Indian Journal of Endocrinology and Metabolism* 18, no. 5 (2014): 683–87.

Griffith, D. M., A. M. Wooley, and J. O. Allen. "'I'm Ready To Eat and Grab Whatever I Can Get': Determinants and Patterns of African American Men's Eating Practices." *Health Promotion Practice* 14, no. 2 (2013): 181–88.

Hernández-Diaz, S., C. E. Boeke, A. T. Romans et al. "Triggers of Spontaneous Preterm Delivery—Why Today?" *Paediatric and Perinatal Epidemiology* 28, no. 2 (2014): 79–87.

Kuroda, T., Y. Onoe, R. Yoshikata, and H. Ohta. "Relationship Between Skipping Breakfast and Bone Mineral Density in Young Japanese Women." *Asian Pacific Journal of Clinical Nutrition* 22, no. 4 (2013): 583–89.

Leidy, H. J., and E. M. Racki. "The Addition of a Protein-Rich Breakfast and Its Effects on Acute Appetite Control and Food Intake in 'Breakfast-Skipping' Adolescents." *International Journal of Obesity* 34 (2010): 1125–33.

Olsta, Julia. "Bringing Breakfast to Our Students: A Program to Increase School Breakfast Participation." *The Journal of School Nursing* 29, no. 4 (2013): 263–70.

Øverby, Nina, and Rune Høigaard. "Diet and Behavioral Problems at School in Norwegian Adolescents." *Food & Nutrition Research* 56 (2012): 17231+.

Pearson, Natalie, Lauren Williams, David Crawford, and Kylie Ball. "Maternal and Best Friends' Influences on Meal-Skipping Behaviours." *British Journal of Nutrition* 108 (2012): 932–38.

Sampasa-Kanyinga, Hugues, Paul Roumeliotis, Claire V. Farrow, and Yuanfeng F. Shi. "Breakfast Skipping Is Associated with Cyberbullying and School Bullying Victimization. A School-Based Cross-Sectional Study." *Appetite* 79 (2014): 76–82.

Sedibe, H. M., K. Kahn, K. Edin et al. "Qualitative Study Exploring Healthy Eating Practices and Physical Activity Among Adolescent Girls in Rural South Africa." *BMC Pediatrics* 14 (2014): 211+.

Web Site

Center for Young Women's Health. http://youngwomenshealth.org.

Drink Sufficient Water

OVERVIEW

You have heard these directives countless times. Drink sufficient water. Stay hydrated. Don't let yourself become too thirsty. Drinking adequate amounts of water is not only important during the sometimes scorching days of summer; it is essential to remain hydrated throughout the year.

According to the European Hydration Institute, water plays a crucial role in the maintenance of life. Water is found in all of the body's cells; about 60 percent of a man's body and 50 to 55 percent of a woman's body is water. Muscles and the brain are about 75 percent water; blood and kidneys are about 81 percent. Water provides cushioning and lubrication to the joints, and it "transports nutrients and carries waste away from the body cells." Water even plays a role in regulating the body's temperature; it redistributes body heat and cools the body by perspiring.[1]

While water requirements vary from person to person, larger people need more water than smaller people, and people who exercise require more water than people who are inactive. Of course, weather conditions influence water needs. People tend to drink more water when temperatures are elevated. Meanwhile, people continuously lose water from breathing, sweating, and the elimination of urine. So, people need a regular intake of water. When the body has an insufficient amount of water to function properly, it is dehydrated. Symptoms of dehydration include muscle weakness, rigidity or tremors, confusion, hallucinations, delirium, abnormal respiration, and in severe cases, death.[2]

It should be parenthetically noted that people who drink too much water may also become ill. Their electrolytes may become imbalanced, a condition known as hyponatremia, which has the potential to be life-threatening.

WHAT THE EXPERTS SAY

Supplementary Water Improves Cognitive Performance in School Children

In a study published in 2012 in *Appetite*, researchers from Italy, Switzerland, and Australia investigated the cognitive effects of children drinking supplemental water during the school day. The cohort consisted of 168 children. All of the children were randomly assigned to receive (93 children) or not receive (75 children) supplemental water. Over the course of a school day, the children in the supplemental group were given 1000 mL of water in two separate bottles, and the researchers assessed the students' cognitive abilities. Urine osmolality (a measure of the concentration of particles in urine) testing was used to evaluate hydration levels. The researchers found that the children with supplemental water drank an average of 624.5 mL of water. Two children did not drink any of their supplemental water, and 19 children drank all of it. The researchers found that the intake of water improved short-term memory. However, the researchers "also found that dehydrated children unexpectedly performed better on verbal analogy tests." According to the researchers, "even though dehydration might effect some cognitive abilities but not others, it is an adverse state that might render the school day more challenging for children."[3]

Intake of Water May Improve Exercise

In a study published in 2014 in *Nutrición Hospitalaria*, researchers from Mexico wanted to learn more about the effects of hydration on performance during spinning, a type of vigorous biking. The cohort consisted of 12 men and nine women; these amateur athletes participated in three controlled, randomly assigned hydration protocols (no fluid, plain water, or sports drink) during three different sessions of 90 minutes of spinning. The researchers found that exercising without the intake of fluids triggered physical stress in men and women. "Both men and women had higher values for body temperature, mean blood pressure and heart rate during the exercise without fluid replacement, confirming that dehydration provokes physical stress." If sufficient fluids are consumed, this physical stress may be avoided. "Consumption of plain water is sufficient for preventing physical stress in both genders, provided that an adequate volume is consumed to replace the loss of body fluid caused by sweating."[4]

Change in Water Intake May Influence Various Moods

In a study published in 2014 in *PLoS ONE*, researchers from France wondered if a change in the intake of water affected various moods in healthy adults. The cohort consisted of 22 people who drank 2.5 liters of water per day and 30 people who drank 1 liter of water per day. There were 11 men and 41 women. During the first two days of the inpatient study, the participants drank as they normally would. Then, during three controlled intervention days, the people who drank 2.5 liters per day were asked to drink 1 liter per day; similarly, the people who drank 1 liter per day were asked to increase their intake to 2.5 liters per day. To reduce the amount of water lost to physical activities, only sedentary activities, such as watching television and reading, were permitted. To assess the moods of the participants, the researchers conducted a number of evaluations. The researchers learned that increasing the water intake of normally low water drinkers prompted a number of beneficial outcomes. They were less fatigued, less confused, and less thirsty. On the other hand, reductions in water intake in people who normally drink larger amounts of water negatively impacted their moods. They reported that they were thirsty, less calm, less content, less vigorous, and had fewer positive emotions. The researchers concluded that "a switch toward an increase in water intake has especially beneficial effects on sleep/wake moods of habitual low-volume drinkers. The switch toward a decrease in water intake has detrimental effects on mood rating of habitual high-volume drinkers, including reduced feelings of calmness, satisfaction and positive emotions."[5]

In a crossover study, published in 2012 in the *Journal of Nutrition*, researchers from France and several locations in the United States examined the association between mild dehydration and moods in healthy young women. The cohort consisted of 25 females; they all participated in three day-long, placebo-controlled experiments. Each day, there were different states of hydration—exercise-induced hydration with no diuretic, exercise-induced hydration with diuretic, and normal state of hydration. A number of different experimental assessments were made. While dehydration did not appear to affect the women's cognitive performance, the researchers found that it had other consequences. When compared to their results when they were adequately hydrated, the mildly dehydrated women had reduced vigor and more fatigue and mood disturbances.

They found it harder to concentrate, and they experienced an increase in their perception of task difficulty. The researchers concluded that "in healthy young women, mild levels of dehydration result in adverse changes in key mood states such as vigor and fatigue as well as increased headaches and difficulty concentrating, without substantially altering key aspects of cognitive performance."[6]

BARRIERS AND PROBLEMS

Though we all hope to be sufficiently hydrated, consuming too few fluids, especially water, is very common. People tend to lead busy lives. Remembering how much water we drink is just one more thing to fit into an overscheduled life. But, a few suggestions may make dehydration less likely.

Try carrying a bottle of water with you. If you prefer, you can fill a glass with ice and water. Having water readily available is particularly important during warmer weather and while exercising. If you need to search for water, it is less likely that you will drink a sufficient amount. People who drink too little water sometimes contend that they don't like the taste of water. Adding lemon and/or lime or a little fruit to water takes only a minute or two. And, it does enhance the taste. One caveat should be noted. Unless you know that your water is unsafe to drink, in the vast majority of cases, it is not necessary to purchase bottled water. In the United States, most public water supplies are tested frequently. That is not the case for bottled water. In fact, some bottled water companies obtain their water from tap water. However, in a study published in 2012 in *Public Health Nutrition*, researchers from Atlanta, Georgia, and College Station, Texas, examined the perceptions of tap water safety in a cohort of 4,184 US adults aged 18 years and older. The researchers found that 13 percent of the respondents believed that their local tap water was not safe to drink and 26.4 percent thought bottled water was safer. These views of tap water varied according to age, income, education, region of the country, and race/ethnicity. These views were most common among "younger adults, lower socio-economic status populations and non-white racial/ethnic groups."[7]

While there are many studies on health problems related to the consumption of inadequate water and other fluids, there are relatively few studies on barriers that help prevent the intake of these fluids. In a study published in 2013 in *BMC Public Health*, researchers from Seattle, Washington, wanted to learn more about the prevention and treatment of heat-related illnesses in Latino farmworkers. One of these concerns is dehydration from the intake of too few fluids, especially water. The researchers conducted three semistructured Spanish-language focus group discussions with a total of 35 Latino farmworkers in Central Washington. Sixty percent of the workers were male; only 19 percent had more than a ninth grade education. All but one of the workers had become ill from heat. Yet, they failed to drink a sufficient amount of water to prevent heat-related illness. While they acknowledged that water was "the healthiest beverage to consume at work," the participants reported drinking soda, energy drinks, and coffee. Why not drink more water? The participants cited a variety of reasons. These ranged from not wanting to interrupt their work to worry about the safety and cleanliness of the water. Some wanted to sweat more in order to lose weight. One person said, "sometimes we don't drink water so we won't have to use the bathroom, because it's too far away."[8]

In a study published in 2013 in *Salud Pública de México* (*Public Health in Mexico*), researchers from Morelos, Mexico, wanted to determine what low-income adults in Cuernavaca, Mexico, knew about the consumption of water. A total of eight focus groups were conducted with either all men or all women; the men and women were between 21 and 59 years old. While some people praised water and said that it was refreshing, people also noted that water caused stomach upset, headaches, and other medical problems. The researchers suggest that these negative notions may create barriers for the consumption of water.[9]

NOTES

1. European Hydration Institute, www.europeanhydrationinstitute.org.

2. Ibid.

3. Roberta Fadda, Gertrude Rapinett, Dominik Grathwohl et al., "Effects of Drinking Supplementary Water at School on Cognitive Performance in Children," *Appetite* 59, no. 3 (2012): 730–37.

4. Arnulfo Ramos-Jiménez, Rosa Patricia Hernández-Torres, Abraham Wall-Medrano et al., "Gender- and Hydration-Associated Differences in the Physiological Response to Spinning," *Nutrición Hospitalaria* 29, no. 3 (2014): 644–51.

5. Nathalie Pross, Agnès Demazières, Nicolas Girard et al., "Effects of Changes in Water Intake on Mood of High and Low Drinkers," *PLoS ONE* 9, no. 4 (2014): e94754.

6. Lawrence E. Armstrong, Matthew S. Ganio, Douglas J. Casa et al., "Mild Dehydration Affects Mood in Healthy Young Women," *Journal of Nutrition* 142 (2012): 382–88.

7. Stephen J. Onufrak, Sohyun Park, Joseph R. Sharkey, and Bettylou Sherry, "The Relationship of Perceptions of Tap Water Safety with Intake of Sugar-Sweetened Beverages and Plain Water Among U. S. Adults," *Public Health Nutrition* 17, no. 1 (2012): 179–85.

8. Michelle Lam, Jennifer Krenz, Pablo Palmández et al., "Identification of Barriers to the Prevention and Treatment of Heat-Related Illness in Latino Farmworkers Using Activity-Oriented, Participatory Rural Appraisal Focus Group Methods," *BMC Public Health* 13 (2013): 1004+.

9. J. Espinosa-Montero, M. F. Aguilar-Tamayo, E. A. Monterrubio-Flores, and S. Barquera-Cervera, "Knowledge About Consumption of Plain Water in Adults of Low Socioeconomic Status of the City of Cuernavaca, México," *Salud Pública de México (Public Health in Mexico)* 55, Supplement 3 (2013): 423–30.

REFERENCES AND RESOURCES

Magazines, Journals, and Newspapers

Armstrong, Lawrence E., Matthew S. Ganio, Douglas J. Casa et al. "Mild Dehydration Affects Mood in Healthy Young Women." *Journal of Nutrition* 142 (2012): 382–88.

Espinosa-Montero, J., M. F. Aguilar-Tamayo, E. A. Monterrubio-Flores, and S. Barquera-Cervera. "Knowledge About Consumption of Plain Water in Adults of Low Socioeconomic Status of the City of Cuernavaca, México." *Salud Pública de México (Public Health in Mexico)* 55, Supplement 3 (2013): 423–30.

Fadda, Roberta, Gertrude Rapinett, Dominik Grathwohl et al. "Effects of Drinking Supplementary Water at School on Cognitive Performance in Children." *Appetite* 59, no. 3 (2012): 730–37.

Holdsworth, J. E.. "The Importance of Human Hydration: Perceptions Among Healthcare Professionals Across Europe." *Nutrition Bulletin* 37 (2012): 16–24.

Lam, Michelle, Jennifer Krenz, Pablo Palmández et al. "Identification of Barriers to the Prevention and Treatment of Heat-Related Illness in Latino Farmworkers Using Activity-Oriented, Participatory Rural Appraisal Focus Group Methods." *BMC Public Health* 13 (2013): 1004+.

Lindseth, Paul D., Glenda N. Lindseth, Thomas V. Petros et al. "Effects of Hydration on Cognitive Function of Pilots." *Military Medicine* 178, no. 7 (2013): 792–98.

Liu, J., X. Hu, Q. Zhang et al. "Knowledge, Attitude, and Practice on Drinking Water of Primary and Secondary Students in Shenzhen." *Wei Sheng Yan Jiu (Journal of Hygiene Research)* 43, no. 3 (2014): 419–22.

Onufrak, Stephen J., Sohyun Park, Joseph R. Sharkey, and Bettylou Sherry. "The Relationship of Perceptions of Tap Water Safety with Intake of Sugar-Sweetened Beverages and Plain Water Among U. S. Adults." *Public Health Nutrition* 17, no. 1 (2012): 179–85.

Pawson, Chris, Mark R. Gardner, Sarah Doherty et al. "Drink Availability is Associated with Enhanced Examination Performance in Adults." *Psychology Teaching Review* 19, no. 1 (2013): 57–66.

Pross, Nathalie, Agnès Demazières, Nicolas Girard et al. "Effects of Changes in Water Intake on Mood of High and Low Drinkers." *PLoS ONE* 9, no. 4 (2014): e94754.

Ramos-Jiménez, Arnulfo, Rosa Patricia Hernández-Torres, Abraham Wall-Medrano et al. "Gender- and Hydration-Associated Differences in the Physiological Response to Spinning." *Nutrición Hospitalaria* 29, no. 3 (2014): 644–51.

Senterre, Christelle, Michèle Dramaix, and Isabelle Thiébaut. "Fluid Intake Survey Among Schoolchildren in Belgium." BMC *Public Health* 14 (2014): 651+.

Web Site

European Hydration Institute. www.europeanhydrationinstitute.org.

Eat Meals as a Family as Often as Possible

OVERVIEW

It may be difficult to imagine, but a few generations ago, families routinely ate meals together. This was especially true for breakfast and dinner. While breakfast might be a little rushed and lunch would likely be away from home, there was time for a more restful dinner. In general, after a long day of work outside the home, the father would return, and the family would sit around the table eating the food prepared by the mother. Each dinner, which included a salad, an entrée, and a dessert, could easily take 20 to 30 minutes or more to consume.

Today, such a daily scenario is hard to imagine. With both parents often working outside the home and with kids' schedules filled with afterschool activities, eating on the run has become fairly common. In fact, in many households, Monday through Friday family dinners are rare; even Saturday and Sunday family dinners may be difficult to coordinate.

Yet, according to researchers, the lack of time for family dinners is a truly unfortunate situation. People who are able to arrange these meals with some degree of regularity appear to obtain a number of benefits. There is even a Cambridge, Massachusetts, organization dedicated to supporting family dinners—the Family Dinner Project.

WHAT THE EXPERTS SAY

According to the Family Dinner Project Web site, "most American families are starved for time to spend together." In fact, "dinner may be the only time of the day when we can reconnect." During a family dinner, family members may "relax, recharge, laugh, tell stories and catch up on the day's ups and downs, while developing a sense of who we are as a family."[1]

The Family Dinner Project Web site notes that the children of families who eat together have lower rates of substance abuse, teen pregnancy, and depression as well as higher grades in school and better levels of self-esteem. Conversation at the dinner table fosters improved vocabulary and resilience. Children and teens who eat with their families have lower rates of obesity and eating disorders. However, it should be noted that meals consumed while watching television do not have the same mental health benefits as those filled with conversation.[2]

Improvements in Nutritional Health

In a study published in 2011 in *Pediatrics*, researchers from the University of Illinois, Urbana-Champaign, conducted a meta-analysis of 17 studies to determine the association between shared family meals and the nutritional health of children and teens. Their analysis included a total of 182,836 children and teens and focused on the three major public health concerns of obesity, unhealthy eating, and disordered eating. The researchers found that the frequency of shared family meals is "significantly related" to the nutritional health of children and teens. "Overall, families that eat five or more meals together have children who are [about] 25% less likely to encounter nutritional health issues than children who eat [less than] one meal with their families." Thus, "shared meals seem to operate as a protective factor for overweight, unhealthy eating, and disordered eating."[3]

In a study published in 2013 in the *Journal of Epidemiology & Community Health*, researchers from the United Kingdom wanted to learn more about how the home environment of children affected their intake of fruits and vegetables. The cohort consisted of 2,383 children with a mean age of 8.3 years; all of the children attended London primary schools. The researchers learned that the children from families that reported "always" eating family meals ate 125 g more fruits and vegetables than families who never ate meals together. Likewise, when compared to parents who rarely or never consumed fruits and vegetables, the daily consumption of fruits and vegetables by parents was associated with higher fruit and vegetable intake of children. Interestingly, when parents cut up the fruits and vegetables, the children ate 44 g more than the children in families where parents did not cup up the fruits and vegetables. The researchers concluded that their findings "illustrate a positive public health message for parents, which could improve their own dietary habits and their children's. The key message from this research is for families to eat fruit and vegetables together at a mealtime."[4]

Helps Control Weight

In a study published in 2011 in *Applied Physiology, Nutrition, and Metabolism*, researchers from Ontario, Canada, investigated the association between the frequency of family meals and body mass index (BMI) in male and female teens. The cohort consisted of 734 male teens and 1,030 female teens with a mean age of 14.12 years. The researchers learned that 62 percent of the overall sample reported participating in family meals every day. Males had a significantly higher participation in daily family meals than females. Yet, the researchers found that a higher frequency of family meals was associated with a lower BMI in female teens but not male teens. "These findings are independent of the potential cofounding effects of parental education, adolescent's age, and snack-food eating."[5]

Fosters Overall Healthy Eating

In a study published in 2013 in *Public Health Nutrition*, researchers from the University of Texas in Austin explored the association between family meals and parental encouragement of healthy eating. The cohort consisted of 2,895 Texas eighth grade students. About half of the children were Hispanic and about one-fourth of them were white. They were divided into three groups—those who ate family meals seven or more times per week, those who ate family meals three to six times per week, and those who ate family meals no more than two times per week. The researchers also created a means to assess how often parents encouraged their children to eat fruits and vegetables, drink water, eat wholegrain bread, eat breakfast, and drink low-fat milk. The researchers found that white students averaged 4.4 family meals during the previous seven days; Hispanic youth had 4.2, and African American youth had 3.7. And, family meal frequency was "significantly associated with encouragement of healthy eating." Moreover, there were no significant differences between the various ethnic groups. According to the researchers, "this suggests that regardless of ethnic differences, parental encouragement may provide the link between family meals and positive dietary benefits for youth."[6]

Reduces Risk of Substance Abuse

In a study published in 2008 in the *Journal of Adolescent Health*, researchers from the University of Minnesota, Minneapolis, reviewed five-year longitudinal associations between family meal patterns and substance abuse in teens. The cohort consisted of 806 Minnesota teens who were interviewed when they had a mean age of 12.8 years and surveyed by mail when they had a mean age of 17.2 years. The researchers found that with the female teens family meals were correlated with significantly lower odds of cigarette smoking, alcohol use, and marijuana use. "Female adolescents reporting regular family meals had odds of cigarette smoking, alcohol use, and marijuana use at follow-up that were approximately half the odds for females who did not report regular family meals at baseline." This relationship was not seen with the male teens. The researchers concluded that "regular family meals in adolescence may have a long-term protective association with the development of substance use over 5 years among female adolescents."[7]

May Help Prevent Disordered Weight Control Behaviors

In a study published in 2013 in *Academic Pediatrics*, researchers from several locations in Massachusetts and Ann Arbor, Michigan, investigated how family meals influence the development of disordered weight control behaviors, such as vomiting, and taking laxatives and diet pills without a prescription. The cohort consisted of 15,641 male and female students in the sixth and eighth grades; a total of 47 Massachusetts middle schools participated. As they had anticipated, the researchers found that the frequency of family meals was associated with a reduced risk of the development of disordered weight control behaviors in both girls and boys. This "protective effect" proved to be "consistent across race/ethnicity and weight status in a large, diverse sample of middle school youth." The researchers advised parents to make time for more family meals. "Health care providers, including clinicians and pediatricians, should consider discussing the multiple beneficial effects associated with family meal frequency with parents and children as part of a family-centered approach to promote healthy weight-related behaviors."[8]

BARRIERS AND PROBLEMS

Most likely, many people do not realize the value of family meals. In today's world, where both parents often work full-time, demanding jobs, it is not uncommon for meals to be rushed, eaten in the car or in front of the television or computer screen. Making time for family meals is just one more thing for overscheduled parents to coordinate . By the end of a long day, parents may be simply grateful to put together some sort of dinner for their hungry children. They know that their daily responsibilities are far from over. Parents may need to clean the dishes, help with homework, and find time to wash and dry a few loads of laundry. Nevertheless, there is some research on dealing with barriers to family meals.

In a study published in 2011 in *Journal of Nutrition Education and Behavior*, researchers from Minneapolis, Minnesota, and San Diego, California, conducted focus groups with working parents of children between the ages of 8 and 10 years. They wanted to learn more about the barriers that parents face concerning family meals; they also wanted to collect ideas on interventions that could facilitate the frequency of these meals. More than half of the parents reported have family dinners at least three times per week. During the work week, the primary reason for not having more family dinners was "time constraints" such as work schedules and the children's extracurricular activities. "Parent comments consistently revealed how difficult it is for parents to prepare meals with time constraints and other responsibilities." Moreover, parents are often multitasking during dinner. So, while they may be nearby, parents are not necessarily interacting with their children. "Parents reported going through the mail, reading their children's homework or school-related notes, cleaning and other household chores."[9]

Another study on the barriers of family meals was published in 2010 in the *Journal of the American Dietetic Association*. The researchers, from the National Institutes of Health in Bethesda, Maryland; the Joslin Diabetes Center in Boston, Massachusetts; and the Virginia Commonwealth University in Richmond, Virginia, conducted 21 focus groups with parents and children between the ages of 8 and 20 years. Both the parents and children agreed that their major barrier to family meals was busy schedules. It is difficult to find the time to sit down together. "Discussions centered around family members' different schedules, including adolescents frequently being away from home. Youth referenced sports and other after-school activities; parents additionally referenced work schedules and teenagers' part-time jobs."[10]

NOTES

1. The Family Dinner Project, http://thefamilydinnerproject.org.

2. Ibid.

3. Amber J. Hammons and Barbara H. Fiese, "Is Frequency of Shared Family Meals Related to the Nutritional Health of Children and Adolescents?" *Pediatrics* 127, no. 6 (2011): e1565–e1574.

4. Meaghan S. Christian, Charlotte E. L. Evans, Neil Hancock et al., "Family Meals Can Help Children Reach Their 5 a Day: a Cross-Sectional Survey of Children's Dietary Intake from London Primary Schools," *Journal of Epidemiology & Community Health* 67, no. 4 (2013): 332–38.

5. Gary S. Goldfield, Marisa A. Murray, Annick Buchholz et al., "Family Meals and Body Mass Index Among Adolescents: Effects of Gender," *Applied Physiology, Nutrition, and Metabolism* 36 (2011): 539–46.

6. Natalie S. Poulos, Keryn E. Pasch, Andrew E. Springer et al., "Is Frequency of Family Meals Associated with Parental Encouragement of Healthy Eating Among Ethnically Diverse Eighth Graders?" *Public Health Nutrition* 17, no. 5 (2013): 998–1003.

7. Marla E. Eisenberg, Dianne Neumark-Sztainer, Jayne A. Fulkerson et al., "Family Meals and Substance Use: Is There a Long-Term Protective Association?" *Journal of Adolescent Health* 43 (2008): 151–56.

8. Monica L. Wang, Karen E. Peterson, Tracy K. Richmond et al., "Family Physical Activity and Meal Practices Associated with Disordered Weight Control Behaviors in a Multiethnic Sample of Middle-School Youth," *Academic Pediatrics* 13, no. 4 (2013): 379–85.

9. Jayne A. Fulkerson, Martha Y. Kubik, Sarah Rydell et al., "Focus Groups with Working Parents of School-Aged Children: What's Needed to Improve Family Meals?" *Journal of Nutrition Education and Behavior* 43, no. 3 (2011): 189–93.

10. Alisha J. Rovner, Sanjeev N. Mehta, Denise L. Haynie et al., "Perceived Benefits, Barriers, and Strategies of Family Meals Among Children with Type 1 Diabetes and Their Parents," *Journal of the American Dietetic Association* 110, no. 9 (2010): 1302–6.

REFERENCES AND RESOURCES

Magazines, Journals, and Newspapers

Christian, Meaghan S., Charlotte E. L. Evans, Neil Hancock et al. "Family Meals Can Help Children Reach Their 5 a Day: A Cross-Sectional Survey of Children's Dietary Intake from London Primary Schools." *Journal of Epidemiology & Community Health* 67, no. 4 (2013): 332–38.

Eisenberg, Marla E., Diane Neumark-Sztainer, Jayne A. Fulkerson et al. "Family Meals and Substance Use: Is There a Long-Term Protective Association?" *Journal of Adolescent Health* 43 (2008): 151–56.

Fink, Sara K., Elizabeth F. Racine, Rebecca E. Mueffelmann et al. "Family Meals and Diet Quality Among Children and Adolescents in North Carolina." *Journal of Nutrition Education and Behavior* 46 (2014): 418–22.

Fulkerson, Jayne A., Martha Y. Kubik, Sarah Rydell et al. "Focus Groups with Working Parents of School-Aged Children: What's Needed to Improve Family Meals?" *Journal of Nutrition Education and Behavior* 43, no. 3 (2011): 189–93.

Goldfield, Gary S., Marisa A. Murray, Annick Buchholz et al. "Family Meals and Body Mass Index Among Adolescents: Effects of Gender." *Applied Physiology, Nutrition, and Metabolism* 36 (2011): 539–46.

Hammons, Amber J. and Barbara H. Fiese. "Is Frequency of Shared Family Meals Related to the Nutritional Health of Children and Adolescents?" *Pediatrics* 127, no. 6 (2011): e1565–e1574.

Larson, Nicole, Jayne Fulkerson, Mary Story et al. 2012. "Shared Meals Among Young Adults are Associated with Better Diet Quality and Predicted by Family Meal Patterns During Adolescence." *Public Health Nutrition* 16, no. 5 (2012): 883–93.

Poulos, Natalie S., Keryn E. Pasch, Andrew E. Springer et al. "Is Frequency of Family Meals Associated with Parental Encouragement of Healthy Eating Among Ethnically Diverse Eighth Graders?" *Public Health Nutrition* 17, no. 5 (2014): 998–1003.

Rovner, Alisha J., Sanjeev N. Mehta, Denise L. Haynie et al. "Perceived Benefits, Barriers, and Strategies of Family Meals Among Children with Type 1 Diabetes and Their Parents: Focus Group Findings." *Journal of the American Dietetic Association* 110, no. 9 (2010): 1302–6.

Wang, Monica L., Karen E. Peterson, Tracy K. Richmond et al. "Family Physical Activity and Meal Practices Associated with Disordered Weight Control Behaviors in a Multiethnic Sample of Middle-School Youth." *Academic Pediatrics* 13, no. 4 (2013): 379–85.

Web Site

The Family Dinner Project. http://thefamilydinnerproject.org.

Eat More Local Foods

OVERVIEW

Until fairly recent times, people only ate locally produced foods. Long distance transportation of food was essentially nonexistent. Food was grown and purchased locally, whether in markets or small stores. By the latter portion of the 19th century, when trains began to travel across the American landscape, that started to change. Over time, our food system has become more industrialized and removed from urban areas.

Still, there have always been people who prefer to eat locally produced food. Eating food that was harvested earlier in the day directly from a farmer must be fresher, tastier, and, sometimes, less costly. Over the past few years, there has been an increasing momentum to consume more local products, especially during the growing seasons. In an article that appeared on the Web site of the University of Vermont, an author listed reasons to buy local food. He noted the fact that local foods, which do not travel long distances, look and taste better, and they are healthier and able to retain more nutrients. Local foods preserve genetic diversity, and they are safer. Moreover, local foods help to support farmers, who contribute more in taxes than they require in services, and they preserve open space and help to build community and the future. "By supporting local farms today, you are helping to ensure that there will be farms in your community tomorrow."[1]

At the same time, the U.S. Department of Agriculture (USDA) reported in 2014 that farmers who sell directly to consumers represent "a very small share" of the national food supply. On average, between 1978 and 2007, only 5.5 percent of all farms sold products directly to consumers. And, that is only 0.3 percent of total farm sales. But, in recent years, that trend has been changing. Increasingly, farmers are finding ways to sell more of their products, especially fruits, vegetables, and nuts, directly to consumers. This is especially true in the Northeast and the West Coast, where there are thousands of summer and winter farmers' markets and community supported agriculture (CSA) groups, programs in which members prepay to receive regular, usually weekly, food products during the growing seasons. The USDA also noted that when farmers sell directly, consumers have access to unusual and heirloom varieties that might be difficult to locate and more fragile products that might be harder to transport.[2]

According to Local Harvest, a nonprofit that "connects people looking for good food with the farmers who produce it," most produce in the United States travels four to seven days before reaching supermarket shelves. Typically, it is shipped 1,500 miles. Of course, produce from other countries travels even longer distances. When food is purchased at large supermarkets, only 18 cents of every dollar goes to the grower. The other 82 cents "go to various unnecessary middlemen."[3]

One cannot help but ask, who are the people buying local food? That was addressed in a cross-sectional analysis published in 2013 in the *Journal of Nutrition Education and Behavior* by researchers from North Carolina, Maryland, and, Utah, who used data from the 2008 North Carolina Child Health Assessment and Monitoring Program. The cohort consisted of 2,932 households with at least one child under the age of 17. The researchers found that during the previous year about half of the participants purchased local fruits and vegetables about once a month, and, they noted that this finding is consistent with a national study on the topic. In addition, families in which children ate more than five servings of fruits and vegetables per day were more likely to buy local produce. African American families were less likely than white or Hispanic families to buy local produce. Moreover, people living in more rural areas bought greater amounts of local produce. Perhaps, the researchers speculated, this is because they live closer to farmers. Although other researchers have found no income differences in buying local food, these researchers learned that those with annual incomes lower than $25,000 bought more local produce than people with annual incomes of $50,000 or more.[4]

WHAT THE EXPERTS SAY

Children Who Grow Their Own Fruits and Vegetables Eat More Produce

In a study published in 2009 in the *Journal of the American Dietetic Association*, researchers from Minnesota wanted to determine if participating in twice-weekly garden-based activities would promote fruit and vegetable intake among 93 fourth to sixth grade children who attended a 12-week YMCA summer camp. Using produce from their garden, the children prepared snacks. In addition, each week the children tasted a fruit and/or vegetable from a farmers market. The researchers found that almost all the children enjoyed the garden and produce-related activities. In fact, some of the children expressed a desire to spend more time working in the garden. Only 5 percent of the children noted that they did not want to participate again the next summer. After completing the program, the children reported a significant increase in the intake of fruits and vegetables. The researchers commented that "participation in the 'seed to table' experience of eating may help promote healthful eating behaviors among youth."[5]

Members of Community Supported Agriculture Programs Eat More Fruits and Vegetables

In a study published in 2012 in *Appetite*, researchers from Phoenix, Arizona, asked members of Arizona's community supported agriculture (CSA) programs to complete an online survey, which included questions on behaviors related to food purchases. The researchers received 115 responses. One section of the survey asked how membership in the CSA influenced the variety and amount of produce that their household consumed. The vast majority of the respondents were white females. Almost 70 percent indicated that they were the primary food purchaser. The researchers learned that 67.5 percent of the respondents noted that since joining the CSA they were eating more fruits and vegetables. An even larger number, 92.1 percent of the members, reported eating a greater variety of fruits and vegetables. The researchers commented that "community supported agriculture (CSA) programs have become a viable source of locally produced foods and represent a new way to increase fruit and vegetable consumptions among individuals."[6]

In a randomized, controlled study published in 2013 in *Preventing Chronic Disease*, researchers based in North Carolina wanted to learn if a CSA "intervention" would increase the inventory and consumption of fruits and vegetables in the homes of low-income women and their children. The researchers recruited

50 low-income women who had children. From May to September of 2012, 25 of the women were offered five educational sessions and a box of fresh produce for 16 weeks; the other 25 women were not offered any sessions and did not receive any fresh produce. Participants in both groups were interviewed by telephone at baseline and after the program was completed. Almost all of the participants in the intervention group found it challenging to attend the educational sessions and pick up the box of produce. Many of them worked multiple jobs, had little workplace flexibility, and needed to rely on public transportation. So, on average, they picked up food only nine of the 16 weeks. Yet, the vast majority indicated that if the program were offered again, they would want to participate. The researchers found that the participants in the intervention group had more variety in their produce intake. The researchers concluded that "CSA is a feasible approach for providing fresh fruits and vegetables to an underresourced community."[7]

Shoppers at Farmers' Markets Eat More Fruits and Vegetables

In a study published in 2013 in *Public Health Nutrition*, researchers from North Carolina examined the association between different shopping patterns and various parameters of health. The cohort consisted of 400 low-income, nonstudent women between the ages of 18 and 44 years who lived in eastern North Carolina. One hundred and fourteen women reported that they shopped at farmers' markets. According to the researchers, they were more likely to consume five or more fruits and vegetables every day.[8]

BARRIERS AND PROBLEMS

Local Food May Not Be the Best Alternative

In an article published in 2010 in the *Proceedings of the Nutrition Society*, a professor at Bangor University, Wales, analyzed the notion that the consumption of local food is more nutritious and better for the environment. The researcher noted that it is widely believed that food that travels longer distances triggers the release of more greenhouse gases. But transportation, the researcher wrote, "is only part of the overall food system." And, different types of transportation vary in the levels of greenhouse gases that they emit. Moreover, there is a seasonality associated with many foods. As a result, during the off-season times, they must be stored, often in a cooled or frozen area. The storage of the food also produces greenhouse gases. And, sometimes, local food is not the best option. For example, in the United Kingdom tomatoes are grown in glasshouses, which are heated with fossil fuel. On the other hand, tomatoes grown in Spain can be grown outside in open fields and then transported to the United Kingdom. Still, the researcher acknowledged that the nutritional quality of fruits and vegetables is the highest right after harvest. "So if local systems could supply fresh food to consumers within a very short time after harvest, then this food would be of high nutritional quality." However, all too often, those conditions do not exist. The researcher commented that his findings "do not offer any support for claims that local food is universally superior to non-local food in terms of its impact on the climate or the health of consumers."[9]

Food Safety Practices May Be Less Than Ideal

In a study published in 2015 in the *Journal of the Science of Food and Agriculture*, researchers from California and Seattle wanted to learn more about the safety of food sold at farmers markets in Los Angeles, Orange County, California, and the greater Seattle area. Researchers collected a total of 133 samples (52 basil, 41 cilantro, and 40 parsley) from 13 different farmers markets. Markets were selected based on their proximity to research labs; the researchers wanted the samples to be analyzed the same day they were purchased. All of the herbs were tested for *Salmonella* and *Escherichia coli* (*E. coli*). One parsley sample was found positive for *Salmonella*, and 24.1 percent of the samples were positive for *E. coli*. The researchers noted that there is a need to determine how this level of contamination compares to other retail sources of these herbs. The researchers noted that in supermarkets fresh herbs are held in refrigerated areas; at farmers markets, they are placed outside, even during very warm summer days. And, they concluded that "the current study, along with future research in this area, will be important in heightening our understanding of the safety of perishable foods sold at farmers' markets."[10]

People Living in "Food Deserts" May Have Limited Access to All Food, Not Just Local Produce

In a study published in 2014 in the *Asian Pacific Journal of Clinical Nutrition*, researchers from Australia examined the food options available for Australian residents who live in remote areas in the western part of the country. The researchers found that while the food costs significantly increased in remote areas, the quality of the food decreased markedly. The healthiest foods, such as fruits and vegetables, tended to cost "disproportionately more." However, oranges, which were grown locally, were rated better. So, these Australians had access to some local food. The researchers suggested that the government provide subsidies for the transport of fresh foods. According to the researchers, it has been shown that reductions in the cost of food have resulted in the consumption of healthier foods.[11]

NOTES

1. University of Vermont, www.uvm.edu.
2. U.S. Department of Agriculture, www.usda.gov.
3. Local Harvest, www.localharvest.org.
4. Elizabeth R. Racine, Elizabeth A. Mumford, Sarah B. Laditka, and Anna E. Lowe, "Understanding Characteristics of Families Who Buy Local Produce," *Journal of Nutrition Education and Behavior* 45, no. 1 (2013): 30+.

5. Stephanie Heim, Jamie Stang, and Marjorie Ireland, "A Garden Pilot Project Enhances Fruit and Vegetable Consumption Among Children," *Journal of the American Dietetic Association* 109 (2009): 1220–26.

6. Alexandra L. MacMillan Uribe, Donna M. Winham, and Christopher M. Wharton, "Community Supported Agriculture Membership in Arizona. An Exploratory Study of Food and Sustainability Behaviours," *Appetite* 59, no. 2 (2012): 431–36.

7. Sara A. Quandt, Janae Dupuis, Caitlin Fish, and Ralph B. D'Agostino, "Feasibility of Using a Community-Supported Agriculture Program to Improve Fruit and Vegetable Inventories and Consumption in an Underresourced Urban Community," *Preventing Chronic Disease* 10 (2013): 130053.

8. Stephanie B. Jilcott Pitts, Qiang Wu, Jared T. McGuirt et al., "Associations Between Access to Farmers' Markets and Supermarkets, Shopping Patterns, Fruit and Vegetable Consumption and Health Indicators Among Women of Reproductive Age in Eastern North Carolina, USA," *Public Health Nutrition* 16, no. 11 (2013): 1944–52.

9. Gareth Edwards-Jones, "Does Eating Local Food Reduce the Environmental Impact of Food Production and Enhance Consumer Health?" *Proceedings of the Nutrition Society* 69 (2010): 582–91.

10. Donna J. Levy, Nicola K. Beck, Alexandra L. Kossik et al., "Microbial Safety and Quality of Fresh Herbs from Los Angeles, Orange County and Seattle Farmers' Markets," *Journal of the Science of Food and Agriculture* 45, no. 13 (2015): 2641–45.

11. Christina Mary Pollard, Timothy John Landrigan, Pernilla Laila Ellies et al., "Geographic Factors as Determinants of Food Security: A Western Australian Food Pricing and Quality Study," *Asian Pacific Journal of Clinical Nutrition* 23, no. 4 (2014): 703–13.

REFERENCES AND RESOURCES

Magazines, Journals, and Newspapers

Edwards-Jones, Gareth. "Does Eating Local Food Reduce the Environmental Impact of Food Production and Enhance Consumer Health?" *Proceedings of the Nutrition Society* 69 (2010): 582–91.

Harrison, Judy A., Julia W. Gaskin, Mark A. Harrison et al. "Survey of Food Safety Practices on Small to Medium-Sized Farms and in Farmers Markets." *Journal of Food Protection* 76, no. 11 (2013): 1989–93.

Heim, Stephanie, Jamie Stang, and Marjorie Ireland. "A Garden Pilot Project Enhances Fruit and Vegetable Consumption Among Children." *Journal of the American Dietetic Association* 109 (2009): 1220–26.

Jilcott Pitts, Stephanie B., Qiang Wu, Jared T. McGuirt et al. "Associations Between Access to Farmers' Markets and Supermarkets, Shopping Patterns, Fruit and Vegetable Consumption and Health Indicators Among Women of Reproduction Age in Eastern North Carolina, USA." *Public Health Nutrition* 16, no. 11 (2013): 1944–52.

Levy, Donna J., Nicola K. Beck, Alexandra L. Kossik et al. "Microbial Safety and Quality of Fresh Herbs from Los Angeles, Orange County and Seattle Farmers' Markets." *Journal of the Science of Food and Agriculture* 95, no. 13 (2015): 2641–45.

Pollard, Christina Mary, Timothy John Landrigan, Pernilla Laila Ellies et al. "Geographic Factors as Determinants of Food Security: A Western Australian Food Pricing and Quality Study." *Asian Pacific Journal of Clinical Nutrition* 23, no. 4 (2014): 703–13.

Quandt, Sara A., Janae Dupuis, Caitlin Fish, and Ralph B. D'Agostino. "Feasibility of Using a Community-Supported Agriculture Program to Improve Fruit and Vegetable Inventories and Consumption in an Underresourced Urban Community." *Preventing Chronic Disease* 10 (2013): 130053.

Racine, Elizabeth R., Elizabeth A. Mumford, Sarah B. Laditka, and Anna E. Lowe. "Understanding Characteristics of Families Who Buy Local Produce." *Journal of Nutrition Education and Behavior* 45, no. 1 (2013): 30+.

Uribe, Alexandra L. MacMillan, Donna M. Winham, and Christopher M. Wharton. "Community Supported Agriculture Membership in Arizona. An Exploratory Study of Food and Sustainability Behaviours." *Appetite* 59, no. 2 (2012): 431–36.

Weinstein, Eleanor, Rodolfo J. Galindo, Martin Fried et al. "Impact of a Focused Nutrition Educational Intervention Coupled with Improved Access to Fresh Produce on Purchasing Behavior and Consumption of Fruits and Vegetables in Overweight Patients with Diabetes Mellitus." *Diabetes Educator* 40, no. 1 (2014): 100–106.

Wheeler, Ashley L. and Karen Chapman-Novakofski. "Farmers' Markets: Costs Compared with Supermarkets, Use Among WIC Clients and Relationship to Fruit and Vegetable Intake and Related Psychosocial Variables." *Journal of Nutrition Education and Behavior* 46, no. 3S (2014): S65–S70.

Web Sites

Local Harvest. www.localharvest.org.
U.S. Department of Agriculture. www.usda.gov.
University of Vermont. www.uvm.edu.

Eat Organically Grown Foods When Possible, Especially for Certain Foods

OVERVIEW

When placed side by side, it may be very difficult to detect any outward differences between conventionally and organically grown fruits and vegetables. While they look very much alike and are filled with vitamins, fiber, and nutrients, during their weeks of maturation, the conventionally grown fruits and vegetables may well have been exposed to synthetic pesticides. Moreover, conventionally grown fruits and vegetables may contain genetically modified organisms. That means that their DNA may have been altered. Though many maintain that pesticides and genetically modified foods are perfectly safe, not everyone agrees. Some contend that pesticides may accumulate in the body, and they may be particularly harmful to pregnant women and the fast-growing bodies of children. Also, it may be too soon to known the long-term effects of genetically modified foods, which are a relatively recent addition to the food supply. On the other hand, farmers who grow organic foods may not use synthetic pesticides or anything that has been genetically modified. If they label their food as organic, then their products must meet strict government standards on how the food is grown, handled, and processed.[1]

WHAT THE EXPERTS SAY

Organically Grown Foods Have More Antioxidants and Less Cadmium and Pesticides

In a study published in 2014 in the *British Journal of Nutrition*, researchers from many countries, who were directed by researchers from Newcastle University in the United Kingdom, wanted to learn if there are significant nutritional differences between organic and nonorganic foods. So, they conducted eight meta-analyses that included 343 peer-reviewed publications. The researchers found more antioxidant activity in the organic food than in the conventionally grown crops. In fact, organic crops had between 18 and 69 percent higher concentrations of antioxidant compounds. Organic food also had more carotenoids and vitamins and about half the amount of cadmium, a toxic heavy metal contaminant. Conventionally grown foods were three or four times more likely to contain pesticide residues than organically grown foods. The researchers wrote that "there is now evidence from a large number of quality studies that consistently show that organic production system result in crops/crop-based compound foods with higher concentrations of antioxidants/(poly)phenolics and lower concentrations of Cd [cadmium] and pesticide residues compared with conventional production systems."[2]

Commenting on this study, Ken Cook, co-founder and president of the non-profit Environmental Working Group, noted that people should no longer question whether organic agriculture is better for the public and the environment. "This study breaks it down for consumers who want science-based evidence on the nutritional benefits of crops grown without pesticides or synthetic fertilizers." Cook added that "there are clear differences between organic and conventional food, and organic comes out on top when it comes to our health and the planet."[3]

Eating Organic School Meals May Promote Healthy Eating Habits

In an observational, cross-sectional study published in 2012 in *Appetite*, researchers from Denmark wanted to learn more about the association between organic school meals and healthy eating patterns in 165 children between the ages of 11 and 13 years. The cohort included students from two schools that served organic food and two schools that did not offer organic food. After all the students completed an online food frequency questionnaire, selected students were chosen to participate in focus group interviews. The researchers found that the students in the schools that offered organic foods purchased their meals more often than the students in the schools with no organic foods. In addition, the students in the schools with organic food "consistently agreed that they had healthier school meals" than the students in the other schools. The researchers found this finding truly remarkable. According to the researchers, "even quite limited exposure to organic school food might have a direct or indirect positive effect on pupils' attitudes toward consumption of organic foods and toward healthy eating."[4]

Organically Grown Foods Reduce the Levels of Pesticides in the Body

In a prospective, randomized, single-blinded, crossover study published in 2014 in *Environmental Research*, researchers from Australia and New Zealand wanted to learn if a diet that consisted primarily of organic food would lower the amount of organophosphate pesticides in the body. (Organophosphate pesticides, which are widely used in conventional agriculture, may have a number of different negative health effects.) The cohort consisted of 13 participants between the ages of 18 and 65 years; their mean age was 42.1 years. During one week of the study, they consumed a diet of conventional foods; during a second week of the study, they consumed a diet with as many organically grown foods as possible. (A minimum intake of 80 percent organic food was required.) Urine tests were conducted to determine the levels of organophosphate pesticides in the body. The researchers found that there were fewer pesticides in the urine after one week of eating organically than after one week of eating a conventional diet. In fact, after only one week, the reduction was "dramatic." The researchers concluded that "the consumption of organic food provides a logical precautionary approach to reducing pesticide exposure."[5]

Consumption of Organically Grown Foods May Improve Overall Health

In a study published in 2012 in the *Journal of the Science of Food and Agriculture*, researchers from the Netherlands investigated "the perceived health effects" experienced by people who eat organic food in the Netherlands. The researchers asked consumers of organic food to complete an online questionnaire, which contained both multiple choice and open-ended questions. They received a total of 566 responses. Almost two-thirds of the respondents reported eating organic foods for more than five years. They cited wanting to eat organic foods to improve their health, support the environment, animal welfare, and taste. About

40 percent of the respondents indicated that they had a health problem before they began to eat organic food. More than three-quarters noted that their health concerns were the primary reason for switching to organic foods.

While about 30 percent of the respondents commented that they had no health effects from the organic foods, the other 70 percent said that they noticed one or more improvements. The most common change was an "improvement in general health and general resistance." Twenty-four percent reported better gastrointestinal health and 19 percent said that their skin, hair, and nails were healthier. Thirty percent said their organic diet had mental health benefits. The researchers concluded that their findings "provided insight into the experienced health effects of consumers of organic food." And, "although the study design does not permit direct conclusions on health effects of organic food, the results can serve as a basis for the generation of new hypotheses."[6]

People Who Regularly Consume Organic Foods Tend to Be Healthier

In a study published in 2013 in *PLoS ONE*, researchers from France assessed the behaviors associated with the consumption of 18 organic food products. The cohort consisted of 54,311 adults who were 18 years and older, with a mean age of 43.7 years. Seventy-seven percent were women. The researchers divided the participants into five clusters. Three of the clusters contained nonconsumers of organic products. A fourth cluster included regular consumers of organic products, and a fifth cluster had occasional users of organic foods. The researchers found that the daily food consumption patterns of the three clusters of people who do not use organic foods to be similar. However, they learned that the organic food consumers had increased consumption of healthier foods, such as whole grains, vegetables, fruit, legumes, and nuts, while they had a lower consumption of less healthful choices such as meat, soda, alcohol, and sweets. In addition, consumers of conventional foods were far more likely to be overweight or obese than consumers of organic foods. In view of the epidemic levels of obesity, this is a potentially life-altering finding. "Since several studies have reported an association between pesticide exposure or residues in the body and obesity and type 2 diabetes . . ., the possibility of a potential role of organic food in preventing excessive adiposity because of it lower content in pesticide residues should be tested in further studies."[7]

BARRIERS AND PROBLEMS

Not that long ago, only a small number of stores contained organic fruits and vegetables. Traditional supermarkets had very limited supplies of such foods. Local convenience stores had none. More recently, however, organic fruits and vegetables are more readily available. They are even sold at some of the biggest chain stores, discount stores, and warehouse stores.

Yet, there remain barriers. Organic fruits and vegetables tend to be more expensive than fruits and vegetables that are grown conventionally. During the colder months, those costs are even higher. Unlike processed foods, fresh fruits and vegetables must be consumed fairly quickly. If not, they will spoil. Families on limited budgets who can barely afford to purchase any fruits and vegetables may avoid the organic section entirely. In addition, the markets where they live may not stock those foods, believing that their customers will not purchase them. It is also possible that people are simply unaware of the value of fruits and vegetables, especially those grown organically. While many people have a serious interest in nutrition, large numbers of people leading hectic lives are just grateful to find the time and resources to feed their families three meals a day.

But, there is a compromise position. Every year, the Environmental Working Group publishes "Clean Fifteen" and "Dirty Dozen" lists. These are conventionally grown foods that are safe to eat and foods that should be avoided when grown conventionally or eaten only when they are grown organically. The 2014 list of "Clean Fifteen" is as follows: asparagus, avocadoes, cabbage, cantaloupe, cauliflower, eggplant, grapefruit, kiwi, mangoes, onions, papayas, pineapples, sweet corn, sweet peas (frozen), and sweet potatoes. The 2014 list of "Dirty Dozen" is as follows: apples, celery, cherry tomatoes, cucumbers, grapes, nectarines (imported), peaches, potatoes, snap peas (imported), spinach, strawberries, sweet bell peppers, and two extra foods, hot peppers, kale/collards.[8] During the warmer seasons, the organic versions of the "Dirty Dozen" may be more reasonably priced; during the colder months, it may be more affordable to purchase some of them in the frozen food aisle.

NOTES

1. Mayo Clinic, www.mayoclinic.org.

2. Marcin Barański, Dominika Średnicka-Tober, Nikolaos Volakakis et al., "High Antioxidant and Lower Cadmium Concentrations and Lower Incidence of Pesticide Residues in Organically Grown Crops: A Systematic Literature Review and Meta-Analysis," *British Journal of Nutrition* 112, no. 5 (2014): 794–811.

3. Environmental Working Group. www.ewg.org.

4. Chen He, Soren Breiting, and Federico J. A. Perez-Cueto, "Effect of Organic School Meals to Promote Healthy Diet in 11–13 Year Old Children. A Mixed Methods Study in Four Danish Public Schools," *Appetite* 59, no. 3 (2012): 866–76.

5. Liza Oates, Marc Cohen, Lesley Braun et al., "Reduction in Urinary Organophosphate Pesticide Metabolites in Adults After a Week-Long Organic Diet," *Environmental Research* 132 (2014): 105–11.

6. Lucy P. L. van de Vijver and Marja E. T. van Vliet, "Health Effects of an Organic Diet—Consumer Experiences in the Netherlands," *Journal of the Science of Food and Agriculture* 92, no. 14 (2012): 2923–27.

7. E. Kesse-Guyot, S. Péneau, C. Méjean et al., "Profiles of Organic Food Consumers in a Large Sample of French Adults: Results from the Nutrinet-Santé Cohort Study," *PLoS ONE* 8, no. 10 (2013): e76998.

8. Environmental Working Group. www.ewg.org.

REFERENCES AND RESOURCES

Magazines, Journals, and Newspapers

Barański, Marcin, Dominika Średnicka-Tober, Nikolaos Volakakis et al. "High Antioxidant and Lower Cadmium Concentrations and Lower Incidence of Pesticide Residues in Organically Grown Crops: A Systematic Literature Review and Meta-Analysis." *British Journal of Nutrition* 112, no. 5 (2014): 794–811.

He, Chen, Soren Breiting, and Federico J. A. Perez-Cueto. "Effect of Organic School Meals to Promote Healthy Diet in 11–13 Year Old Children. A Mixed Methods Study in Four Danish Public Schools." *Appetite* 59, no. 3 (2012): 866–76.

Kesse-Guyot, E., S. Péneau, C. Méjean et al. "Profiles of Organic Food Consumers in a Large Sample of French Adults: Results from the Nutrinet-Santé Cohort Study." *PLoS ONE* 8, no. 10 (2013): e76998.

Oates, Liza, Marc Cohen, Lesley Braun et al. "Reduction in Urinary Organophosphate Pesticide Metabolites in Adults After a Week-Long Organic Diet." *Environmental Research* 132 (2014): 105–11.

Spangler, Crystal, Margaret L. Brandeau, Grace E. Hunter et al. "Are Organic Foods Safer or Healthier Than Conventional Alternatives? A Systematic Review." *Annals of Internal Medicine* 157 (2012): 348–66.

Turgut, Cafer, Hakan Ornek, and Teresa J. Cutright. "Determination of Pesticide Residues in Turkey's Table Grapes: The Effect of Integrated Pest Management, Organic Farming, and Conventional Farming." *Environmental Monitoring and Assessment* 173 (2011): 315–23.

Vallverdú-Queralt, Anna, Olga Jáuregui, Alexander Medina-Remón et al. "Evaluation of a Method to Characterize the Phenolic Profile of Organic and Conventional Tomatoes." *Journal of Agricultural and Food Chemistry* 60 (2012): 3373–80.

van de Vijver, Lucy P. L. and Marja E. T. van Vliet. "Health Effects of an Organic Diet—Consumer Experiences in the Netherlands." *Journal of the Science of Food and Agriculture* 92, no. 14 (2012): 2923–27.

Web Sites

Environmental Working Group. www.ewg.org.
Mayo Clinic. www.mayoclinic.org.
Organic Consumers Association. www.organicconsumers.org.

Eat the Recommended Amount of Fruits and Vegetables

OVERVIEW

You have heard it said hundreds of times. Eat your fruits and vegetables. According to the World Health Organization (WHO), millions of people die each year because of inadequate consumption of fruits and vegetables. The WHO contends that a daily intake of only five portions of fruits and vegetables (400 g) could help reduce the risk of cardiovascular disease, cancer, and cognitive problems, such as memory loss. Fruits and vegetables are an incredibly rich source of vitamins and minerals, dietary fiber, flavonoids, plant sterols, and antioxidants.[1]

In an article published in 2014 in *Critical Reviews in Food Science and Nutrition*, a researcher from Madrid, Spain wrote that the association between diet and overall health has been recognized since ancient times. More recently, there have been a host of epidemiological studies that have shown that diets rich in fruits and vegetables lower the risk of chronic illnesses, such as cancer and cardiovascular disease, and they reduce the risk of premature mortality. The researcher concluded that "phytochemicals in fruits and vegetables might be a promising tool for the prevention and/or amelioration of a wide range of diseases."[2]

Meanwhile, in a 2012 article in *Advances in Nutrition*, researchers from Valhalla, New York, noted that diets high in fruits and vegetables are "widely recommended for their health promoting properties." Fruits and vegetables have been valued for high amounts of vitamins, minerals, electrolytes, and fiber. Their high amounts of phytochemicals "function as antioxidants, phytoestrogens, and anti-inflammatory agents." On average, half of a typical meal should consist of fruits and vegetables; most people in the United States don't even come close to eating this amount.[3] In "Youth Risk Behavior Surveillance—United States, 2013," a survey completed by the Centers for Disease Control and Prevention and reported in the June 13, 2014, issue of *Morbidity and Mortality Weekly Report*, researchers noted that during the seven days before their survey, "5.0% of the high school students had not eaten fruit or drunk 100% fruit juices and 6.6% had not eaten vegetables."[4] Moreover, there may be disagreements between government officials and nutritionists on what constitutes a serving. "Published studies on 3 methods for counting fruits and vegetables in 4th grade students found that different counting methods yielded significantly different tallies of fruit and vegetable intake."[5]

WHAT THE EXPERTS SAY

Consumption of Fruits and Vegetables Appears to Extend the Lifespan

In a study published in 2015 in the *European Journal of Nutrition*, researchers from Norway, Sweden, and Finland examined the association between the consumption of berries, fruits, and vegetables, and all causes of mortality among close to 10,000 Norwegian men during four decades (1968 to 2008). Information on dietary consumption was obtained from questionnaires. During a median of 20.3 years of follow-up with a total of 207,506 person-years, 92 percent of the men died. The median age at death was 78.7 years. The researchers found that when compared with the men who ate berries, fruits, and vegetables less than 27 times per month, the men who ate these foods more than 27 times per month had a 8 to 10 percent decreased risk of dying during follow-up. The consumption of fruits was inversely associated with the risk of dying from cancer, and the total consumption of berries, fruits, and vegetables was inversely related to the risk of dying from a stroke. The researchers concluded that the "increased consumption of vegetables, fruits, and berries was associated with a delayed risk of all-cause mortality and of mortality due to cancer and stroke."[6]

Fruit and Vegetable Consumption Appears to Reduce the Rate of All Types of Mortality

In a study published in 2014 in the *Journal of Epidemiology & Community Health*, researchers based in England wanted to learn if the consumption of fruits and vegetables would reduce the rate of mortality in the general English population. The cohort consisted of 65,226 people, 35 years of age and older, who were included in the 2001 to 2008 Health Surveys for England. Participants in this survey were interviewed in person; the initial interview was followed by a second visit with a nurse who took measurements, such as waist circumference and blood pressure, and collected biological samples, such as blood. During the median follow-up of 7.7 years, 4,399 deaths were recorded. The researchers found a strong association between consumption of fruits and vegetables and mortality. Those who ate seven or more portions per day of fruits and vegetables had the lowest risk of mortality from any cause. Moreover, these researchers found that vegetables appeared to have a greater effect per portion than fruit. The researchers concluded that "a robust association exists between fruit and vegetable consumption and mortality."[7]

Fruits and Vegetables May Reduce the Risk of Stroke

In a prospective study published in 2013 in *Atherosclerosis*, researchers from Sweden and Finland examined the association between consumption of fruits and vegetables and risk for stroke in Swedish men and women. The researchers followed 40,291 men and 34,670 women, between the ages of 45 and 83 years, who were free of stroke, coronary artery disease, and cancer when they completed food frequency questionnaires in 1997. During a mean follow-up of 10.2 years, there were 40 cases of stroke. Of these, 3,159 were cerebral infarctions, which are blockages of the flow of blood in the brain. The researchers found an inverse association between total fruit and vegetable consumption and stroke risk. This association was "most pronounced up to a consumption of around five servings per day." The researchers concluded that their findings "lend further support to the recommendation to increase fruits and vegetable consumption."[8]

Fruits and Vegetables May Reduce the Incidence of Coronary Heart Disease

In a study published in 2010 in *PLoS ONE*, researchers from the Netherlands investigated the association between consumption of raw and processed fruits and vegetables and coronary heart disease. The cohort was drawn from two locations in the Netherlands; there were a total of 20,069 men and women between the ages of 20 and 65 years. At baseline, all the participants were free of cardiovascular disease. Information on the consumption of 178 food items was obtained from food frequency questionnaires. During a mean follow-up time of 10.5 years, 245 incident cases of coronary heart disease were documented. Of these, 34 were fatal. The researchers found that the participants with a high intake of raw or processed fruits and vegetables had a 34 percent lower risk of coronary heart disease than the participants with a low intake of these fruits and vegetables. The researchers noted that their findings "suggest that a high consumption [of] fruit and vegetables, whether consumed raw or processed, may protect against CHD [coronary heart disease] incidence."[9]

BARRIERS AND PROBLEMS

Healthier Foods, Such as Fruits and Vegetables, Tend to Be More Expensive

It is very clear that large numbers of people have a diet that includes few fruits and vegetables. While they are probably aware that they should be eating more fruits and vegetables, to them, it is easier and more convenient to consume prepared or processed foods. And, fruits and vegetables may well be pricey. According to an article published in 2014 in *PLoS ONE*, there are ever-increasing price gaps between more healthful and less healthful foods. Researchers from the United Kingdom used data from the U.K. Department of Health National Diet and Nutrition Survey to trace the price trends of more and less healthful foods from 2002 to 2012. Each of the 94 foods studied was placed in one of five groups; one of these groups was fruits and vegetables. All the foods were classified as either "more healthy" or "less healthy." Though healthier foods and drinks have always been more expensive than less healthy alternatives, the researchers found that over the 10-year period of the study, the size of the price gap had increased 28.6 percent. Thus, the healthier foods were even less affordable than they had previously been, making it more likely that people will eat the less healthy foods. The researchers noted that their findings "suggest that we should consider not only the issue of people being able to afford to eat enough food to avoid hunger but also being able to eat enough food which is healthy."[10]

Teens May Not Have the Healthiest Habits

In a cross-sectional study published in 2014 in *Przegl Epidemiol*, researchers based in Poland wanted to estimate the prevalence of healthy behaviors, such as eating fruits and vegetables, among adolescents. Their cohort consisted of 574 teens who were 13 years old. In two separate questions, the teens were asked how many times per week they ate fruits and vegetables. Almost half of the teens reported eating fruits and vegetables at least once per day; there was no significant difference between the male and female teens.[11] Still, that intake is significantly lower than the WHO recommendations mentioned early in this entry.

NOTES

1. World Health Organization, www.who.int.
2. Arantxa Rodriguez-Casado, "The Health Potential of Fruits and Vegetables Phytochemicals: Notable Examples," *Critical Reviews in Food Science and Nutrition* (2014).
3. Joanne L. Slavin and Beate Lloyd, "Health Benefits of Fruits and Vegetables," *Advances in Nutrition* 3 (2012): 506–16.
4. Centers for Disease Control and Prevention, "Youth Risk Behavior Surveillance—United States, 2013," *Morbidity and Mortality Weekly Report* 63, no. 4 (2014). http://www.cdc.gov/mmwr/pdf/ss/ss6304.pdf.
5. Slavin and Lloyd, "Health Benefits."
6. Anette Hjartåker, Markus Dines Knudsen, Steinar Tretli, and Elisabete Weiderpass, "Consumption of Berries, Fruits and Vegetables and Mortality Among 10,000 Norwegian Men Followed for Four Decades," *European Journal of Nutrition* 54 (2015): 599–608.
7. Oyinlola Oyebode, Vanessa Gordon-Dseagu, Alice Walker, and Jennifer S. Mindell, "Fruit and Vegetable Consumption and All-Cause, Cancer and CVD Mortality: Analysis of Health Survey for England Data," *Journal of Epidemiology & Community Health* 68 (2014): 856–62.
8. Susanna C. Larsson, Jarmo Virtamo, and Alicja Wolk, "Total and Specific Fruit and Vegetable Consumption and Risk of Stroke: A Prospective Study," *Atherosclerosis* 227 (2013): 147–52.
9. Linda M. Oude Griep, Johanna M. Geleijnse, Daan Kromhout et al., "Raw and Processed Fruit and Vegetable Consumption and 10-Year Coronary Heart Disease Incidence in a Population-Based Cohort Study in the Netherlands," *PLoS ONE* 5, no. 10 (2010): e13609.
10. Nicholas R. V. Jones, Annalijn I. Conklin, Marc Suhrcke, and Pablo Monsivais, "The Growing Price Gap Between More and Less Healthy Foods: Analysis of a Novel Longitudinal UK Dataset," *PLoS ONE* 9, no. 10 (2014): e109343.
11. Maria Jodkowska, Anna Oblacińska, and Izabela Tabak, "How Well Do Polish Teenagers Meet Health Behaviour Guidelines?" *Przegl Epidemiol* 68 (2014): 65–70.

REFERENCES AND RESOURCES

Magazines, Journals, and Newspapers

Aune, D., D. S. M. Chan, A. R. Vieira et al. "Fruits, Vegetables and Breast Cancer Risk: A Systematic Review and Meta-Analysis of Prospective Studies." *Breast Cancer Research and Treatment* 134 (2012): 479–93.

Fulton, Sharon L., Michelle C. McKinley, Ian S. Young et al. 2014. "The Effect of Increasing Fruit and Vegetable Consumption on Overall Diet: A Systematic Review and Meta-Analysis." *Critical Reviews in Food Science and Nutrition*

Gardiner, Breeana, Miranda Blake, Raeleigh Harris et al. "Can Small Stores Have a Big Impact? A Qualitative Evaluation of a Store Fruit and Vegetable Initiative." *Health Promotion Journal of Australia* 24 (2013): 192–98.

Hjartåker, Anette, Markus Dines Knudsen, Steinar Tretli, and Elisabete Weiderpass. "Consumption of Berries, Fruits and Vegetables and Mortality Among 10,000 Norwegian Men Followed for Four Decades." *European Journal of Nutrition* 54 (2015): 599–608.

Jodkowska, Maria, Anna Oblacińska, and Izabela Tabak. "How Well Do Polish Teenagers Meet Health Behaviour Guidelines?" *Przegl Epidemiol* 68 (2014): 65–70.

Jones, Nicholas R. V., Annalijn I. Conklin, Marc Suhrcke, and Pablo Monsivais. "The Growing Price Gap Between More and Less Healthy Foods: Analysis of a Novel Longitudinal UK Dataset." *PLoS ONE* 9, no. 10 (2014): e109343.

Larsson, Susanna C., Jarmo Virtamo, and Alicja Wolk. "Total and Specific Fruit and Vegetable Consumption and Risk of Stroke: A Prospective Study." *Atherosclerosis* 227 (2013): 147–52.

Mytton, O. T., K. Nnoaham, H. Eyles et al. "Systematic Review and Meta-Analysis of the Effect of Increased Vegetable and Fruit Consumption on Body Weight and Energy Intake." *BMC Public Health* 14 (2014): 886+.

Oude Griep, Linda M., Johanna M. Geleijnse, Daan Kromhout et al. "Raw and Processed Fruit and Vegetable Consumption and 10-Year Coronary Heart Disease Incidence in a Population-Based Cohort Study in the Netherlands." *PLoS ONE* 5, no. 10 (2010): e13609.

Oyebode, Oyinlola, Vanessa Gordon-Dseagu, Alice Walker, and Jennifer S. Mindell. "Fruit and Vegetable Consumption and All-Cause Cancer and CVD Mortality: Analysis of Health Survey for England Data." *Journal of Epidemiology & Community Health* 68 (2014): 856–62.

Rodriguez-Casado, Arantxa. "The Health Potential of Fruits and Vegetables Phytochemicals: Notable Examples." *Critical Reviews in Food Sciences and Nutrition* 34, no. 7 (May 2016): 1097–1107.

Slavin, Joanne L., and Beate Lloyd. "Health Benefits of Fruits and Vegetables." *Advances in Nutrition* 3 (2012): 506–16.

Storey, Maureen, and Patricia Anderson. "Income and Race/Ethnicity Influence Dietary Fiber Intake and Vegetable Consumption." *Nutrition Research* 34 (2014): 844–50.

Young, Candace R., Jennifer L. Aquilante, Sara Solomon et al. "Improving Fruit and Vegetable Consumption Among Low-Income Customers at Farmers Markets: Philly Food Bucks, Philadelphia, Pennsylvania, 2011." *Preventing Chronic Disease* 10 (2013): E166.

Web Sites

Centers for Disease Control and Prevention. www.cdc.gov.
World Health Organization. www.who.int.

Eliminate or Greatly Reduce the Trans Fats in Your Diet

OVERVIEW

The vast majority of trans fats are vegetable oils that that have been transformed into solid fats, such as hard margarine and shortening. This is accomplished by adding hydrogen to vegetable oil, a process that is known as hydrogenation. Foods that contain this hydrogenated oil have a longer shelf life and greater flavor stability. (Only a small number of trans fats are found naturally, primarily in animal-based foods.) And, trans fats, which are also known as partially hydrogenated oils or trans fatty acids, are found in a vast array of processed foods including baked goods, such as pie crusts, biscuits, and pizza dough; fried foods, such as French fries; candies; ready-to-eat frostings; crackers; and snack foods such as microwave popcorn. There are even trans fats in some dietary supplements.[1]

WHAT THE EXPERTS SAY

Trans Fats Negatively Impact the Cardiovascular System

In a trial published in 2014 in *Nutrition, Metabolism & Cardiovascular Diseases*, researchers from Columbia University Medical Center/New York-Presbyterian Hospital in New York City examined the association between intake of trans fats and levels of LDL ("bad" cholesterol) in the blood. The cohort consisted of 400 family members of patients who were hospitalized for cardiovascular disease; all the family members participated in a one-year randomized controlled primary prevention lifestyle intervention. During the baseline calculations, the researchers found "a significant positive correlation" between the intake of trans fats and LDL levels. They also learned that the majority of the participants were less than 65 years old, female, white, obese/overweight, and physically inactive. At the end of the year, the researchers found some of the participants had reduced their intake of trans fats. These participants had lower levels of LDL than the participants who continued to consume the same amount of trans fats. The researchers recommended that "healthcare providers should reinforce the beneficial impact of a healthy diet, and in particular modifications in trans fat intake on improving lipid profiles."[2]

In a randomized, crossover trial published in 2009 in *Atherosclerosis*, researchers from the Jean Mayer USDA Human Nutrition Research Center on Aging at Tufts University in Boston recruited 37 postmenopausal women aged 50 or older. Although all of the women were healthy, they had elevated LDL serum levels. The trial consisted of two 35-day diet phases and a 14-day washout period. Food was consumed both onsite and offsite; all offsite food was provided by the trial. The food contained either corn oil or partially hydrogenated soybean oil. Thirty participants completed the entire trial. When compared to the partially hydrogenated soybean oil–enriched diet, the researchers found that the women on the corn oil diet had improvements in a number of important cardiovascular values, such as lower levels of fasting total cholesterol and LDL. The researchers concluded that "substituting partially hydrogenated soybean oil with an unmodified vegetable oil (corn oil) favorably affects cardiovascular risk factors in moderately hypercholesterolemic postmenopausal women in both the fasting and non-fasting state."[3]

Trans Fats May Increase the Risk of Cancer

In a study published in 2013 in the *Journal of Nutrition*, researchers from the Mayo Clinic in Rochester, Minnesota, evaluated the association between intake of trans fats and risk of developing non-Hodgkin lymphoma, a type of cancer that grows in the body's lymphatic system. The cohort consisted of 603 people with non-Hodgkin lymphoma and 1,007 matched controls. The researchers learned that the intake of trans fats was "positively associated" with the overall risk of non-Hodgkin lymphoma. They concluded that "diets high in TFAs . . . were positively associated with NHL risk."[4]

In a study published in 2008 in the *American Journal of Epidemiology*, researchers from the University of North Carolina in Chapel Hill reviewed the association between the consumptions of trans fats and the development of colorectal adenomas, polyps that may grow into colorectal cancer. The researchers used data from a cross-sectional investigation of 622 people who underwent complete colonoscopies, a procedure in which a physician, usually a gastroenterologist, views the entire large colon with a lighted instrument. Of these, 173 were cases and 449 were controls. When the researchers compared the participants who consumed the least amount of trans fats to those who consumed the most trans fats (an average of about 6.5 grams per day), the researchers found that the high consumers had a significantly greater number of colorectal adenomas. In fact, their risk increased by 86 percent. The researchers noted that "the prevalence of colorectal adenomas was positively associated with high *trans*-fatty acid consumption."[5]

Trans Fats May Increase the Risk of Attention Deficit/ Hyperactivity Disorder

In a study published in 2012 in *Acta Paediatrica*, researchers from Seoul, Korea, wanted to learn if there was an association between intake of trans fats and the risk for attention deficit/hyperactivity disorder (ADHD). Teens with this medical problem have difficulty focusing on specific tasks, and they tend to be overactive and impulsive. The cohort consisted of 485 female teens who were in their first or second year of a girls' high school in Seoul. The researchers assessed the girls' intake of food during the previous 12 months as well as their intake of oils and vitamins and minerals. They also determined that 12 of the girls had ADHD and 464 did not. The researchers found that the female teens with ADHD had "significantly higher" trans fats intake levels that those without ADHD. And, they concluded that their findings "suggested that female adolescents with ADHD had significantly higher TFAs [trans fatty acids] intake than those without ADHD."[6]

Trans Fats May Increase the Risk of Depression

In a study published in 2011 in *PLoS ONE*, researchers from Spain and the Netherlands investigated the relationship between the intake of different oils and the risk of depression. The cohort consisted of 5,038 men and 7,021 women, with a mean age at recruitment of 37.5 years. During a follow-up period of 6.1 years, researchers identified 657 new cases of depression. The researchers found an association between intake of trans fats and a "higher risk" for depression. And, the risk was statistically significant. "The magnitude of this association was robust and persisted after several degrees of control for confounding and several sensitivity analyses."[7]

BARRIERS AND PROBLEMS

For decades, a seemingly limitless number of food products contained trans fats. And, most people consumed them. In the years before mandatory labeling, it was usually impossible to know what type of oil was used to make those scrumptious blueberry muffins or those mouth-watering potato chips. But, there are also other reasons that people gravitate toward eating foods with trans fats. Trans fats are often found in fast foods, which are relatively inexpensive and convenient. Foods with trans fats cost significantly less than foods with a good quality oil, such as extra virgin olive oil. And, foods with trans fats, especially those that contain sugar and salt, tend to be tasty, hard to resist, and alluring to consumers, particularly those who are really hungry.

Nevertheless, as reports of the harmful effects of trans fats gained attention and as strict labeling laws were passed, more people began reading labels and searching for trans fat–free alternatives. Moreover, there have been prominent organizations and respected people advocating restrictions on their use. For example, in 2013, the *Bulletin of the World Health Organization* published an article on the effectiveness of policies that reduce the use of trans fats in the United States, Brazil, Canada, Costa Rica, Denmark, the Republic of Korea, and the Netherlands. (The World Health Organization has supported the complete elimination of trans fats from the world's food supply.) Though the policies put in place to curb the use of trans fats varied, the researchers found that they were all effective. "National and local bans were the most effective." Not surprisingly, mandatory regulation had a greater effect than voluntary regulation. And, labeling requirements in the United States and Canada have also made "significant progress."

Still, making these changes is not an easy process. It is not uncommon for "countries, states and cities [to] lack the political will to introduce the necessary legislation." Generally, there is opposition from the food and agriculture industries. In addition, different government departments and/or agencies may attempt to control or disrupt the process. The article mentioned what happened in Cleveland, Ohio. The leadership of the city introduced legislation to ban trans fats. But, the city's effort was blocked by the state government. The city sued the state government and won. Trans fats are banned in Cleveland.[8]

In a 2014 article in *Scientific American*, Walter Willett, a Harvard-based physician who also earned a doctoral degree in public health, noted that the inventors of trans fats earned a 1912 Nobel Prize for their discovery. Obviously, at the time it was believed to be a wonderful addition to the diet. Decades later, trans fats were found to have a litany of negative consequences. And, the effort to reduce their use has resulted in marked change. Willett estimated that by 2012 about "75 percent of trans fats had been removed from the U. S. food supply." Still, the 25 percent of trans fats still in the food supply cause an estimated 7,000 premature deaths each year. Change is happening, but too slowly for many. "We should not get too carried away," Willett said. "It is sobering that it has taken more than a century for this moment to arrive."[9]

Though it may be difficult, try to preplan your meals and snacks. Choose selections that do not contain trans fats. Be very careful when ordering food from fast food establishments. Fast foods frequently contain trans fats. Make substitutions in recipes. For example, use butter instead of margarine in piecrusts. Find local restaurants and bakeries that refuse to use trans fats. Patronize those businesses. Let them know that you support their opposition to trans fats. In the beginning, these changes may be a little challenging; in time, they will become relatively easy to follow.

NOTES

1. U.S. Food and Drug Administration, www.fda.gov.

2. M. Garshick, H. Mochari-Greenberger, and L. Mosca, "Reduction in Dietary Trans Fat Intake Is Associated with Decreased LDL Particle Number in a Primary Prevention Population," *Nutrition, Metabolism & Cardiovascular Diseases* 24 (2014): 100–106.

3. Sonia Vega-López, Nirupa R. Matthan, Lynne M. Ausman et al., "Substitution of Vegetable Oil for Partially-Hydrogenated Fat Favorably Alters Cardiovascular Disease Risk Factors in Moderately Hypercholesterolemic Postmenopausal Women," *Atherosclerosis* 207 (2009): 208–12.

4. Bridget Charbonneau, Helen M. O'Connor, Alice H. Wang et al., "*Trans* Fatty Acid Intake Is Associated with Increased Risk and n3 Fatty Acid Intake with Reduced Risk of Non-Hodgkin Lymphoma," *Journal of Nutrition* 143, no. 5 (2013): 672–81.

5. Lisa C. Vinikoor, Jane C. Schroeder, Robert C. Millikan et al., "Consumption of *Trans*-Fatty Acid and Its Association with Colorectal Adenomas," *American Journal of Epidemiology* 168, no. 3 (2008): 289–97.

6. Jung-Ha Kim, Chung-Mo Nam, Jae-Won Kim et al., "Relationship Between Attention-Deficit/Hyperactivity Disorder and Trans Fatty Acids Intake in Female Adolescents," *Acta Paediatrica* 101, no. 9 (2012): e431–e433.

7. Almudena Sánchez-Villegas, Lisa Verberne, Jokin De Irala et al., "Dietary Fat Intake and the Risk of Depression: The SUN Project," *PLoS ONE* 6, no. 1 (2011): e16268.

8. Shauna M. Downs, Anne Marie Thow, and Stephen R. Leeder, "The Effectiveness of Policies for Reducing Dietary Trans Fat: A Systematic Review of the Evidence," *Bulletin of the World Health Organization* 91 (2013): 262–269H.

9. Walter Willett, "The Case for Banning Trans Fats," *Scientific American* 310, no. 3 (2014): 13.

REFERENCES AND RESOURCES

Magazines, Journals, and Newspapers

Barcelos, R. C. S., L. T. Vey, H. J. Segat et al. "Cross-Generational *Trans* Fat Intake Exacerbates UV Radiation-Induced Damage in Rat Skin." *Food and Chemical Toxicology* 69 (2014): 38–45.

Charbonneau, Bridget, Helen M. O'Connor, Alice H. Wang et al. "*Trans* Fatty Acid Intake Is Associated with Increased Risk and n3 Fatty Acid Intake with Reduced Risk of Non-Hodgkin Lymphoma." *Journal of Nutrition* 143, no. 5 (2013): 672–81.

Downs, Shauna M., Anne Marie Thow, and Stephen R. Leeder. "The Effectiveness of Policies for Reducing Dietary Trans Fat: A Systematic Review of the Evidence." *Bulletin of the World Health Organization* 91 (2013): 262–269H.

Garshick, M., H. Mochari-Greenberger, and L. Mosca. "Reduction in Dietary Trans Fat Intake Is Associated with Decreased LDL Particle Number in a Primary Prevention Population." *Nutrition, Metabolism & Cardiovascular Diseases* 24 (2014): 100–106.

Golomb, Beatrice A., Marcella A. Evans, Halbert L. White, and Joel E. Dimsdale. "Trans Fat Consumption and Aggression." *PLoS ONE* 7, no. 3 (2012): e32175.

Hu, Jinfu, Carlo La Vecchia, Margaret de Groh et al. "Dietary Transfatty Acids and Cancer Risk." *European Journal of Cancer Prevention* 20, no. 6 (2011): 530–38.

Kiage, James N., Peter D. Merrill, Suzanne E. Judd et al. "Intake of *Trans* Fat and Incidence of Stroke in the REasons for Geographic and Racial Differences in Stroke (REGARDS) Cohort." *American Journal of Clinical Nutrition* 99, no. 5 (2014): 1071–76.

Kim, Jung-Ha, Chung-Mo Nam, Jae-Won Kim et al. "Relationship Between Attention-Deficit/Hyperactivity Disorder and Trans Fatty Acids Intake in Female Adolescents." *Acta Paediatrica* 101, no. 9 (2012): e431–e433.

Kris-Etherton, Penny M., Michael Lefevre, Ronald P. Mensink et al. "*Trans* Fatty Acid Intakes and Food Sources in the U.S. Population: NHANES 1999–2002." *Lipids* 47 (2012): 931–40.

Sánchez-Villegas, Almudena, Lisa Verberne, Jokin De Irala et al. "Dietary Fat Intake and the Risk of Depression: The SUN Project." *PLoS ONE* 6, no. 1 (2011): e16268.

Vega-López, Sonia, Nirupa R. Matthan, Lynne M. Ausman et al. "Substitution of Vegetable Oil for a Partially-Hydrogenated Fat Favorably Alters Cardiovascular Disease Risk

Factors in Moderately Hypercholesterolemic Postmenopausal Women." *Atherosclerosis* 107 (2009): 208–12.

Vinikoor, Lisa C., Jane C. Schroeder, Robert C. Millikan et al. 2008. "Consumption of *Trans*-Fatty Acid and Its Association with Colorectal Adenomas." *American Journal of Epidemiology* 168, no. 3 (2008): 289–97.

Willett, Walter. "The Case for Banning Trans Fats." *Scientific American* 310, no. 3 (2014): 13.

Web Site

U.S. Food and Drug Administration. www.fda.gov.

Incorporate Healthier Snacks into Your Diet

OVERVIEW

It is not uncommon for people to become hungry in between meals. Eating a small snack may be just what is needed to remain satiated. According to a 2014 article in *Physiology & Behavior*, snacking is a widespread activity. "Snacking, defined as eating outside of main meals, is a very common behavior, as established by numerous cross-sectional and longitudinal studies carried out in various areas of the world."[1]

But, not all snacks have equal nutritional value. In fact, some snacks, such as those with trans fats (see the entry on trans fats), negatively impact the body, especially if they are a frequent part of the diet. On the other hand, simple snacks, such as a piece of fruit, are low in calories and full of nutrients. However, fruit is not always readily available. And, people who are really hungry may reach for a snack that is filled with fat, sugar, and salt. It is well known that those types of snacks negatively impact the body and contribute to the development of body fat and excess weight.

WHAT THE EXPERTS SAY

It May Be Possible to Prompt People to Eat Healthier Snacks

In a study published in 2014 in *Eating Behaviors*, researchers from Australia examined their ability to use certain prompts to encourage the eating of healthier snacks. (This process is known as attentional bias modification.) The cohort consisted of 146 undergraduate women between the ages of 18 and 25 years; the women were randomly assigned to one of two groups. One group was trained to direct their attention to healthy snacks; the other was trained to focus on unhealthy snacks. The researchers found that the women trained to direct their attention to healthy snacks ate more of the healthy snacks than those trained to concentrate on unhealthy snacks. The researchers concluded that "the present study demonstrated that it is possible to experimentally induce an attentional bias for healthy food, which translates into relatively greater healthy snack consumption in young women." But, the researchers acknowledged that their findings do not indicate whether these preferences "can be sustained over time."[2]

After School Programs Are Able to Make Cost-Effective, Healthy Snacks Available

In a study published in 2014 in the *Journal of School Health*, researchers from the University of South Carolina in Columbia wondered if the snacks served in after-school programs could be improved in a cost-effective manner. Why is this important? According to the researchers, throughout the United States, after-school programs care for over eight million children. The cohort consisted of four large after-school programs, serving about 500 children between the ages of 5 and 12 years. During the 18-week preintervention phase, the students were fed low-nutrient-density salty snacks, sugar-sweetened drinks, and desserts; during the 7-week postintervention phase, the students ate fruits and vegetables, with no sugar-sweetened beverages or desserts. Thanks to the involvement of a grocery chain that discounted food prices, the after-school programs actually improved the healthfulness of their snacks while reducing their costs. The researchers noted that their findings "demonstrated that engaging community grocery stores in a collaborative partnership to provide discounted prices on healthful snacks can result in sizeable price reductions for fruits and vegetables." The researchers added that these changes could be replicated in other locations, and such partnerships could have an impact on the millions of children who attend these programs.[3]

A similar study was published in 2012 in *Preventing Chronic Disease*. Researchers based at the Harvard Prevention Research Center at Harvard University assessed the cost of food and drinks served at 32 YMCA after-school programs in four U.S. cities. They wanted to learn if healthier snacks were more costly and to identify less expensive wholesome options. The researchers found that the more nutritious snacks were about 50 percent more expensive than the less nourishing ones. For example, foods with trans fats were less expensive than those without trans fats. Fruits and vegetables are also pricier. But, the researchers deciphered ways to save money. A glass of tap water coupled with a banana costs the same as 100 percent apple juice. Tap water with cheese slices costs even less than 1 percent chocolate milk. The researchers concluded that their "findings demonstrated that a range of healthful foods and snack combinations can be served at a similar or lower price than less healthful options. In light of the obesity epidemic and the increasing number of children attending after-school programs, these findings may help programs to purchase and offer more healthful, affordable snacks."[4]

It Appears That Container Size Plays a Role in Snack Food Intake

In a study published in 2012 in *Appetite*, researchers from Belgium wanted to learn more about the association between container size and the amount of snack food that is consumed. The cohort consisted of 88 undergraduate students who regularly ate a snack in the afternoon. While they watched a television show, all of the participants were served M&M's for consumption in cubicles. They were given either a medium portion in a small container or a medium portion in a large container or a large portion in a large container. The researchers found the participants who consumed the food in the large container ate considerably more. According to the researchers, "the important message emerging from this research is that CS [container size] influences food intake for high-energy food *even* when PS [portion size] is kept constant." So, people eat more when food is placed in larger containers. "As a matter of fact, calories intake increased by more than 100% when increasing CS by 300%."[5] The message from this trial is clear. Place your snack in a smaller container.[6]

There Are Ways to Improve the Snacks That Are Offered in School Cafeterias

In a qualitative study published in 2013 in the *International Journal of Preventive Medicine*, researchers from Iran evaluated the types of snacks middle-school students obtained from their cafeterias. They also suggested ways in which the schools could improve these snacks. The cohort consisted of 240 students between the ages of 12 and 15 years from 12 middle schools in Tehran. Information was obtained during small focus-group discussions. Because adolescents spend so much of their day at school, the cafeteria becomes "one of the major sources of providing their daily nutritional needs." Interestingly, over half the students thought that snack consumption was "necessary." The students reported some of the benefits of snacking, such as providing energy and increasing intelligence, and they said that their most frequently consumed snacks were "cookies, fruits, bread and cheese, sandwiches, chocolate milk, fruit juices, and potato chips." Students purchased these foods because they were the items that the cafeteria sold. The researchers advised making more nutritional choices available. "Providing favorable, nutritious and healthy snacks, available in cafeterias, is an approach that may affect their food habits."[7]

BARRIERS AND PROBLEMS

Of course, in an ideal world everyone would always have access to healthy snacks. They would be readily available and easily affordable. And, in an even more perfect world, everyone would consistently prefer healthy snacks to the more fatty, salty, and tasty options. But, as we all know, less nutritious snacks tend to be sold just about everywhere, and they are often less expensive. There is some research on barriers to eating healthier snacks.

In a study published in 2014 in *Childhood Obesity*, researchers from Winston-Salem, North Carolina, wanted to learn more about the type of snacks that were available at youth sports games such as baseball. Observations were made at a youth baseball field in a small town in northwest North Carolina. There were six teams of boys between the ages of 8 and 11 years. A total of 12 games were randomly observed throughout the six-week season. By the end of the observation period, food and beverage information was obtained for 179 adults and 83 children who attended the games as well as 51 youth players. The results contained 102 snacks and 82 beverages. The team snacks, which were provided by parents, included French fries, chips, crackers, popcorn, candy, and cookies. Parents also arrived with healthier alternatives such as granola bars and peanuts. Team members drank water, regular and diet soda, sugar-sweetened sport drinks, and milk shakes. The vast majority of the food consumed by spectators was purchased from a concession stand; generally, the offerings had no nutritional value. "Most food consumed by both parents and children were considered unhealthy snack items." The researchers concluded that the ballpark "could be considered an obesigenic [fosters excessive weight] environment, despite the focus on physical activity and sport participation."[8]

A study published in 2009 in *Cadernos de Saúde Pública* (*Reports in Public Health*) also addressed barriers to healthy snacking. In this study, researchers from Brazil conducted four focus groups with 25 teens between the ages of 10 and 19 years. During their discussions, the teens mentioned a few obstacles to healthy snacking. They noted that snacks with less nutritional value are sold in many locations, and they tend to taste better. And, these snacks did not require any preparation, which made them easy to consume when there is a time crunch. Moreover, the snacks available at school were generally of low nutritional quality. According to the researchers, "the main barriers cited were focused on personal and social aspects, such as: the temptation, the taste of food, the influence of parents and the lack of time and options for healthy snacks at school."[9]

In a study published in 2011 in the *Journal of School Health*, researchers from several locations in the United States wanted to learn more about the foods sold in vending machines in 106 schools in the St. Paul-Minneapolis, Minnesota, metropolitan area. The 829 vending machines surveyed contained a total of 5,085 food and 8,442 beverage items. Ninety-three percent of the foods consisted of salty snacks, candy bars, and baked goods; only 18 percent of the beverages "met the established criteria for healthy beverages." Clearly, this is a problematic situation. The researchers recommended "increasing the availability of fresh fruit and vegetables, whole grain products, and low-fat dairy products such as string cheese or yogurt." This "would go a long way in offering healthful, nutrient-rich snack options for youth at school."[10]

NOTES

1. France Bellisle, "Meals and Snacking, Diet Quality and Energy Balance," *Physiology & Behavior* 134 (2014): 38–43.

2. Naomi Kakoschke, Eva Kemps, and Marika Tiggemann, "Attentional Bias Modification Encourages Healthy Eating," *Eating Behaviors* 15 (2014): 120–24.

3. Michael W. Beets, Falon Tilley, Gabrielle Turner-McGrievy et al., "Community Partnership to Address Snack Quality and Cost in After-School Programs," *Journal of School Health* 84, no. 8 (2014): 543–48.

4. Rebecca S. Mozaffarian, Analisa Andry, Rebekka M. Lee et al., "Price and Healthfulness of Snacks in 32 YMCA After-School Programs in Four US Metropolitan Areas, 2006–2008," *Preventing Chronic Disease* 9 (2012): E38.

5. David Marchiori, Olivier Corneille, and Olivier Klein, "Container Size Influences Snack Food Intake Independently of Portion Size," *Appetite* 58 (2012): 814–17.

6. Ibid.

7. Fatemeh Esfarjani, Fatemeh Mohammadi, Roshanak Roustaee, and Majid Hajifaraji, "Schools' Cafeteria Status: Does It Affect Snack Patterns? A Qualitative Study," *International Journal of Preventive Medicine* 4, no. 10 (2013): 1194–99.

8. Megan B. Irby, Marcie Drury-Brown, and Joseph A. Skelton, "The Food Environment of Youth Baseball," *Childhood Obesity* 10, no. 3 (2014): 260–65.

9. Natacha Toral, Maria Aparecida Conti, and Betzabeth Slater, "Healthy Eating According to Teenagers: Perceptions, Barriers, and Expected Characteristics of Teaching Materials," *Cadernos de Saúde Pública (Reports in Public Health)* 25, no. 11 (2009): 2386–94.

10. Keryn E. Pasch, Leslie A. Lytle, Annie C. Samuelson et al., "Are School Vending Machines Loaded with Calories and Fat: An Assessment of 106 Middle and High Schools," *Journal of School Health* 81, no. 4 (2011): 212–18.

REFERENCES AND RESOURCES

Magazines, Journals, and Newspapers

Beets, Michael W., Falon Tilley, Gabrielle Turner-McGrievy et al. "Community Partnership to Address Snack Quality and Cost in After-School Programs." *Journal of School Health* 84, no. 8 (2014): 543–48.

Bellisle, France. "Meals and Snacking, Diet Quality and Energy Balance." *Physiology & Behavior* 134 (2014): 38–43.

Esfarjani, Fatemeh, Fatemeh Mohammadi, Roshanak Roustaee, and Majid Hajifaraji. "Schools' Cafeteria Status: Does it Affect Snack Patterns? A Qualitative Study." *International Journal of Preventive Medicine* 4, no. 10 (2013): 1194–99.

Gonzalez-Suarez, Consuelo B., Karen Lee-Pineda, Nenita D. Caralipio et al. "Is What Filipino Children Eat Between Meals Associated with Body Mass Index?" *Asia-Pacific Journal of Public Health* 27, no. 2 (2015): NP650–NP661.

Irby, Megan B., Marcie Drury-Brown, and Joseph A. Skelton. "The Food Environment of Youth Baseball." *Childhood Obesity* 10, no. 3 (2014): 260–65.

Kakoschke, Naomi, Eva Kemps, and Marika Tiggemann. "Attentional Bias Modfication Encourages Healthy Eating." *Eating Behaviors* 15 (2014): 120–24.

Marchiori, David, Olivier Corneille, and Olivier Klein. "Container Size Influences Snack Food Intake Independently of Portion Size." *Appetite* 58 (2012): 814–17.

Mozaffarian, Rebecca S., Analisa Andry, Rebekka M. Lee et al. "Price and Healthfulness of Snacks in 32 YMCA After-School Programs in Four US Metropolitan Areas, 2006–2008." *Preventing Chronic Disease* 9 (2012): E38.

Pasch, Keryn E., Leslie A. Lytle, Anne C. Samuelson et al. "Are School Vending Machines Loaded with Calories and Fat: An Assessment of 106 Middle and High Schools." *Journal of School Health* 81, no. 4 (2011): 212–18.

Piernas, Carmen, and Barry M. Popkin. "Trends in Snacking Among U.S. Children." *Health Affairs* 29, no. 3 (2010): 398–404.

Toral, Natacha, Maria Aparecida Conti, and Betzabeth Slater. "Healthy Eating According to Teenagers: Perceptions, Barriers, and Expected Characteristics of Teaching Materials." *Cadernos de Saúde Pública (Reports in Public Health)* 25, no. 11 (2009): 2386–94.

Web Site

American Academy of Nutrition and Dietetics. www.eatright.org.

Limit Fast Food Intake

OVERVIEW

Fast food, or food that is prepared and served quickly, is a relatively new addition to the restaurant world. Until the middle of the 20th century, there were few fast food restaurants. It was around that time that McDonald's appeared on roadsides in the United States. The food, which was made according to a set formula created by the corporate offices, was widely available and inexpensive. People flocked to these establishments and more appeared on the scene. Soon, additional fast food chains emerged. Burger King, Wendy's, and Kentucky Fried Chicken restaurants were built in cities and towns throughout the country. It did not take long for the restaurants to add drive-up windows, which made it possible to purchase a meal without leaving the car. Instead of eating at a dining table, eating on the go became fairly common. Entire families were able to eat their fast food meals while driving in cars. Without question, fast food became an integral part of the contemporary diet.

According to the National Center for Health Statistics, a division of the U.S. Department of Health and Human Services, from 2007 to 2010, on average, 11.3 percent of an individual's total daily calories were obtained from fast food. While the percentage did not differ significantly between men and women, older people ate less fast food, only 6 percent. Younger non-Hispanic black adults obtained one-fifth of their calories from fast food. Among adults, researchers observed that the more people weighed, the higher the consumption of fast food. The heaviest people consumed the highest percentage of calories from fast food.[1]

WHAT THE EXPERTS SAY

Research Studies Support the Association between Fast Food Intake and Excessive Weight Gain

In a study published in 2012 in *Obesity Surgery*, researchers from San Antonio, Texas, wanted to learn more about behavioral factors associated with severe obesity in patients scheduled to have bariatric surgery. (Bariatric surgery includes a variety of surgical procedures used to reduce the food intake of people who are obese.) The cohort consisted of 270 people who were surveyed before undergoing surgery. The researchers divided the patients into three groups according to body mass index (BMI), a key measure of obesity: obese (BMI 30–39.99), morbidly obese (BMI 40.00–49.99), and super morbidly obese (BMI 50.00+). The obese category had 54 patients; the morbidly obese had 149 patients; and, the super morbidly obese had 76 patients. About 49 percent of the group was Hispanic. With an average age of 43.5 years, 23.7 percent of the patients were males. Almost half of the sample reported that they exercised at least once per week, and the average rate of fast food consumption was 2.68 times per week. The researchers learned that the consumption of fast food "emerged as a key determinant of higher levels of obesity." They found a direct correlation between higher rates of fast food consumption and increases in the super morbidly obese category. The researchers discussed that this relationship may be explained by the types of food sold at fast food establishments, including "oversized portions, high energy density, high processed, high fat content, and large amounts of refined starch and added sugars." The researchers underscored the extraordinary health care costs associated with extreme forms of obesity and stressed the need to find ways to break this eating pattern.[2]

In a descriptive, cross-sectional study published in 2014 in the *Journal of Clinical and Diagnostic Research*, researchers from India examined the association between body mass index and the consumption of fast food, soft drinks, and the level of physical activity in 147 first-year medical students. The data were collected using a questionnaire. The researchers found that more than 90 percent of the students ate fast food. Of these, 47 students (34.05 percent) were overweight or obese. Interestingly, despite their medical school status, "more than 60% of the students were unaware about the fact that fast food was unhealthy." Over half the students drank soft drinks with their fast food, and this practice was more common with the obese and overweight students than the normal weight students. The researchers concluded that their findings found a "significant relationship" between fast food consumption and BMI.[3]

Fast Food May Increase the Risk for Metabolic Syndrome

In a prospective study published in 2013 in the *European Journal of Nutrition*, researchers from Iran investigated whether the consumption of fast food influenced rates of metabolic syndrome, a medical disorder in which there are increased levels of waist fat, high blood pressure, and elevated levels of cholesterol. The cohort consisted of 1,476 men and women with a mean age of 37.8 years. At baseline, none of the participants had been diagnosed with metabolic syndrome. After three years, 249 of the participants were diagnosed with this disorder. The researchers found that the younger participants were more likely to be in the highest quartile of fast food consumption. And, fast food consumption was significantly associated with an increased occurrence of metabolic syndrome. "Energy intake, dietary energy density, intake of total fat, saturated trans fat and cholesterol, as main dietary risk factors of metabolic syndrome, increased with consumption of fast food."[4]

Fast Food Appears to Increase the Risk of Type 2 Diabetes and Coronary Heart Disease

In a study published in 2012 in *Circulation*, researchers from Minneapolis, Pittsburgh, and Singapore examined the association between consumption of Western-style fast food and the incidence of type 2 diabetes and coronary heart disease mortality in China. The cohort consisted of men and women 45 to 74 years old who were enrolled in the Singapore Chinese Health Study between 1993 and 1998. The type 2 diabetes group originally included 43,176 participants. During follow-up interviews from 1999 to 2004, there were 2,252 cases of diabetes. The coronary heart disease group initially included 52,584 participants, By December 31, 2009, there were 1,397 deaths. The researchers found that Chinese Singaporeans who had a relatively frequent intake of Western fast food had a higher risk of developing type 2 diabetes and dying from heart disease than those who ate little or no Western fast food. And, they concluded that "Chinese Singaporeans with relatively frequent intake of Western-style fast food items have a modestly increased risk of developing type 2 diabetes mellitus and a strong and graded risk of dying as a result of CHD [coronary heart disease]."[5]

Taxing Fast Food May Reduce Intake

In an article published in 2012 in *BMJ*, researchers from the United Kingdom proposed taxing "unhealthy foods and drinks." According to these researchers, taxing fast foods and other similar products should increase their price and, subsequently, reduce their consumption. The researchers cited evidence from natural experiments, controlled trials of price change in closed environments, and modeling studies. Of course, the researchers also acknowledged that the taxes would have the greatest impact on the poorer members of society. On the other hand, when people with fewer economic resources eat less unhealthful food, their general health should improve. The researchers concluded that "health related food taxes could improve health." Moreover, "existing evidence suggests that taxes are likely to shift consumption in the desired direction."[6]

BARRIERS AND PROBLEMS

It is generally agreed that people know that fast food is not a better option. But, it is inexpensive and convenient. So, abstaining is difficult.

When Fast Food Is Readily Available, People Will Eat More

Without a doubt, most people would agree that it is almost impossible to avoid fast food restaurants. And, generally, one does not need to travel very far to purchase fast food. In fact, in a cross-sectional study published in 2014 in *Applied Physiology, Nutrition, and Metabolism*, researchers from Ontario, Canada, examined the fast food consumption of students who lived and attended school in a neighborhood with a moderate to high number of fast food restaurants. The cohort consisted of 6,099 Canadian students between the ages of 11 and 15 years from 255 school neighborhoods. The researchers found that the students from neighborhoods with higher numbers of fast food restaurants were more likely "to be excessive fast-food consumers" than students from neighborhoods with no fast food restaurants. The researchers concluded that "the fast-food retail environment within which youth live and go to school is an important contributor to their eating behaviours."[7]

Fast Food Restaurants Maintain That They Sell the Food Their Customers Want to Eat

In a qualitative study published in 2014 in BMC *Public Health*, researchers from Scotland conducted nine interviews with managers and one interview with a senior employee of fast food shops near secondary schools (students ages 12 to 17 years) in low-income areas in the Scottish cities of Aberdeen, Edinburgh, and Glasgow. They wanted to learn why the restaurants didn't offer more healthful menu options. Since managers of chain restaurants have limited control over the food selection, chain restaurants were not included in the study. The researchers found that the respondents maintained that they prepared foods that the customers wanted to consume. They were only responding to customer demand, and they believed "that the customers in their area, especially school children, would not be persuaded to purchase healthier foods." In addition, healthier options were considered unrealistic, "because vendors perceived that they wouldn't be able to charge enough to make a profit." They said that they were already struggling to make a profit. The researchers commented that "cost and profitability were major concerns among food vendors, especially in regards to introducing healthier options."[8]

Fast Food May Be Addictive

In an article published in 2011 in *Current Drug Abuse Reviews*, researchers from San Francisco explored the possibility that fast food is addictive. According to these researchers, on any given day, about one-third of Americans eat fast food. Fast food is primarily consumed by children, teens, and young adults; people with fewer financial resources consume far more fast food than those with more resources. While the researchers noted that there is not sufficient scientific evidence to prove that fast food is addictive, there are similarities between drug and food addiction. As with drugs, people may crave fast food and experience withdrawal-type symptoms went they stop eating it. Specifically, they may derive satisfaction from foods high in sugar, fat, and salt. Once a person becomes obese, he or she may become dependent on fast food. And, people may easily gravitate to fast food in response to stress or attempts to lose weight. "These individuals are more likely to meet the criteria for substance dependence."[9]

NOTES

1. National Center for Health Statistics, www.cdc.gov/nchs.

2. Ginny Garcia, Thankam S. Sunil, and Pedro Hinojosa, "The Fast Food and Obesity Link: Consumption Patterns and Severity of Obesity," *Obesity Surgery* 22, no. 5 (2012): 810–18.

3. T. Shah, G. Purohit, S. P. Nair et al., "Assessment of Obesity, Overweight and Its Association with the Fast Food Consumption in Medical Students." *Journal of Clinical and Diagnostic Research* 8, no. 5 (2014): CC05–CC07.

4. Z. Bahadoran, P. Mirmiran, F. Hosseini-Esfahani, and F. Azizi, "Fast Food Consumption and the Risk of Metabolic Syndrome After 3-Years of Follow-Up: Tehran Lipid and Glucose Study," *European Journal of Clinical Nutrition* 67, no. 12 (2013): 1303–9.

5. Andrew O. Odegaard, Woon Puay Koh, Jian-Min Yuan et al., "Western-Style Fast Food Intake and Cardiometabolic Risk in an Eastern Country," *Circulation* 126 (2012): 182–88.

6. Oliver Mytton T., Dushy Clarke, and Mike Rayner, "Taxing Unhealthy Food and Drinks to Improve Health," *BMJ* 344 (2012): e2931.

7. Rachel E. Laxer and Ian Janssen, "The Proportion of Excessive Fast-Food Consumption Attributable to the Neighbourhood Food Environment Among Youth Living Within 1 km of Their School," *Applied Physiology, Nutrition, and Metabolism* 39, no. 4 (2014): 480–86.

8. Michelle Estrade, Smita Dick, Fiona Crawford et al., "A Qualitative Study of Independent Fast Food Vendors Near Secondary Schools in Disadvantaged Scottish Neighbourhoods," *BMC Public Health* 14 (2014): 793+.

9. Andrea K. Garber and Robert H. Lustig, "Is Fast Food Addictive?" *Current Drug Abuse Reviews* 4, no. 3 (2011): 146–62.

REFERENCES AND RESOURCES

Magazines, Journals, and Newspapers

Bahadoran, Z., P. Mirmiran, F. Hosseini-Esfahani, and F. Azizi. "Fast Food Consumption and the Risk of Metabolic Syndrome After 3-Years of Follow-Up: Tehran Lipid and Glucose Study." *European Journal of Clinical Nutrition* 67, no. 12 (2013): 1303–9.

Estrade, Michelle, Smita Dick, Fiona Crawford et al. "A Qualitative Study of Independent Fast Food Vendors Near Secondary Schools in Disadvantaged Scottish Neighbourhoods." *BMC Public Health* 14 (2014): 793+.

Garber, Andrea K., and Robert H. Lustig. "Is Fast Food Addictive?" *Current Drug Abuse Reviews* 4, no. 3 (2011): 146–62.

Garcia, Ginny, Thankam S. Sunil, and Pedro Hinojosa. "The Fast Food and Obesity Link: Consumptions Patterns and Severity of Obesity." *Obesity Surgery* 22, no. 5 (2012): 810–18.

Hollands, Simon, M. Karen Campbell, Jason Gilliland, and Sisira Sarma. "Association Between Neighbourhood Fast-Food and Full-Service Restaurant Density and Body Mass Index: A Cross-Sectional Study of Canadian Adults." *Canadian Journal of Public Health* 105, no. 3 (2014): e172–e178.

Laxer, Rachel E., and Ian Janssen. "The Proportion of Excessive Fast- Food Consumption Attributable to the Neighbourhood Food Environment Among Youth Living Within 1 km of Their School." *Applied Physiology, Nutrition, and Metabolism* 39, no. 4 (2014): 480–86.

Mytton, Oliver T., Dushy Clarke, and Mike Rayner. "Taxing Unhealthy Food and Drinks to Improve Health." *BMJ* 344 (2012): e2931.

Odegaard, Andrew O., Woon Puay Koh, Jian-Min Yuan et al. "Western-Style Fast Food Intake and Cardiometabolic Risk in an Eastern Country." *Circulation* 126 (2012): 182–88.

Shah, T., G. Purohit, S. P. Nair et al. "Assessment of Obesity, Overweight and Its Association with the Fast Food Consumption in Medical Students." *Journal of Clinical and Diagnostic Research* 8, no. 5 (2014): CC05–CC07.

Tobin, K. J. "Fast-Food Consumption and Educational Test Scores." *Child: Care, Health and Development* 39, no. 1 (2013): 118–24.

Web Site

National Center for Health Statistics. www.cdc.gov/nchs.

Limit the Intake of Caffeine and Energy Drinks

OVERVIEW

Caffeine is a chemical compound that is naturally found in the leaves and seeds of many plants and may also be artificially produced. Though caffeine is bitter, when it is highly processed, as it usually is, the bitter taste is muted. Found in many foods and drinks, such as coffee, chocolate, sodas, energy drinks, caffeinated water, and some medications, caffeine is considered a drug because it acts as a stimulant to the central nervous system and causes an increase in alertness, mood elevation, and energy boost. But, it may also trigger anxiety, dizziness, headaches, and jitters. Consuming a food or drink with caffeine later in the day or at night may result in insomnia or abnormal sleep patterns. People vary in their responses to caffeine. An amount that might keep one person up all night may have little effect on another person. Normally, smaller people react more than larger people to the same amount of caffeine. People easily develop a sensitivity to caffeine. So, as time passes, they may need to consume more caffeine for the same effects.

Caffeine is a mild diuretic, which means that it causes a person to urinate slightly more than usual. Most people will probably not notice the difference. Still, in hot weather or during longer workouts or sports practices or games, it is a good idea not to eat or drink too much food with caffeine. Some people maintain that caffeine triggers migraines; others contend that the consumption of caffeine during the early stages of a migraine stops the progression of the disorder. Caffeine causes the body to lose calcium, and, over time, that may result in bone loss. Caffeine has also been known to exacerbate certain heart problems.[1]

For teens, energy drinks are a frequent source of caffeine. Energy drinks, which contain between 50 and 500 mg of caffeine per can, have become very popular. In a 2015 study published in the *Canadian Journal of Public Health*, researchers from Ontario, Canada, wanted to determine the rates of energy drink use among secondary school students. The cohort consisted of 23,610 secondary students in Ontario. The researchers determined that nearly one in five of the students reported consuming an energy drink at least once a week. Of those who reported consuming energy drinks, the majority consumed energy drinks one or two days per week. However, 1 in 10 consumed energy drinks six or seven days each week. Males were more likely than females to use energy drinks. The researchers commented that their findings found that "Regular use of energy drinks was common among this sample of students."[2]

WHAT THE EXPERTS SAY

Caffeine-Consuming Children and Adolescents Demonstrate Altered Sleep Behavior and Sleep Depth

In a study published in 2015 in *Brain Sciences*, researchers from Switzerland and Colorado noted that caffeine is the most commonly consumed psychoactive drug throughout the world. Increasingly, it is becoming popular among children and teens. While it is known that caffeine may interfere in sleep quality among adults, the researchers wanted to learn if it interferes with sleep quality among children and teens. Using a sleep electroencephalogram (EEG), the researchers examined the sleep patterns of 32 children and teens between the ages of 10 and 16.9 years. Sixteen of the subjects reported the habitual consumption of at least two servings of caffeine per day for the past three years. The caffeine consumers were compared to the teens who denied regular caffeine intake. During the trial, the subjects were advised to follow their usual use or non-use of caffeine. The researchers learned that the caffeine consumers went to bed almost a full hour later than the non-caffeine consumers and spent 53 fewer minutes in bed. In addition, there was some indication that regular caffeine consumption was associated with reduced sleep depth. The researchers commented that "because deep sleep is involved in recovery processes during sleep, further research is needed to understand whether a caffeine-induced loss of sleep depth interacts with neuronal network refinement processes that occur during the sensitive period of adolescent development."[3]

Adolescent Intake of Caffeine Appears to Be Associated with Poorer Academic Achievement

In a study published in 2011 in the *Journal of Adolescence*, researchers from Ireland and Iceland wanted to learn more about the association between the use of caffeine by teens and academic achievement. The researchers noted that, on a typical day, about 75 percent of adolescent teens consume one or more beverages containing caffeine. The cohort consisted of 7,377 Icelandic teens, who were surveyed on several topics including caffeine use. While their primary source of caffeine was cola drinks, their second source was energy drinks. Caffeine appeared to have an independent negative effect on academic achievement. The researchers said that this finding "runs counter to popular beliefs that caffeine had performance-enhancing properties." The researchers wondered if the poorer functioning could be explained by symptoms of caffeine withdrawal such as sleepiness, lethargy, lack of attention, and decreased cognitive performance. "Improvements in performance following caffeine consumption [could be] explained by reversal of such withdrawal effects."[4]

There Appears to Be an Association between Energy Drink Consumption and Alcohol Dependence

In a study published in 2011 in the journal *Alcoholism: Clinical & Experimental Research*, researchers based in College Park, Maryland, examined the association between the consumption of energy drinks and alcohol dependence. Data were obtained from 1,097 fourth-year college students who attended a large university. They ranged in age from 20 to 23 years, and almost half were men. The participants were asked a series of questions about their use of energy drinks during the previous 12 months. They were also questioned about their alcohol intake. Slightly over 10 percent of the students were classified as high-frequency energy drink users; a little over half were classified as low-frequency energy drink users. When compared to the low-frequency energy drink users, the high-frequency energy drink users drank alcohol more frequently and in higher quantities, and the researchers determined that these participants were at increased risk for a dependence on alcohol. Their increased use of alcohol was associated with alcohol-related consequences, such as blacking out, missing class because of a hangover, and hangover-related limitations while completing usual activities. The researchers wondered if the heavier drinkers relied on energy drinks to help them function normally. And, they concluded that more research is needed "to clarify the mechanisms by which energy drink consumption might be related to increased risk for alcohol-related problems."[5]

Caffeine Consumption in Secondary School Teens Is Associated with Anxiety and Depression

In a study published in 2015 in the *Journal of Psychopharmacology*, researchers from the United Kingdom examined the association between the consumption of caffeine by secondary school teens and self-assessed stress, anxiety, and depression. They used cross-sectional data from the Cornish Academies Project, a large-scale longitudinal program of research on school performance, general health, and stress, anxiety, and depression in secondary school students from the southwest of England. The researchers found that the consumption of coffee was the "major contributor" to the teens' overall intake of caffeine. Initially, the researchers found associations between caffeine consumption and stress, anxiety, and depression. After further testing, the association between caffeine consumption and stress disappeared. And, the testing found that males and females had different response levels. For example, at the multivariate level, the consumption of caffeine was associated with anxiety in males but not females. In addition, though there was an association between caffeine intake and depression in males and females, the threshold for appearing was lower in males than in females. The researchers commented that their findings may "be a concern for public health and school policy."[6]

BARRIERS AND PROBLEMS

Many Teens Want to Use Energy Drinks That May Improve Their Cognitive Functioning, At Least Temporarily

In a randomized, double-blind, placebo-controlled, crossover study published in 2013 in *Appetite*, researchers from the United Kingdom, Australia, and California wanted to learn more about the effects of an energy drink shot on cognitive function and mood over a six-hour period of time. The trial compared the acute effects of the energy drink with a matching placebo in 94 healthy volunteers between the ages of 18 and 55 years. The night before each testing day, the volunteers were told to sleep between three and six hours. So, the researchers considered the volunteers "partially sleep-deprived." When compared to the placebo subjects, the energy drink significantly improved six validated cognitive functions as well as self-rated alertness. The benefits of four of the cognitive functions were still evident after six hours. The volunteers who received placebos experienced declines in their cognitive performance. The energy drink "helped maintain attentional focus, concentration, information processing and vigilance over the six hour period." The energy drink shot "facilitated performance on a range of everyday tasks in partially sleep deprived volunteers."[7]

Price and Labeling Information May Discourage Some Teens from Purchasing Energy Drinks

In a study published in 2016 in the *Journal of Nutrition Education and Behavior*, researchers from Buffalo, New York, investigated the effect energy drink pricing and labeling have on sales. Does increasing the price lower the chances that a teen will purchase an energy drink? Does providing more information on the label have a similar effect? The cohort consisted of 36 (18 males and 18 females) participants between the ages of 15 and 30 years with an average age of 20.4 years. They were all classified as energy drink consumers (drinking more than two energy drinks per week) or nonconsumers (drinking less than one energy drink per month). The participants visited a laboratory-based convenience store three times. In between visits, prices and labeling were altered. The researchers found that increasing the price of the energy drinks decreased the rates in which they were purchased. When the price was increased by 100 percent, no one who regularly used these drinks purchased them. "This suggests that ED [energy drink] consumers are sensitive to price manipulations and that increasing the price of these drinks may decrease ED purchasing among youth." When the price rose, adolescent consumers purchased other caffeinated products. Moreover, when the labels contained warnings about caffeine content, teens appeared to reduce their intake. The researchers commented that their findings "have implications for potential regulations that may discourage ED purchasing, especially among adolescents."[8]

NOTES

1. The Nemours Foundation, www.kidshealth.org.

2. J. L. Reid, D. Hammond, C. McCrory et al., "Use of Caffeinated Energy Drinks Among Secondary School Students in Ontario: Prevalence and Correlates of Using Energy Drinks and Mixing With Alcohol," *Canadian Journal of Public Health* 106, no. 3 (2015): e101–e108.

3. Andrina Aepli, Salome Kurth, Noemi Tesler et al., "Caffeine Consuming Children and Adolescents Show Altered Sleep Behavior and Deep Sleep," *Brain Sciences* 5 (2015): 441–55.

4. Jack E. James, Álfgeir Logi Kristjánsson, and Inga Dóra Sigfúsdóttir, "Adolescent Substance Use, Sleep, and Academic Achievement: Evidence of Harm Due to Caffeine," *Journal of Adolescence* 34 (2011): 665–73.

5. Amelia M. Arria, Kimberly M. Caldeira, Sarah J. Kasperski et al., "Energy Drink Consumption and Increased Risk for Alcohol Dependence," *Alcoholism: Clinical & Experimental Research* 35, no. 2 (2011): 365–75.

6. Gareth Richards and Andrew Smith. "Caffeine Consumption and Self-Assessed Stress, Anxiety, and Depression in Secondary School Children," *Journal of Psychopharmacology* 29, no. 12 (2015): 1236–47.

7. Keith A. Wesnes, Marilyn L. Barrett, and Jay K. Udani, "An Evaluation of the Cognitive and Mood Effects of An Energy Shot Over a 6h Period in Volunteers. A Randomized, Double-Blind, Placebo Controlled, Cross-Over Study," *Appetite* 67 (2013): 105–13.

8. Jennifer L. Temple, Amanda M. Ziegler, and Leonard H. Epstein, "Influence of Price and Labeling on Energy Drink Purchasing in an Experimental Convenience Store," *Journal of Nutrition Education and Behavior* 48, no. 7 (2016): 54–59e1.

REFERENCES AND RESOURCES

Magazines, Journals, and Newspapers

Aepli, Andrina, Salome Kurth, Noemi Tesler et al. "Caffeine Consuming Children and Adolescents Show Altered Sleep Behavior and Deep Sleep." *Brain Sciences* 5 (2015): 441–55.

Arria, Amelia M., Kimberly M. Caldeira, Sarah J. Kasperski et al. "Energy Drink Consumption and Increased Risk for Alcohol Dependence." *Alcoholism: Clinical & Experimental Research* 35, no. 2 (2011): 365–75.

Beckford, Kelsey, Carley A. Grimes, and Lynn J. Riddell. "Australian Children's Consumption of Caffeinate, Formulated Beverages: A Cross-Sectional Analysis." *BMC Public Health* 15 (2015): 70.

Ibrahim, N. K., and R. Iftikhar. "Energy Drinks: Getting Wings but at What Health Cost?" *Pakistan Journal of Medical Sciences* 30, no. 6 (2014): 1415–19.

James, Jack E., Álfgeir Logi Kristjánsson, and Inga Dóra Sigfúsdóttir. "Adolescent Substance Use, Sleep, and Academic Achievement: Evidence of Harm Due to Caffeine." *Journal of Adolescence* 34 (2011): 665–73.

Miyake, E. R., and N. R. Marmorstein. "Energy Drink Consumption and Later Alcohol Use Among Early Adolescents." *Addictive Behavior* 43 (2015): 60–65.

Reid, J. L., D. Hammond, C. McCrory et al. "Use of Caffeinated Energy Drinks Among Secondary School Students in Ontario: Prevalence and Correlates of Using Energy Drinks and Mixing With Alcohol." *Canadian Journal of Public Health* 106, no. 3 (2015): e101–e108.

Richards, Gareth, and Andrew Smith. "Caffeine Consumption and Self-Assessed Stress, Anxiety, and Depression in Secondary School Children." *Journal of Psychopharmacology* 29, no. 12 (2015): 1236–47.

Temple, Jennifer L., Amanda M. Ziegler, and Leonard H. Epstein. "Influence of Price and Labeling on Energy Drink Purchasing in An Experimental Convenience Store." *Journal of Nutrition Education and Behavior* 48, no. 2 (2016): 54–59e1.

Wesnes, Keith A., Marilyn L. Barrett, and Jay K. Udani. 2013. "An Evaluation of the Cognitive and Mood Effects of An Energy Shot Over a 6h Period in Volunteers. A Randomized, Double-Blind, Placebo Controlled, Cross-Over Study." *Appetite* 67 (2013): 105–13.

Web Sites

Psychology Today. www.psychologytoday.com.
The Nemours Foundation. www.kidshealth.org.

Limit Processed Food

OVERVIEW

While it is healthier to eat a clean diet of real foods, such as fresh fruits and vegetables—actual apples and fresh spinach—most people eat foods that have been mixed together and processed in some way. Often, the mixing together becomes complicated. Refined and artificial ingredients are added. The ingredient labeling may become an endless list of foods and other substances that are nearly impossible to pronounce. There are a countless number of these types of processed foods that are now available in most markets.

To make them tastier, processed foods often contain higher amounts of sugar and high fructose corn syrup. They tend to be high in calories, trans fats, and refined carbohydrates, and low in fiber. When purchasing any processed food, look for options with fewer ingredients. At least those processed foods will have fewer unhealthful ingredients. However, it is always best to treat processed foods as an occasional option, never a common mainstay.

WHAT THE EXPERTS SAY

There Appears to Be an Association between the Consumption of Processed Food and Depression

In a case-controlled study published in 2015 in the *Journal of Pediatric and Adolescent Gynecology*, researchers wanted to learn more about the association between the dietary patterns of adolescent females and depression. The study, which was conducted from April 2011 to December 2012, had a cohort of 849 females between the ages of 12 and 18 years, with a mean age of 15 years. After assessments were conducted of the participants' dietary patterns for the previous 12 months, the researchers learned that 116 or 13.6 percent of the teens had depressive symptoms. The researchers found a significant positive association between depressive symptoms and consumption of instant and processed foods, including ramen noodles, hamburger, pizza, and fried food. In contrast, the researchers observed that the nondepressive teens had higher intakes of green vegetables and fruits. According to the researchers, "this is the first report in

which high intake of fast foods and processed foods and low intake of green vegetables and fruits were associated with increased risk of depression in Korean
adolescent girls."[1]

Processed Foods Tend to Contain Higher Amounts of Sodium

In a cross-sectional study that was published in 2015, researchers from Brazil
investigated the levels of sodium found in the snacks consumed by children and
adolescents in Brazil. Sodium content and snack sizing were assessed in 2,945
processed foods sold at a supermarket that is part of a large chain in Brazil. Data
were collected from October to December 2011. The researchers learned that
21 percent of the foods had high levels of sodium, 35 percent had medium levels,
and 43 percent had low levels. Processed foods tended to have higher levels of
sodium. In fact, the prepared/semiprepared food subgroup had sodium values up
to 2,390 mg/serving, well over what the maximum intake should be for an entire
day. The researchers noted that high sodium levels found in some of the snacks
could be reduced, as they have been reduced in other similar snacks. "This situation suggests the potential to reduce Na [sodium] content in most of the processed foods assessed, especially those classified as high Na."[2]

Eating Processed Foods Seems to Be Associated
with Weight Gain

In a study published in 2015 in the journal *Health Affairs*, researchers from
Singapore and Durham, North Carolina, wanted to identify foods and beverages
that were associated with weight gain in children and teens. For their data, the
researchers used a cohort from the Avon Longitudinal Study of Parents and
Children in the United Kingdom that consisted of 15,444 children born in southwest England. With 4,646 children from that cohort, the researchers quantified
associations between 27 food and beverage groups and excess weight gain in three-
year periods among youth ages 7, 10, and 13 years. Several foods were associated
with excess weight gain. These included processed foods such as breaded or bat-
tered poultry, coated fish, processed meats, desserts, and sweets. The researchers
noted that students should be encouraged to eat foods that will not add excess
weight, such as those with less processing. "A strategy that encourages them to eat
foods that are associated with weight loss, such as whole grains, uncoated poultry,
and vegetables may be effective in controlling hunger and restricting total energy
intake."[3]

In a study published in 2015 in the journal *Preventive Medicine*, researchers
from Brazil, Boston, and the United Kingdom investigated the association between the consumption of ultraprocessed foods and obesity among Brazilian teens
and adults. The researchers used cross-sectional food consumption data on 30,243
people aged 10 years and older. Slightly over half were women. Forty-one percent

of the participants were overweight and 12 percent were obese. Food items were classified according to their amount of processing. Ultraprocessed foods contained little or no whole food. In the cohort studied, 30 percent of the total food intake came from ultraprocessed foods. Those in the highest quintile of ultraprocessed food consumption had significantly higher body mass index and higher odds of being obese and having excess weight than those in the lowest quintile of ultra-processed food consumption. The researchers also learned that almost one-third of the energy consumed in Brazil came from ultraprocessed foods; many of the portions are far larger than they should be and the food has little if any nutritional value. And, the health of women who eat ultraprocessed foods is more negatively impacted than the health of men. "Growing evidence suggests that women are more predisposed to adverse metabolic effects of rapidly digested, carbohydrate-rich foods than men, which might explain larger effects of ultra-processed foods on adiposity in women." The researchers noted that their findings "supported the role of ultra-processed foods consumption in the obesity epidemic in Brazil."[4]

Consumption of Processed Foods Appears to Be Associated with Metabolic Syndrome in Adolescents

In a study published in 2011 in the journal *Public Health Nutrition*, researchers from Brazil wanted to learn more about the association between consumption of ultraprocessed foods and metabolic syndrome, a disorder characterized by obesity, hypertension, alternation in glucose metabolism, low HDL ("good") cholesterol, and wider waist circumference. The researchers used data from the CAMELIA (cardio-metabolic-renal) project, which included surveys with 210 adolescents conducted from July 2006 to December 2007. Metabolic syndrome was diagnosed in 6.7 percent of the teens, who were between 12 and 19 years. When their food intake was analyzed, it was determined that the teens with metabolic syndrome had a higher average daily intake of energy, carbohydrates, and ultraprocessed foods than the teens without metabolic syndrome. According to the researchers, "a balanced diet, emphasizing the intake of minimally processed foods and a low consumption of ultra-processed foods, should be encouraged and incorporated into the habits of teenagers."[5]

BARRIERS AND PROBLEMS

Students Who Attend Schools Located Near Fast Food Outlets Eat More Processed Food

In a study published in 2015 in the *Asia Pacific Journal of Clinical Nutrition*, researchers from Korea examined the impact of fast food outlets selling processed foods near 342 elementary and secondary schools in the Gyeonggi province of Korea. Specifically, they wanted to learn more about the relationship between the dietary health of the children and teens and the density of fast food outlets in that area of Korea. Would children and teens who had increased access to the outlets eat more processed foods? The researchers used a questionnaire to gather data on the dietary intake of 243 sixth and eighth grade students at eight schools. They classified schools in the upper 20 percent of fast food outlets as having high density and in the lower 20 percent as having low density. The high-density group had 8 to 12 fast food outlets within a 15-minute walk from the school; the low-density group had no more than one outlet within the same distance. The researchers determined that the students in the low-density areas visited fast food outlets less often than the students in the high-density areas. The difference was statistically significant. As a result, students in the high-density areas ate far more processed food. The researchers advised schools and parents in high-density areas to offer the students "more active education on the selection of foods and formation of proper dietary habits at school and at home."[6]

To Emerging Adults, Taste Is the Most Important Influence on Food Selection, and Processed Food Tends to Be Tasty

In a study published in 2015 in the *Journal of Human Nutrition and Dietetics*, researchers from Australia wanted to learn more about the outside of the home food selection patterns of older teens and young adults. Their cohort consisted of 112 emerging adult university students between the ages of 19 and 24 years. All of the participants completed an online survey which assessed demographics, perceived stress, dieting, physical activity, and influences on food selection. Body mass index and waist circumference, both indicators of adiposity, were measured. The researchers found that taste was the most important influence on food selection. Taste was following by convenience (availability), cost, nutrition/health value, smell, and stimulatory properties (alertness). Processed foods tend to be tasty, convenient, and budget friendly, but they are definitely not healthful. Emerging adults should be eating more nonprocessed food. "Health promotion strategies addressing tertiary education food environments should focus on ensuring the ready availability of tasty and nutritious foods at a low cost."[7]

Processed Foods Tend to Be the Most Readily Available Packaged Products

In a study published in 2016 in *Public Health Nutrition*, researchers from New Zealand wanted to determine more about the availability of ultraprocessed foods in four major supermarkets in Auckland New Zealand in 2011 and 2013. Using data obtained from the NutriTrack database, which collected data on 6,020 packaged food and beverage products in 2011 and 13,406 packaged food products in 2013, the researchers determined that the vast majority of packaged foods were ultraprocessed. In 2011, 84 percent of the packaged foods and in 2013, 83 percent of the packaged foods were ultraprocessed. While ultraprocessed foods are readily available, they contain few, if any, nutrients. And, the consumption of these processed foods seems to decrease the quality of the diet. The researchers commented that "the high availability of ultra-processed foods is a major concern."[8]

NOTES

1. Tae-Hee Kim, Ji-young Choi, Hae-Hyeog Lee, and Yongsoon Park, "Associations between Dietary Pattern and Depression in Korean Adolescent Girls," *Journal of Pediatric and Adolescent Gynecology* 28, no. 6 (2015): 533–37.

2. M. V. Kraemer, R. C. Oliveira, D. A. Gonzalez-Chica, and R. P. Proença, "Sodium Content on Processed Foods for Snacks," *Public Health Nutrition* 19, no. 6 (April 2016): 967–75.

3. Di Dong, Marcel Bilger, Rob M. van Dam, and Eric A. Finkelstein, "Consumption of Specific Foods and Beverages and Excess Weight Gain Among Children and Adolescents," *Health Affairs* 34, no. 11 (2015): 1940–48.

4. M. L. Louzada, L. G. Baraldi, E. M. Steele et al., "Consumption of Ultra-Processed Foods and Obesity in Brazilian Adolescents and Adults," *Preventive Medicine* 81 (2015): 9–15.

5. L. F. Tavares, S. C. Fonseca, M. L. G. Rosa, and E. M. Yokoo, "Relationship between Ultra-Processed Foods and Metabolic Syndrome in Adolescents from a Brazilian Family Doctor Program," *Public Health Nutrition* 15, no. 1 (2011): 82–87.

6. Soonnam Joo, Seyoung Ju, and Hyeja Chang, "Comparison of Fast Food Consumption and Dietary Guideline Practices for Children and Adolescents by Clustering of Fast Food Outlets around Schools in the Gyeonggi Area of Korea," *Asia Pacific Journal of Clinical Nutrition* 24, no. 2 (2015): 299–307.

7. L. Hebden, H. N. Chan, J. C. Louie et al., "You Are What You Choose to Eat: Factors Influencing Young Adults' Food Selection Behaviour," *Journal of Human Nutrition and Dietetics* 28, no. 4 (2015): 401–8.

8. Claire M. Luiten, Ingrid H. M. Steenhuis, Helen Eyes et al., "Ultra-Processed Foods Have the Worst Nutrient Profile, Yet They Are the Most Available Packaged Products in a Sample of New Zealand Supermarkets." *Public Health Nutrition* 19, no. 3 (2016): 530–38.

REFERENCES AND RESOURCES

Magazines, Journals, and Newspapers

Dong, Di, Marcel Bilger, Rob M. van Dam, and Eric A. Finkelstein. "Consumption of Specific Foods and Beverages and Excess Weight Gain Among Children and Adolescents." *Health Affairs* 34, no. 11 (2015): 1940–48.

Hebden, L., H. N. Chan, J. C. Louie et al. "You Are What You Choose To Eat: Factors Influencing Young Adults' Food Selection Behaviour." *Journal of Human Nutrition and Dietetics* 28, no. 4 (2015): 401–8.

Joo, Soonnam, Seyoung Ju, and Hyeja Chang. "Comparison of Fast Food Consumption and Dietary Guideline Practices for Children and Adolescents by Clustering of Fast Food Outlets around Schools in the Gyeonggi Area of Korea." *Asia Pacific Journal of Clinical Nutrition* 24, no. 2 (2015): 299–307.

Kim, Tae-Hee, Ji-young Choi, Hae-Hyeog Lee, and Yongsoon Park. "Associations between Dietary Pattern and Depression in Korean Adolescent Girls." *Journal of Pediatric and Adolescent Gynecology* 28, no. 6 (2015): 533–37.

Kraemer, M. V., R. C. Oliveira, D. A. Gonzalez-Chica, and R. P. Proença. "Sodium Content on Processed Foods for Snacks." *Public Health Nutrition* 19, no. 6 (April 2016) 967–75.

Louzada, M. L., L. G. Baraldi, E. M. Steele et al. "Consumption of Ultra-Processed Foods and Obesity in Brazilian Adolescents and Adults." *Preventive Medicine* 81 (2015): 9–15.

Luiten, Claire M., Ingrid H. M. Steenhuis, Helen Eyles et al. "Ultra-Processed Foods Have the Worst Nutrient Profile, Yet They Are the Most Available Packaged Products in a Sample Of New Zealand Supermarkets." *Public Health Nutrition* 19, no 3 (2016): 530–38.

Powell, L.M., B. T. Nguyen, and W. H. Dietz. "Energy and Nutrient Intake from Pizza in the United States." *Pediatrics* 135, no. 2 (2015): 322–30.

Punitha, V. C., A. Amudhan, P. Sivaprakasam, and V. Rathanaprabu. "Role of Dietary Habits and Diet in Caries Occurrence and Severity among Urban Adolescent School Children." *Journal of Pharmacy & BioAllied Sciences* 7, Supplement 1 (2015): S296–S300.

Tavares, L. F., S. C. Fonseca, M. L. G. Rosa, and E. M. Yokoo. "Relationship between Ultra-Processed Foods and Metabolic Syndrome in Adolescents from a Brazilian Family Doctor Program." *Public Health Nutrition* 15, no. 1 (2011): 82–87.

Web Site

Body Ecology. www.bodyecology.com.

Limit Sodium and Salt Intake

OVERVIEW

People of all ages require some amount of sodium, an essential mineral and electrolyte, in their bodies. The many everyday heart and muscular functions carried out by the body cannot be completed without a small amount of sodium. Sodium is also needed for nerve cell transmission and to keep bones strong. But, most people, including teens and young adults, consume far more sodium than the body requires. The problem is not only a result of the sodium obtained from the shaker on the table. Rather, it is a direct result the high amounts of sodium frequently found in prepared and processed foods.

Like adults, teens require about 1,500 milligrams of sodium per day. Most of the sodium in the diet is derived from ordinary salt. Salt contains about 40 percent sodium and 60 percent chloride. That means that a teaspoon of salt has 2,000 milligrams of sodium. Americans consume about 3,400 milligrams of sodium per day, far more than they require. Children two years of age and older should consume no more than 2,300 mg/day. African American children and children with medical problems, such as high blood pressure, diabetes, or chronic kidney disease, should consume less than 1,500 mg/day. While a teen is far more likely to have a diet that has too much salt, salt deficiencies may occur. Thus, a teen who plays a sport on a hot day may lose salt in sweat. Or, a teen who becomes ill with fever, diarrhea, and/or vomiting may have low levels of sodium. During these special circumstances, a sports drinks may be used to replenish the lost sodium. But, most sports drinks contain higher amounts of sugar and calories. So, they should not be part of the daily diet.

WHAT THE EXPERTS SAY

There Is an Association between Sodium Intake and Blood Pressure Readings in U.S. Children and Adolescents

In a study published in 2012 in the journal *Pediatrics*, researchers based at the Centers for Disease Control and Prevention in Atlanta, Georgia, investigated the association between the intake of sodium and elevated levels of blood pressure in children and teens. They also reviewed the role that weight may play in this association. The cohort consisted of 6,235 children and adolescents between the ages of 8 and 18 years who participated in the National Health and Nutrition Examination Survey from 2003 to 2008. All of the subjects provided at least one 24-hour dietary recall at the examination center, and 91 percent provided a second recall during a telephone interview conducted 3 to 10 days later. During visits to the examination center, blood pressure measurements were taken up to three times. The researchers found that the study subjects consumed an average of 3,387 mg/day of sodium, and the average sodium intake appeared to increase with age. Thirty-seven percent of the subjects were either overweight or obese. Each 1,000 mg/day was associated with an increase in the systolic blood pressure (top blood pressure number). High sodium intake was also associated with the risk for pre–high blood pressure and high blood pressure. Sodium consumption was higher among males than among female subjects and higher among those of normal weight than among those who were overweight or obese. But, the high intake of sodium may affect overweight and obese children and adolescents more than those with normal weight, making them more at risk for pre–high blood pressure and high blood pressure. The researchers commented that "evidence-based interventions that help participants reduce their sodium intake, increase physical activity, and attain or maintain a healthy weight may help reduce the greater than expected prevalence of HBP [high blood pressure] and other cardiovascular disease risk factors among children and adolescents."[1]

There May Be an Independent Association between the Intake of Salt and Obesity

In a study published in 2015 in the journal *Hypertension*, researchers from the United Kingdom and China wanted to learn more about the association between the intake of salt and obesity. They used data obtained from the U.K. National Diet and Nutrition Survey 2008/2009 to 2011/2012 that included 458 children and 785 adults who had completed 24-hour urine collections. Energy intake was calculated from a four-day diary. The researchers found that salt intake was higher in people who are overweight or obese. In fact, a one gram/day increase in salt intake was associated with a 28 percent increase in the risk of obesity in children and a 26 percent increase in the risk of obesity in adults. Higher salt intake was also significantly related to higher body fat mass in children and adults. The researchers commented, "Salt intake is a potential risk factor for obesity independent of energy intake," and that their findings have important public health implications. People trying to lose weight should reduce their intake of salt. "Salt reduction could also reduce obesity risk."[2]

People Are Consuming Excess Amounts of Salt

In a study published in 2015 in the journal *Nutrients*, researchers from China wanted to determine sources of dietary salt as well as quantify the actual amount of salt people were consuming. Nine hundred and three families, including 1,981 adults and 971 children, participated in a one-week salt estimation trial. The children were students in schools in urban and suburban Beijing. The researchers found that, on average, the daily dietary salt intake of family members in Beijing was 11 grams for children and teens and 15.2 grams for adults, and 10.2 grams for people 60 years and older. These amounts are at least twice the Word Health Organization's recommendation of no more than 5 grams/day. Slightly over 60 percent of the salt was consumed at home; the remaining salt was consumed outside the home, specifically in cafeterias and restaurants. Suburban residents consumed more salt than urban residents, and men consumed more salt than women. The researchers concluded that "more targeted interventions aimed at altering domestic cooking habits and commercial cooking methods to use less salt should be undertaken to reduce the harm and risk posed by a high salt diet."[3]

BARRIERS AND PROBLEMS

Teens Tend to Obtain High Levels of Sodium from the Snacks They Eat, and That Is Associated with Elevated Blood Pressure

In a study published in 2015 in the *European Journal of Clinical Nutrition*, researchers from Italy wanted to learn more about the association between the intake of sodium in snacks and blood pressure levels in teens. The cohort consisted of

1,200 randomly selected teens between the ages of 11 and 13 years who were first-year middle school students. The researchers used a food frequency questionnaire to evaluate the teens' weekly consumption of snacks. Trained researchers obtained blood pressure readings. Four hundred of the teens also completed a dietary 24-hour food-recall questionnaire. The researchers learned that the teens obtained about half of their total sodium from snacks. In addition, there was a positive significant association between blood pressure and both the sodium intake from snacks and the frequency of the consumption of salty snack foods.[4]

People May Be Confused by Sodium Information on Nutrition Labels

In a study published in 2015 in the journal *Preventing Chronic Disease*, researchers from the Centers for Disease Control and Prevention conducted an assessment of consumers' use of sodium information on U.S. nutrition labels. The cohort consisted of 3,729 people aged 18 years or older who participated in two national cross-sectional mail panel surveys in 2010. The researchers determined that 19.3 percent of the respondents were confused about the amounts of sodium in the food that they were eating. Close to 60 percent of the respondents noted that the person who shops for their food purchases foods labeled low salt or low sodium, and, hoping to lower their intake of sodium, almost half reported checking labels for sodium content. Consumers with a high school education or less were more likely than college graduates to report that they were confused about sodium content on labels. Adults aged 71 years or older, non-Hispanic blacks, and people with diabetes were also more likely to be confused about sodium labeling. The researchers suggested that food manufacturers should produce food products that are lower in sodium and include low sodium information on the front of packages. "Doing so will offer greater choice and availability for the majority of consumers who want to buy low sodium products."[5]

Restaurant Meals May Contain High Amounts of Sodium

In a study published in 2014 in *Preventing Chronic Illness*, researchers from the Centers for Disease Control and Prevention addressed the high amounts of sodium that are often contained in restaurant meals. Why is this important? In 2011, Americans dined outside the home almost five times per week. Obviously, eating so many meals with high amounts of sodium increases the risk of a number of medical problems, especially high blood pressure. According to these researchers, there are a number of commonly eaten foods that tend to be high in sodium. These include sandwiches, pizza, hamburgers, chicken, Mexican entrees, and salads. The situation is further complicated by the fact that restaurant patrons often underestimate the sodium, calorie, and fat content of the food they eat. "Because consumers have less control over the way in which meals are prepared outside the home, it is challenging to simply look at a meal and discern the amount of sodium that it contains."[6]

Many Children Appear to Prefer the Taste of Saltier Foods

In a study published in 2013 in the online journal *PLoS ONE*, researchers from France noted that there has been little research on the role that salt plays in the willingness of children to eat certain foods. The researchers recruited 75 children between the ages of 8 and 11 years to participate in five lunches in their school cafeteria. The green beans and pasta had two different amounts of added salt. The children's intake of all lunch items was measured, and the children ranked the foods according to preferences and saltiness. While the primary reason the children ate was hunger, the second most important factor was the enjoyment of the food. And, the children preferred the food with more salt. A reduction in the salt content of green beans decreased their intake by 21 percent, and an increase in the salt content in pasta increased their intake by 24 percent. "Taking into account children's preferences for salt . . . may lead to excessive added salt."[7]

NOTES

1. Q. Yang, Z. Zhang, E. V. Kuklina et al., "Sodium Intake and Blood Pressure Among US Children and Adolescents," *Pediatrics* 130, no. 4 (2012): 611–19.

2. Yuan Ma, Feng J. He, and Graham A. MacGregor, "High Salt Intake: Independent Risk Factor for Obesity?" *Hypertension* 66, no. 4 (2015): 843–49.

3. Frang Zhao, Puhong Zhang, Lu Zhang et al., "Consumption and Sources of Dietary Sat in Family Members in Beijing," *Nutrients* 7 (2015): 2719–30.

4. V. Ponzo, G.P. Ganzit, L. Soldati et al., "Blood Pressure and Sodium Intake from Snacks in Adolescents," *European Journal of Clinical Nutrition* 69, no. 6 (2015): 681–86.

5. Jessica Lee Levings, Joyce Maalouf, Xin Tong, and May E. Cogswell, "Reported Use and Perceived Understanding of Sodium Information on US Nutrition Labels," *Preventing Chronic Disease* 12 (2015): 140522.

6. Jessica Lee Levings and Janelle Peralez Gunn, "From Menu to Mouth: Opportunities for Sodium Reduction In Restaurants," *Preventing Chronic Disease* 11 (2014): 130237.

7. Sofia Bouhlal, Claire Chabanet, Sylvie Issanchou, and Sophie Nicklaus, "Salt Content Impacts Food Preferences and Intake Among Children," *PLoS ONE* 8, no. 1 (2013): e53971.

REFERENCES AND RESOURCES

Magazines, Journals, and Newspapers

Bouhlal, Sofia, Claire Chabanet, Sylvie Issanchou, and Sophie Nicklaus. "Salt Content Impacts Food Preferences and Intake Among Children." *PLoS ONE* 8, no. 1 (2013): e53971.

He, Feng J., Yangfeng Wu, Xiang-Xian Feng et al. "School Based Education Programme to Reduce Salt Intake in Children and Their Families (School-EduSalt): Custer Randomised Controlled Trial." *BMJ* 350 (2015): h770.

Hoeft, Kristin S., Claudia Guerra, M. Judy Gonzalez-Vargas, and Judith C. Barer. "Rural Latino Caregivers' Beliefs and Behaviors Around Their Children's Salt Consumption." *Appetite* 87 (2015): 1–9.

Levings, Jessica Lee, Joyce Maalouf, Xin Tong, and Mary E. Cogswell. "Reported Use and Perceived Understanding of Sodium Information on US Nutrition Labels." *Preventing Chronic Disease* 12 (2015): 140522.

Levings, Jessica Lee, and Janelle Peralez Gunn. "From Menu to Mouth: Opportunities for Sodium Reduction in Restaurants." *Preventing Chronic Disease* 11 (2014): 130237.

Ma, Yuan, Feng J. He, and Graham A. MacGregor. "High Salt Intake: Independent Risk Factor for Obesity?" *Hypertension* 66, no. 4 (2015): 843–49.

Ponzo, V., G. P. Ganzit, L. Soldati et al. "Blood Pressure and Sodium Intake from Snacks in Adolescents." *European Journal of Clinical Nutrition* 69, no. 6 (2015): 681–86.

Yang, Q., Z. Zhang, E. V. Kuklina et al. "Sodium Intake and Blood Pressure Among US Children and Adolescents." *Pediatrics* 130, no. 4 (2012): 611–19.

Zhao, Frang, Puhong Zhang, Lu Zhang et al. "Consumption and Sources of Dietary Salt in Family Members in Beijing." *Nutrients* 7 (2015): 2719–30.

Web Site

American Heart Association. www.heart.org.

Read Food Labels

OVERVIEW

For many people, shopping for food is just one more thing to do in an already time-pressed day. Often, the goal is simply to purchase the food as quickly as possible. So, why should anyone set aside additional time to read food labels? Some people have medical conditions that require the elimination of certain foods, so reading labels is a mandatory component of shopping for them. For example, people with peanut allergies must be certain that their food contains no peanuts and was not prepared near any peanuts, which could result in cross-contamination. Similarly, people with celiac disease, an autoimmune disorder, need to avoid foods with gluten found in wheat, barley, rye, and oats (via cross-contamination). Eating foods with gluten may trigger a host of different medical concerns including anemia, diarrhea, bloating, and infertility. People may also have a food intolerance. It is not uncommon for adults to lack the ability to digest milk; people with a milk intolerance may wish to avoid foods containing milk and milk products.

There are still more reasons for people to read food labels. The millions of people who are trying to lose weight may wish to eat foods that have fewer calories. Those who are trying to lower their blood pressure may want foods lower in sodium, also known as salt, sodium benzoate, and disodium. And, those who want to eliminate trans fats, which are discussed in another entry, may be searching for partially hydrogenated oil and hydrogenated oil on the label. It is interesting to note that a food may be labeled trans fat–free even if it contains up to a half gram of trans fats per serving.

When discussing food labels, it is important to realize that the ingredients are listed in descending order. As a result, the first few listed ingredients are the ones that are most important. Thus, if the first ingredient is sugar, then the food contains more sugar than any other ingredient.

It may be hard for people to believe, but the U.S. Food and Drug Administration (FDA) did not become seriously involved with food labeling until the 1980s. Then, the passage of the Nutrition Labeling and Education Act of 1990 launched the first Nutrition Facts label. According to the FDA, improved food labeling would "reduce consumer confusion about labels, help consumers make better food choices and encourage innovation by giving manufacturers an incentive to improve the nutrition profiles of foods." The law went into effect on May 8, 1994. Since then, all packaged food must have food labels. In 2006, the FDA required the listing of trans fats on labels. Early in 2014, the FDA proposed more changes to the Nutrition Facts label. The FDA wants to increase the calorie and serving size information as well as shift the location of the Percent Daily Value column to the left. In addition, the FDA wants the serving sizes to reflect the amount of food that people actually eat or drink. Other changes include requiring manufacturers to indicate the amount of "nutrients of public health significance" and "added sugar."[1]

WHAT THE EXPERTS SAY

Reading Food Labels Appears to Be Associated with Healthier Eating in Korean Men

In a study published in 2014 in the *Korean Journal of Family Medicine*, researchers from Korea investigated the association between the reading of nutrition labels in Korea and the actual food that people ate. The researchers noted that previous studies have found that females and people with higher levels of income and education tend to read these labels more frequently. Their cohort consisted of 13,924 people derived from data from the fourth KNHANES, a national Korean data project. The subjects were divided into two groups—those who read labels (slightly less than 25 percent) and those who didn't. The mean age of the label readers was 37.6 years; the mean age of the nonreaders was 46.3 years. People who thought they were obese or who had a chronic illness such as hypertension or diabetes were more likely to read the labels. Female label readers had a lower intake of calories and carbohydrates; male label readers had an increased consumption of calcium, vitamin C, and fiber. The researchers concluded that their results are "important." According to the researchers, "this study . . . has used data that represents the adult population in Korea to confirm the association between the use of nutrition labels and actual nutrition intake."[2]

Health-Conscious People Are More Likely to Read Food Labels

In a study published in 2011 in *Public Health Nutrition*, researchers from Switzerland wanted to learn more about factors that determine who uses food labels. Questionnaires were sent to a sample of households in German-speaking sections of Switzerland. Residents completed and returned 1,162 questionnaires, a response rate of 38 percent. While 13 percent of the respondents reported that they never used labels, only 5 percent said that they always used them. Knowledge about nutrition and the belief that healthy eating is a cornerstone to good health were pivotal predictors of food label reading. "Respondents who considered health, healthy eating, and the nutritional value of food as important reported more frequent label use than respondents who did not place importance on these aspects." On the other hand, disease-related aspects seemed to play a lesser role in predicting the use of labels. The researchers noted that their findings "implied that people rather use labels because they are interested in health and healthy eating and not primarily because they are afraid of falling ill."[3]

Frequent Food Label Use Is Associated with Healthier Dietary Intake in College Students

In a study published in 2012 in the *Journal of the Academy of Nutrition and Dietetics*, researchers from Minneapolis, Minnesota, investigated the association between the reading of food labels and quality of diet in a diverse group of college age students. The cohort consisted of 1,201 students; 598 attended a two-year community college and 603 attended a public four-year university. The students had a mean age of 21.5 years. The researchers classified 35 percent of the students as "frequent label readers." When compared to the students who infrequently read food labels, the frequent label readers had healthier dietary behaviors, such as eating more fiber and limiting their consumption of fast food, and they demonstrated more knowledge about nutrition. The researchers concluded that "reading nutrition labels appears to be a mechanism through which college students who value healthy meal preparation make healthy dietary decisions." Moreover, "even among those who do not believe it is important to prepare healthy meals, nutrition label use is linked with healthier dietary intake, suggesting that label use among college relates to healthful dietary intake independently of attitude toward healthy meals."[4]

BARRIERS AND PROBLEMS

Of course, there are barriers to reading food labels. And, there is a research study that found a serious underutilization of food ingredient labels, even by people who should be more motivated. In a cross-sectional trial published in 2013 in the *Pakistan Journal of Biological Sciences*, researchers from Iran wanted to assess the knowledge women have about nutrition and food labels. The cohort consisted of 380 women who were interviewed in person in 2012 at four large supermarkets. Only 49.7 percent of the women were considered healthy; the majority had chronic illnesses, especially high blood pressure. Yet, only 32.9 percent of the women "always use nutritional labels." Of the women who read labels, they were most often looking for low calorie counts and reduced amounts of fat; they were least likely to be looking for foods with low levels of sugar. And, despite the high rates of elevated blood pressure, women tended not to look at the levels of sodium, which is known to raise blood pressure. In addition, the women who read the food labels had more knowledge about nutrition and higher levels of education.[5]

Other researchers have investigated additional barriers and problems related to the use of food labels.

Food Labels Are Not Always Read Correctly or Understood Properly, and Some People Have No Interest in Them

In a study published in 2014 in the *Journal of the Academy of Nutrition and Dietetics*, researchers from Los Angeles and Tucson, Arizona, wanted to learn if the Latino population of two East Los Angeles neighborhoods read and utilized food labels. The researchers noted that there have been few studies on this topic. Studies that have been completed have found "low levels of awareness of the labels as well as language barriers that hinder comprehension." The cohort consisted of 269 people aged 18 years or older who lived within certain block clusters; all the participants identified themselves as "Latino." More than three-quarters of the participants were female. The researchers found that the participants scored poorly. There was "no statistically significant association between Nutrition Facts label utilization and adequate comprehension." Thus, "those who reported using the Nutrition Facts label more often did not have a higher performance of reading and interpreting the label correctly." Thus, while the participants may well be reading the labels, they are incorrectly interpreting the information.[6]

In a study published in 2012 in *Appetite*, researchers from Israel investigated the ability of 120 young adults, with a mean age of 24.1 years, to comprehend the information written on food labels. All the participants were attending an international travel immunization clinic. Most of them, 77.5 percent, indicated that they read food labels. Women, people with higher levels of education, and those who regularly exercise were more likely to read the labels. During the study, the participants were asked to answer questions about information on the labels of 10 products. The overall median comprehension score was 6 out of 10. "The subjects thought they understood the food labels better than they actually did; 43.9 percent stated that they understood them very well, whereas only 27.2 percent achieved high scores." The researchers commented that "this inadequate comprehension of food labels represents a missed opportunity to provide essential information necessary for healthy food choices at the individual level."[7]

In a study published in 2014 in *Public Health Nutrition*, researchers from New Zealand conducted in person semistructured interviews with 10 women and six men, who were grocery shoppers between the ages of 28 and 63 years. The researchers wanted to determine how they did or did not use food labels and other behaviors to control their intake of sodium. The researchers learned that their food purchases were primarily a function of "practical considerations."

The most important element in choosing a product was "price." But, brand familiarity also played a role. No one reported using nutrition information. Although 13 participants recalled that they had seen such information, nine noted that they did not "pay particular attention to it." At the same time, the participants reported that they "paid attention to eating healthy food." And, according to them, because they ate well, they did not need to read food labels.

During a portion of the interview, the participants were asked specific questions about their intake of salt. They appeared to have little understanding of the relationship between salt and health problems. "Ironically, participants were more concerned they might be consuming inadequate quantities of salt, which they believed could be bad for their health." The researchers concluded that New Zealand consumers need more food and nutrition education.[8]

In a cross-sectional study published in 2014 in *Public Health Nutrition*, researchers from India wanted to learn more about what Indian consumers knew about food labels. As a result, they conducted interviews with 1,832 consumers at supermarket sites. They also led focus groups; each had between four and nine participants. The researchers learned that more than 12 percent of all consumers reported purchasing prepackaged foods every day. Over 44 percent said that they bought prepackaged food once weekly. While the participants noted that they checked labels for brand name, manufacturing date, and expiration date, they generally did not review nutrition information. They were concerned primarily with "safety aspects of foods." The technical information on the label was deemed too difficult to comprehend. The researchers concluded that "there is a need to take up educational activities and/or introduce new forms of labeling."[9]

Information on the Food Label May Be Incorrect

In a study published in 2014 in *Nutrients*, researchers from Calgary and Toronto, Canada, tested the accuracy of food labels in Canada. During a four-year period, 1,010 foods and beverages from supermarkets, bakeries, and restaurants across Canada were analyzed at the Canadian Food Inspection Agency. The inspectors compared the sodium levels, calories, and the amounts of saturated fat, trans fat, and sugar listed on the labels to what they found in their laboratory analyses. The researchers determined that 169 items or 16.7 percent of the tested products had laboratory values that exceeded the label's stated amount by more than 20 percent. Sodium had the highest number of inaccuracies; trans fats had the lowest. The researchers noted that "Canadians' ability to make informed nutritional decisions is grounded in the assumption that the NFt [Nutrition Facts table] is accurate and reliable." Likewise, NFt inaccuracies could have serious implications for the many consumers who use this data to make healthy dietary choices and for decision makers developing and evaluating national nutrition policies.[10]

NOTES

1. U.S. Food and Drug Administration, www.fda.gov.

2. Min-Gyou Kim, Seung-Won Oh, Na-Rae Han et al., "Association Between Nutrition Label Reading and Nutrient Intake in Korean Adults: Korea National Health and Nutritional Examination Survey, 2007–2009 (KNHANES IV)," *Korean Journal of Family Medicine* 35, no. 4 (2014): 190–98.

3. Rebecca Hess, Vivianne H. M. Visschers, and Michael Siegrist, "The Role of Health-Related, Motivational and Sociodemographic Aspects in Predicting Food Label Use: A Comprehensive Study." *Public Health Nutrition* 15, no. 3 (2012): 407–14.

4. Dan J. Graham and Melissa N. Laska, "Nutrition Label Use Partially Mediates the Relationship Between Attitude Toward Healthy Eating and Overall Dietary Quality Among College Students," *Journal of the Academy of Nutrition and Dietetics* 112, no. 3 (2012): 414–18.

5. Afsane Ahmadi, Pariya Torkamani, Zahra Sohrabi, and Fariba Ghahremani, "Nutrition Knowledge: Application and Perception of Food Labels Among Women," *Pakistan Journal of Biological Sciences* 16, no. 24 (2013): 2026–30.

6. Mienah Sharif, Shemra Rizzo, Michael L. Prelip et al., "The Association Between Nutrition Fact Label Utilization and Comprehension Among Latinos in Two East Los Angeles Neighborhoods," *Journal of the Academy of Nutrition and Dietetics* 114, no. 12 (2014): 1915–22.

7. Miri Sharf, Ruti Sela, Gary Zentner et al., "Figuring Out Food Labels. Young Adults' Understanding of Nutritional Information Presented on Food Labels Is Inadequate," *Appetite* 58 (2012): 531–34.

8. Rachael McLean and Janet Hoek, "Sodium and Nutrition Labelling: A Qualitative Study Exploring New Zealand Consumers' Food Purchasing Behaviours," *Public Health Nutrition* 17, no. 5 (2014): 1138–46.

9. Sudershan R. Vemula, SubbaRao M. Gavaravarapu, Vishnu Vardhana Rao Mendu et al., "Use of Food Label Information by Urban Consumers in India—A Study Among Supermarket Shoppers," *Public Health Nutrition* 17, no. 9 (2014): 2104–14.

10. Laura Fitzpatrick, JoAnne Arcand, Mary L'Abbe et al., "Accuracy of Canadian Food Labels for Sodium Content of Food," *Nutrients* 6, no. 8 (2014): 3326–35.

REFERENCES AND RESOURCES

Magazines, Journals, and Newspapers

Ahmadi, Afsane, Pariya Torkamani, Zahra Sohrabi, and Fariba Ghahremani. "Nutrition Knowledge: Application and Perception of Food Labels Among Women." *Pakistan Journal of Biological Sciences* 16, no. 24 (2013): 2026–30.

Chen, Xiaoli, Lisa Jahns, Joel Gittelsohn, and Youfa Wang. "Who Is Missing the Message? Targeting Strategies to Increase Food Label Use Among US Adults." *Public Health Nutrition* 15, no. 5 (2011): 760–72.

Deville-Almond, J., and K. Halliwell. "Understanding and Interpreting Nutrition Information on Food Labels." *Nursing Standard* 28, no. 29 (2014): 50–57.

Fitzpatrick, Laura, JoAnne Arcand, Mary L'Abbe et al. "Accuracy of Canadian Food Labels for Sodium Content of Food." *Nutrients* 6, no. 8 (2014): 3326–35.

Graham, Dan J., and Melissa N. Laska. "Nutrition Label Use Partially Mediates the Relationship Between Attitude Toward Healthy Eating and Overall Dietary Quality Among College Students." *Journal of the Academy of Nutrition and Dietetics* 112, no. 3 (2012): 414–18.

Hess, Rebecca, Vivianne H. M. Visschers, and Michael Siegrist. "The Role of Health-Related, Motivational and Sociodemographic Aspects in Predicting Food Label Use: A Comprehensive Study." *Public Health Nutrition* 15, no. 3 (2012): 407–14.

Kim, Min-Gyou, Seung-Won Oh, Na-Rae Han et al. "Association Between Nutrition Label Reading and Nutrient Intake in Korean Adults: Korea National Health and Nutritional Examination Survey, 2007–2009 (KNHANES IV)." *Korean Journal of Family Medicine* 35, no. 4 (2014): 190–98.

McLean, Rachael, and Janet Hoek. "Sodium and Nutrition Labelling: A Qualitative Study Exploring New Zealand Consumers' Food Purchasing Behaviours." *Public Health Nutrition* 17, no. 5 (2014): 1138–46.

Ratnayake, W. M. Nimal, Eleonora Swist, Rana Zoka et al. "Mandatory *Trans* Fat Labeling Regulations and Nationwide Product Reformulations to Reduce *Trans* Fatty Acid Content in Foods Contributed to Lowered Concentrations of *Trans* Fat in Canadian Women's Breast Milk Samples Collected in 2009–2011." *American Journal of Clinical Nutrition* 100, no. 4 (2014): 1036–40.

Sharf, Miri, Ruti Sela, Gary Zentner et al. "Figuring Out Food Labels. Young Adults' Understanding of Nutritional Information Presented on Food Labels Is Inadequate." *Appetite* 58 (2012): 531–34.

Sharif, Mienah, Shemra Rizzo, Michael L. Prelip et al. "The Association Between Nutrition Fact Label Utilization and Comprehension Among Latinos in Two East Los Angeles Neighborhoods." *Journal of the Academy of Nutrition and Dietetics* 114, no. 12 (2014): 1915–22.

Vemula, Sudershan R., SubbaRao M. Gavaravarapu, Vishnu Vardhana Rao Mendu et al. "Use of Food Label Information by Urban Consumers in India—A Study Among Supermarket Shoppers." *Public Health Nutrition* 17, no. 9 (2014): 2104–14.

Web Sites

American Heart Association. www.heart.org.

U.S. Food and Drug Administration. www.fda.gov.

Reduce Your Intake of Refined Sugar

OVERVIEW

There are two main types of simple sugars, which are carbohydrates. Monosaccharides have one sugar, and disaccharides have two monosaccharides that are bonded together. (This is in contrast to polysaccharides, which have three or more sugars and are called complex carbohydrates.) Monosaccharides work faster than disaccharides; they are easily digested and give the body a quick energy boost. Before being useful to the body, dissccharides must be converted into their two monosaccharide components. Glucose, fructose, and galactose are common monosaccarides; sucrose, lactose, and maltose are common dissccharides. Sugars are found naturally in milk products (lactose) and fruits (fructose). Most of the sugar in the American diet is from adding sugar products to foods. When people discuss reducing the intake of sugar, they are normally not advising a reduction in the intake of milk or fruit. Rather, they are suggesting a reduction in the added sugar.

It is very clear that refined sugar, or sugar that has been processed from raw sugar to remove impurities and colors, is an integral part of our daily lives. And, it is not only found in the sugar bowl that may sit on the kitchen table. Refined sugar, which is also known as table sugar or pure sucrose, is ubiquitous. Just about any processed food that we eat contains sugar, and sugar is found in sodas, sweetened drinks, desserts, and baked goods.

There are actually a few different types of refined sugar. The most common type of refined sugar is granulated sugar. This is the sugar people add to coffee and tea, and it is used for cooking and baking. A second type of refined sugar is called sanding sugar. It has a coarser texture than granulated sugar. When used in baking, it retains a grainy feel. A third type of refined sugar, super-refined sugar, is used in sugary beverages and pie meringues. Finally, powered sugar, which is also known as confectioner's sugar, is smoother than the other types of refined sugar and is used in icings and dessert toppings.[1]

In addition, not all sugars are equally sweet. Fructose is one of the sweetest sugars. It is followed, respectively, by sucrose, glucose, galactose, maltose, and lactose.[2]

According to the Sugar Association, a teaspoon of sugar, which is pure sucrose, has 15 calories. During processing, it is not chemically altered or bleached. The addition of molasses adds flavor and color to brown sugar. Darker versions of brown sugar contain more molasses than lighter versions. Moreover, the Sugar Association maintains that "sugar is a healthy part of a diet." Carbohydrates, such as sugar, "are the preferred sources of the body's fuel for brain power, muscle energy and every natural process that goes on in every functioning cell."[3]

Obviously, not everyone extolls the healthfulness of sugar. Many have associated it with a host of different medical problems such as obesity, type 2 diabetes, cardiovascular concerns, and other serious illnesses.

WHAT THE EXPERTS SAY

There Is Evidence of an Association between Sugar Intake and Type 2 Diabetes

In a study published in 2013 in *PLoS ONE*, researchers from Palo Alto, Berkeley, and San Francisco wanted to learn if the intake of sugar plays a role in the prevalence of type 2 diabetes in different populations. Data from 175 countries were included in the calculations. The researchers found an association between 150 kcal/person/day increase in sugar availability (about the amount of sugar in one can of soda/day) and an increase in diabetes prevalence by 1.1 percent. This association occurred between 2000 and 2010. So, during this time, the more sugar in the food supply of each country, the higher the incidence of type 2 diabetes in the population. Countries with declining amounts of sugar, such as Bangladesh, South Korea, Albania, and Nigeria, witnessed reductions in the rates of type 2 diabetes. The researchers concluded that their findings "lend credence to the notion that further investigations into sugar availability and/or consumption are warranted to further elucidate the pathogenesis of diabetes at an individual level and the drivers of diabetes at a population level."[4]

In Addition to Type 2 Diabetes, Sugar May Be Associated with Insulin Resistance and Metabolic Syndrome

In a study published in 2011 in *Clinical and Translational Science*, researchers from Nashville, Tennessee, and Davis, California, investigated the association between the consumption of the dietary sugar known as fructose and the incidences of insulin resistance and metabolic syndrome. (Insulin resistance is a medical problem in which the cells fail to respond normally to the actions of the hormone insulin, and metabolic syndrome is a cluster of conditions such as excess body fat around the waist, high blood sugar levels, high blood pressure, and abnormal cholesterol levels, which increase the risk for cardiovascular problems and diabetes.) The researchers noted that there have been numerous studies that have demonstrated that diets that are high in fructose induce insulin resistance in rodents. But, they wanted to come closer to a human model. So, they studied high fructose diets in rhesus monkeys, which, as primates, are more metabolically akin to humans. The cohort consisted of 29 adult male rhesus monkeys between the ages of 12 and 20 years. For 12 months, they were fed a diet with 30 percent of the total energy from fructose. By the end of the study all of the monkeys had developed symptoms of metabolic syndrome. Four of the monkeys had type 2 diabetes. Unlike many studies, this trial had no control group. As a result, researchers could not determine how many cases of metabolic syndrome were actually caused by fructose. Nevertheless, the researchers concluded that they "successfully demonstrated that, like in humans, consumption of a high-fructose diet in rhesus monkeys produces many of the components of the metabolic syndrome."[5]

Sugar in Sugar-Sweetened Beverages May Contribute to Weight Gain

In a study published in 2014 in *PLoS ONE*, researchers from Australia and Thailand wanted to learn if consumption of sugar-sweetened beverages in a large group of Thai university students contributed to weight gain. Why is this a problem? "Thailand is now a major producer of sugar which Thais have consumed in increasing quantities over the last few decades." And, the consumption of sugar-sweetened beverages "has played a substantial part in this increase in Thailand."

The researchers conducted their analyses from 59,283 respondents, with a median age of 30 years, who returned two separate questionnaires administered in 2005 and 2009. The researchers learned that most of the respondents consumed sugar-sweetened beverages 3 times or less per month; only a small minority drank them every day. Males were more likely than females to be frequent drinkers of these beverages. The researchers found that the higher frequency of sugar-sweetened beverage consumption in 2005 was associated with weight gain in 2009. Sugar-sweetened beverage consumption in 2005 "was the strongest predictor of future weight gain among the physical activity and energy-dense diet variables available in our survey." Still, the researchers were pleased to report that the overall consumption of these drinks declined during the study period. In fact, the proportion of people drinking three or more sugar-sweetened drinks per week dropped from 23 percent in 2005 to 16 percent in 2009. The researchers concluded that their findings support their hypothesis that drinking sugar-sweetened beverages "in even moderate amounts leads in the mid-to-longer term to increases in weight; that increasing intake increases this effect; and perhaps most importantly, that diminishing it reduces weight gain."[6]

In an article published in 2013 in *BMJ*, researchers from New Zealand conducted a systematic review and meta-analysis of randomized controlled trials and cohort studies on the association between the intake of dietary sugars and body weight in adults and children. Their data consisted of 30 trials and 38 cohort studies. The researchers found that, in adults, a reduced intake of dietary sugars was associated with a decrease in body weight, and an increase in sugar intake "was associated with comparable weight increase." And the researchers added that they "were able to show a consistent effect when comparing groups with the highest intakes of sugars with those with the lowest intakes." While the findings were somewhat uniform for adults, the "evidence was less consistent in children."[7]

Sugar-Sweetened Beverages May Increase the Risk of Cavities in Adults

In a study published in 2014 in the *Journal of Dentistry*, researchers from the United Kingdom and Finland examined the association between the frequency of the adult consumption of sugar-sweetened beverages and the incidence of cavities (caries) over a four-year period. The cohort consisted of 939 adults, with a mean age of 48.2 years. At baseline, the participants submitted information on a number of factors, including their intake of sugar-sweetened beverages. Clinical oral examinations were conducted at baseline and at a four-year follow-up. The researchers found that those who consumed higher numbers of sugary drinks had more cavities. "The findings suggest that drinking SSB [sugar-sweetened beverages] on a daily basis will lead to greater caries risk in adults and that such risk will increase even further with increasing frequency of daily consumptions." Not surprisingly, the researchers concluded that "SSB consumption is detrimental to dental health."[8]

Sugar May Negatively Impact Cardiovascular Health

In a study published in 2014 in *JAMA Internal Medicine*, researchers from Boston and Atlanta noted that researchers have found an association between intake of added sugar and cardiovascular risk factors. They wanted to learn if sugar was associated with death from cardiovascular disease. The cohort consisted of self-reported data from three groups of people representing a cross-section of America; there were about 40,000 people in the cohort. Excluded from the study were people who were already diagnosed with diabetes, heart disease, or cancer. The researchers found that compared to people who obtained only 8 percent of their total daily calories from sugar, those who obtained 17 to 21 percent of their daily calories from sugar increased their risk of death from cardiovascular disease by 38 percent. "The positive association between added sugar intake and CVD [cardiovascular disease] mortality remained significant after adjusting for the conventional CVD risk factors, such as blood pressure and total serum cholesterol." And, it is not that difficult to add significant amounts of sugar to the diet. The researchers mentioned that "one 60-ml can of regular soda contains about 35 g of sugar (140 calories)." The researchers concluded that most adults in the United States "consume more added sugar than is recommended for a healthy diet."[9]

In a prospective study published in 2009 in the *American Journal of Clinical Nutrition*, researchers from several Boston locations examined the association between the consumption of sugar-sweetened beverages and the risk of coronary heart disease in women. The cohort consisted of 88,520 women for the Nurses' Health Study; they ranged in age from 34 to 59 years. During 24 years of follow-up, there were 3,105 incident cases of coronary heart disease. After the researchers adjusted for nondietary risk factors for coronary heart disease, they found "a significant positive association" between the consumption of sugar-sweetened beverages and coronary heart disease. According to the researchers, their findings "provide further rationale for limiting the consumption of SSBs."[10]

BARRIERS AND PROBLEMS

As sugar is found in so many foods, it is nearly impossible to have a sugar-free diet. Sugar is often an ingredient in bakery products, soft drinks, flavored yogurt, and candy. And, sugar is not always listed as "sugar" on ingredient labels. There are dozens of names for sugar. These include malt, cane, maltose, glucose, dextrose, sorbitol, high fructose corn syrup, corn sweetener, fruit juice concentrate, and mannitol. The American Heart Association recommends that women consume no more than 100 calories per day (6 teaspoons) and men consume no more than 150 calories per day (9 teaspoons) of added sugar.[11] As a result, people need to devote time to reading labels.

Still, reducing added sugar in the diet is a daunting task. The literature on this topic offers a few suggestions. In a 2012 article in *Health Affairs*, researchers from New York City and San Francisco advised levying a penny-per-ounce tax on sugar-sweetened beverages. According to these researchers, data compiled by the beverage industry determined that in 2009 Americans consumed 13.8 billion gallons of sugar-sweetened beverages. To lower this level of consumption, a number of states have proposed initiating a penny-per-ounce tax. So, a 12-ounce can of regular soda would cost an extra 12 cents. It has been estimated that such a tax would reduce the consumption of these drinks by 15 percent in adults between the ages of 25 and 64 years. "The tax would have a greater impact on consumption and weight among younger adults and men, who consume more sugar-sweetened beverages at baseline, than among older adults and women." The researchers compared the health benefits of a tax on sugar-sweetened beverages to the tax on tobacco products, which has markedly reduced their use. "In addition to generating substantial revenue, which can be used to fund health services or other infrastructure, the proposed penny-per-ounce excise tax on sugar-sweetened beverages is predicted to greatly reduce the adverse health and cost burdens of obesity, diabetes, and cardiovascular disease among US adults."[12]

And, it may not be as difficult as some believe to reduce or eliminate the consumption of sugar-filled beverages. In a randomized trial published in 2013 in *PLoS ONE*, researchers from Australia and the Netherlands tested the response of children to substituting sugar-free beverages for sugar-sweetened beverages. The cohort consisted of 203 children between the ages of 7 and 11 years. For about 1 1/2 years, during their morning snack time in school, Dutch children were given either a noncaloric, artificially sweetened drink or a sugar-sweetened drink. One hundred and forty-six or 72 percent of the children completed the study. The researchers found no statistically significant difference in satiety between the two groups of children; both groups of children were similarly pleased with their drinks. The researchers concluded that "the sugar content of the drinks did not have a measurable effect on satiety."[13]

Still, People Appear to Be Predisposed to Like Sweet Foods

In a two-day, single-blind study published in 2014 in *PLoS ONE*, researchers from Philadelphia examined sweet and salty taste preferences in 101 children between the ages of 5 and 10 years and 76 of their mothers. The researchers found that children preferred higher concentrations of sucrose in water than their mothers. Though the differences were relatively small, boys preferred even higher concentrations of sucrose solutions than did the girls. The researchers noted that the preference for sugar appears to have "a biological basis." As a result, encouraging children to eat a diet lower in sugar "requires a social, political, and economic food environment that supports and promotes this behavior change."[14]

Sugar May Act Like a Drug

In a startling article published in 2013 in *Current Opinion in Clinical Nutrition and Metabolic Care*, researchers from France reviewed research studies that investigated the comparison of the addiction to drugs to the addiction to foods with high amounts of added sugar. The researchers acknowledged that such an analogy may at first seem "absurd." However, like drugs, foods that have high amounts of sugar may alter brain activity. "People now often report seeking and consuming sweet foods for their drug-like psychoactive and mood-altering effects." The researchers concluded that "there is now strong evidence" that foods that contain large amounts of added sugar "can induce reward and craving that are at least comparable to addictive drugs."[15]

NOTES

1. LIVESTRONG, www.livestrong.com.

2. Elmhurst College, www.elmhurst.edu.

3. The Sugar Association, www.sugar.org.

4. Sanjay Basu, Paula Yoffe, Nancy Hills, and Robert H. Lustig, "The Relationship of Sugar to Population-Level Diabetes Prevalence: An Econometric Analysis of Repeated Cross-Sectional Data," *PLoS ONE* 8, no. 2 (2013): e57873.

5. Andrew A. Bremer, Kimber L. Stanhope, James L. Graham et al., "Fructose-Fed Rhesus Monkeys: A Nonhuman Primate Model of Insulin Resistance, Metabolic Syndrome, and Type 2 Diabetes," *Clinical and Translational Science* 4, no. 4 (2011): 243–52.

6. Lynette Lim, Cathy Banwell, Chris Bain et al., "Sugar Sweetened Beverages and Weight Gain over Four Years in a Thai National Cohort—A Prospective Analysis," *PLoS ONE* 9, no. 5 (2014): e95309.

7. Lisa Te Morenga, Simonette Mallard, and Jim Mann, "Dietary Sugars and Body Weight: Systematic Review and Meta-Analyses of Randomised Controlled Trials and Cohort Studies," *BMJ* 346 (2013): e7492.

8. Eduardo Bernabé, Miira M. Vehkalahti, Aubrey Sheiham et al., "Sugar-Sweetened Beverages and Dental Caries in Adults: A Four-Year Prospective Study," *Journal of Dentistry* 42 (2014): 952–58.

9. Quanhe Yang, Zefeng Zhang, Edward W. Gregg et al., "Added Sugar Intake and Cardiovascular Diseases Mortality Among US Adults," *JAMA Internal Medicine* 174, no. 4 (2014): 516–24.

10. Teresa T. Fung, Vasanti Malik, Kathryn M. Rexrode et al., "Sweetened Beverage Consumption and Risk of Coronary Heart Disease in Women," *American Journal of Clinical Nutrition* 89, no. 4 (2009): 1037–42.

11. American Heart Association, www.heart.org.

12. Y. Claire Wang, Pamela Coxson, Yu-Ming Shen et al., "A Penny-Per-Ounce Tax on Sugar-Sweetened Beverages Would Cut Health and Cost Burdens of Diabetes," *Health Affairs* 31, no. 1 (2012): 199–207.

13. Janne C. de Ruyter, Martijn B. Katan, Lothar D. J. Kuijper et al., "The Effect of Sugar-Free Versus Sugar-Sweetened Beverages on Satiety, Liking and Wanting: An 18 Month Randomized Double-Blind Trial in Children," *PLoS ONE* 8, no. 10 (2013): e78039.

14. Julie A. Mennella, Susana Finkbeiner, Sarah V. Lipchock et al., "Preferences for Salty and Sweet Tastes are Elevated and Related to Each Other During Childhood," *PLoS ONE* 9, no. 3 (2014): e92201.

15. Serge H. Almed, Karine Guillem, and Youna Vandaele, "Sugar Addiction: Pushing the Drug-Sugar Analogy to the Limit," *Current Opinion in Clinical Nutrition and Metabolic Care* 16, no. 4 (2013): 434–39.

REFERENCES AND RESOURCES

Magazines, Journals, and Newspapers

Almed, Serge H., Karine Guillem, and Youna Vandaele. "Sugar Addiction: Pushing the Drug-Sugar Analogy to the Limit." *Current Opinion in Clinical Nutrition and Metabolic Care* 16, no. 4 (2013): 434–39.

Basu, Sanjay, Paula Yoffe, Nancy Hills, and Robert H. Lustig. "The Relationship of Sugar to Population-Level Diabetes Prevalence: An Econometric Analysis of Repeated Cross-Sectional Data." *PLoS ONE* 8, no. 2 (2013): e57873.

Bernabé, Eduardo, Miira M. Vehkalahti, Aubrey Sheiham et al. "Sugar-Sweetened Beverages and Dental Caries in Adults: A Four-Year Prospective Study." *Journal of Dentistry* 42 (2014): 952–58.

Bremer, Andrew A., Kimber L. Stanhope, James L. Graham et al. "Fructose-Fed Rhesus Monkeys: A Nonhuman Primate Model of Insulin Resistance, Metabolic Syndrome, and Type 2 Diabetes." *Clinical and Translational Science* 4, no. 4 (2011): 243–52.

de Ruyter, Janne C., Martijn B. Katan, Lothar D. J. Kuijper et al. "The Effect of Sugar-Free Versus Sugar-Sweetened Beverages on Satiety, Liking and Wanting: An 18 Month Randomized Double-Blind Trial in Children." *PLoS ONE* 8, no. 10 (2013): e78039.

Fuchs, Michael A., Kari Sato, Donna Niedzwiecki et al. "Sugar-Sweetened Beverage Intake and Cancer Recurrence and Survival in CALGB89803 (Alliance)." *PLoS ONE* 9, no. 6 (2014): e99816.

Fung, Teresa T., Vasanti Malik, Kathryn M. Rexrode et al. "Sweetened Beverage Consumption and Risk of Coronary Heart Disease in Women." *American Journal of Clinical Nutrition* 89, no. 4 (2009): 1037–42.

Lim, Lynette, Cathy Banwell, Chris Bain et al. "Sugar-Sweetened Beverages and Weight Gain over Four Years in a Thai National Cohort—A Prospective Analysis." *PLoS ONE* 9, no. 5 (2014): e95309.

Mennela, Julie A., Susana Finkbeiner, Sarah V. Lipchock et al. "Preferences for Salty and Sweet Tastes are Elevated and Related to Each Other During Childhood." *PLoS ONE* 9, no. 3 (2014): e92201.

Te Morenga, Lisa, Simonette Mallard, and Jim Mann. "Dietary Sugars and Body Weight: Systematic Review and Meta-Analyses of Randomised Controlled Trials and Cohort Studies." *BMJ* 346 (2013): e7492.

Wang, Y. Claire, Pamela Coxson, Yu-Ming Shen et al. "A Penny-Per-Ounce Tax on Sugar-Sweetened Beverages Would Cut Health and Cost Burdens of Diabetes." *Health Affairs* 31, no. 1 (2012): 199–207.

Yang, Quanhe, Zefeng Zhang, Edward W. Gregg et al. "Added Sugar Intake and Cardiovascular Diseases Mortality Among US Adults." *JAMA Internal Medicine* 174, no. 4 (2014): 516–24.

Web Sites

American Heart Association. www.heart.org.
Elmhurst College. www.elmhurst.edu.
LIVESTRONG.COM. www.livestrong.com.
The Sugar Association. www.sugar.org.

Exercise and Physical Activity

Make Time for Frequent Exercise

OVERVIEW

Today, teens lead incredibly busy, often overscheduled, lives. Between their schoolwork, after-school activities, homework, and part-time jobs, there may be little time for frequent exercise. Yet, just as the consumption of regular meals is integral to proper growth and development, so is the setting aside time for exercise at least five or six days per week, preferably every day.

Regular exercise is good for all parts of the body. It supports the skin and bones and improves sleep and mood. It may boost your brainpower, enabling you to learn faster and retain more. Exercise reduces anxiety and depression, often seen during the teen years, and it supports the immune system, helping to reduce the number of colds teens easily transmit to one other. And, exercise is useful in the maintenance of a normal weight. For example, four miles of fast walking may burn about 400 calories. If you walk seven days a week, that's 2,800 calories. If you do not have the time to walk four miles, try walking two or three miles or divide your walks. Remember, some exercise is better than no exercise.

Even children, teens, and young adults who have faced serious medical problems, such as surgery for congenital heart disease, may benefit from physical activity. In a randomized, controlled trial published in 2014 in the *Journal of Adolescent Health*, researchers from the Netherlands examined the role of exercise in 93 patients between the ages of 10 and 25 years who had surgery at young ages for congenital heart disease. The participants were randomly assigned to participate in an exercise program of three one-hour sessions per week (or two sessions, if they were already exercising) or to be in a control group. The control group members were told to continue with their regular exercise programs. The researchers believed that it would have been "unethical" to ask them to avoid exercising altogether. At baseline and follow-up, all the participants completed questionnaires. Forty-eight patients in the exercise group and 32 patients in the control group completed all the questionnaires. There were also semistructured interviews with the children, teens, and young adults, as well as the parents. When compared to the control group, the participants who were aged 10 to 15 years in the exercise group had significant improvements in cognitive functioning and parent-reported social functioning. On the other hand, the exercise did not appear to improve the quality of life for those between the ages of 16 and 25 years. The researchers wondered if the quality of life of this second group was already high. Or, perhaps more age-appropriate exercises, "involving more 'normal' sports participation with health peers," might have yielded different results.[1]

WHAT THE EXPERTS SAY

Exercise Appears Useful for Relieving Depressive Symptoms

In a study published in 2011 in the *British Journal of Health Psychology*, researchers from Ireland wanted to learn more about the association between exercise and depression. Their cohort consisted of 104 sedentary males between the ages of 18 and 40 years. The men were randomly assigned to participate in either a team or individual sport; the members of the control group did not take part in any sports. At baseline, they all completed a questionnaire. The participants were asked to attend a maximum of 20 55-minute exercise sessions over a 10-week period of time. A researcher monitored each session. Members of the control group were asked to refrain from exercise. Researchers collected data at week 5, week 10, and eight weeks after the trial ended. Eighty-four men completed the trial and were included in the analysis. When compared to the men in the control group, the men in both types of exercise had fewer symptoms of depression. The pre-to-post depressive symptoms scores decreased by 45 percent in the men who exercised in a group and by 52 percent in the men who exercised alone. The researchers noted the need for more research on this topic. "Because exercise-based interventions have the potential to reach young men, further research is warranted to examine the effectiveness, feasibility, sustainability, and cost of this type of intervention as a first line source of support for this difficult target group."[2]

Another study on exercise and depression was published in 2014 in the *International Journal of Behavioral Medicine*. For six years, researchers from Finland examined the association between changes in the frequency, intensity, and duration of physical activity in 1,959 men and women between the ages of 24 and 39 years. The participants completed questionnaires during medical examinations in 2001 and 2007. The researchers found that higher levels of physical activity were consistently associated with lower levels of depressive symptoms. "Both men and women who participated regularly in more frequent, higher intensity, longer duration, and higher overall of PA [physical activity] during the 6 years had a lower risk for depressive symptoms compared to those who were inactive."[3]

Exercise Seems to Be Useful for People with High Levels of Stress, Such As Police Officers

In a study published in 2013 in the *Journal of Occupational Health*, researchers from Switzerland and Lebanon investigated the association between exercise and the chronic stress often experienced by police officers. The cohort consisted of 344 male and 116 female police officers, who worked in the German-speaking section of northwestern Switzerland; they all completed multiple questionnaires. The researchers found that the officers who reported high levels of fitness revealed better mental health and better sleeping. But, there was a caveat. "Perceived fitness revealed a stress-buffering effect, but only among officers who reported good sleep." So, exercise did indeed help with stress only in those officers who were also good sleepers.[4]

Exercise Reduces Mortality in Black Adults

In a study published in 2014 in the *American Journal of Epidemiology*, researchers based at the National Cancer Institute in Bethesda, Maryland, reviewed the association between physical activity, sedentary behavior, and mortality rates in a large number of black adults. The cohort consisted of participants, between the ages of 40 and 79 years, enrolled in the Southern Community Cohort Study between 2002 and 2009, a total of 63,308 people. About 70 percent of the respondents were black and about two-thirds reported household incomes of less than $25,000. During the 6.4 years in which the participants were followed, there were 3,613 and 1,394 deaths in blacks and whites, respectively. This study included adults in urban and rural areas in Florida, Alabama, Mississippi, Louisiana, Arkansas, Tennessee, Georgia, South Carolina, North Carolina, Virginia, West Virginia, and Kentucky.

Black adults who reported the highest level of physical activity had the lowest risk of death from all causes. When compared to the blacks with the least amount of activity, they had a 24 percent lower risk of death from all causes, a 19 percent lower risk of death from cardiovascular disease, and a 24 percent lower risk of death from cancer. In whites, a higher level of physical activity was associated with a lower risk of death from all causes, but not cancer. Both blacks and whites who led sedentary lives increased their risk of all causes of death by 20 to 25 percent. The researchers concluded that their findings presented "much needed empirical evidence supporting the hypothesis that more overall physical activity is associated with a lower mortality risk and that prolonged time in sedentary behavior is associated with an increased mortality risk in both black and white adults."[5]

Exercise Improves Cardiac Health in African Americans

In a study published in 2013 in the journal *Medicine & Science in Sports & Exercise*, researchers from Minnesota and Mississippi investigated the association between exercise and cardiovascular diseases in African Americans. Using data from the Atherosclerosis Risk in Communities study, the cohort consisted of 3,707 African Americans and 10,018 whites between the ages of 45 and 64 years. From 1987 to 2008, levels of physical activity were determined through the administration of questionnaires. The researchers found an inverse association between physical activity and cardiovascular disease, heart failure, and coronary heart disease in both African Americans and whites and with strokes in African Americans. So, those who were the most physically active tended to have fewer cardiovascular problems. The researchers concluded that their findings supported the belief that "regular physical activity is important for CVD [cardiovascular disease] risk reduction, including reductions in stroke and HF [heart failure]." According to the researchers, their results "provide strong new evidence that this risk reduction applies to African Americans as well as Caucasians and support the idea that some physical activity is better than none."[6]

BARRIERS AND PROBLEMS

Canadians with Type 2 Diabetes Do Not Get Enough Exercise

In a study published in 2014 in the *International Journal of Behavioral Medicine*, researchers from Canada wanted to learn more about why Canadians with type 2 diabetes do not obtain a sufficient amount of exercise. According to the researchers, the Canadian Diabetes Association's 2013 Clinical Practice Guidelines recommended that people with type 2 diabetes obtain a minimum of 150 minutes of moderate to vigorous exercise a week; this exercise should be spread over at least three days. The researchers targeted men and women with type 2 diabetes between the ages of 35 and 55 years living in private homes in Quebec, Canada. They were randomly selected from the Quebec Health Insurance Board data. Two hundred participants completed baseline questionnaires. One month later, they self-reported their level of physical activity. The researchers found that, at baseline, the men and women participated in physical activities of moderate intensity totaling at least 30 minutes a day about two to three times per month. After one month, the same men and women were active about once a week. Obviously, this was an improvement, but it was still far below the recommendations. So, while the men and women knew they should exercise more, they were not exercising. The researchers concluded that there is a need to design "counseling messages to promote leisure-time physical activity among individuals with type 2 diabetes."[7]

In a study published in 2012 in *Preventive Medicine*, researchers from the United Kingdom wanted to identify barriers and facilitators to exercise and physical activity among older South Asians. Their analysis included 11 papers on 10 separate studies. The researchers learned that a number of factors influenced exercise and physical activities, including communication, relationships, beliefs, and the environment. In many instances, communication is a key problem. Healthcare professionals had not communicated the importance of physical activities and provided information on frequency, duration, and intensity. A second factor was a relationship issue or the lack of peer support—other people who were able to help them adhere to an exercise program. A third element was the belief that people naturally become less active as they age. And, still another obstacle was environmental or the lack of access to an appropriate gym facility and/or inclement weather, making it difficult to walk outside. The researchers concluded that "synthesizing qualitative data relating to people's views and experiences can assist in guiding the development of interventions to increase PA [physical activity]."[8]

Different Exercises May Vary in Usefulness

In a cross-sectional study published in 2014 in the journal *Perceptual and Motor Skills*, researchers from Switzerland compared the benefits of four types of exercise (aerobic exercise, ball sports, dancing, and weight lifting) on stress and depression in 201 medical students and 250 exercise and health sciences students. The researchers began with the hypothesis that all four types of exercise would be useful for dealing with stress and depression. Students completed questionnaires asking about stress, depressive symptoms, and exercise. The researchers found that the students with elevated stress levels were helped by the frequent participation in ball sports and dancing. No such effect was seen in students with lower levels of stress. Aerobic exercise did not appear to reduce stress levels. And, weight lifting was only effective in students with low stress levels. The researchers noted that "among Swiss university students, certain exercises may have better potential to moderate the relationship between perceived stress and depressive symptoms than others." So, why was exercise not more useful for the more stressed students? The researchers added that "one could argue that highly stressed students are at a higher risk of making everything stressful, including exercise."[9]

Running Strenuously May Not Be Good for the Body

In a study published in 2015 in the *Journal of the American College of Cardiology*, researchers from Denmark and Kansas City, Missouri, compared people who are sedentary to those who run lightly, moderately, or strenuously. The cohort consisted of 1,098 healthy joggers between the ages of 20 to 86 and 413 healthy people, between the ages of 21 and 92 years, who were mostly sedentary. The people were followed for 12 years. During that time, there were 28 deaths among joggers and 128 deaths among sedentary non-joggers. The researchers found that during the years of the trial, the light joggers were far less likely to die than the strenuous joggers and the sedentary people. In fact, the strenuous joggers had a rate of mortality that was not statistically different than the people who were more sedentary. The researchers commented that this "suggests the existence of an upper limit for exercise doing that is optimal for health benefits."[10]

NOTES

1. Karolijn Dulfer, Nienke Duppen, Irene M. Kuipers et al., "Aerobic Exercise Influences Quality of Life of Children and Youngsters with Congenital Heart Disease: A Randomized Controlled Trial," *Journal of Adolescent Health* 55 (2014): 65–72.

2. Nadine McGale, Siobhain McArdle, and Paul Gaffney, "Exploring the Effectiveness of an Integrated Exercise/CBT Intervention for Young Men's Mental Health," *British Journal of Health Psychology* 16 (2011): 457–71.

3. Xiaolin Yang, Mirja Hirvensalo, Mirka Hintsanen et al., "Longitudinal Associations Between Changes in Physical Activity and Depressive Symptoms in Adulthood: The Young Finns Study," *International Journal of Behavioral Medicine* 21 (2014): 908–17.

4. Markus Gerber, Michael Kellmann, Catherine Elliot et al., "Perceived Fitness Protects Against Stress-Based Mental Health Impairments Among Police Officers Who Report Good Sleep," *Journal of Occupational Health* 55 (2013): 376–84.

5. Charles E. Matthews, Sarah S. Cohen, Jay H. Fowke et al., "Physical Activity, Sedentary Behavior, and Cause-Specific Mortality in Black and White Adults in the Southern Community Cohort Study," *American Journal of Epidemiology* 180, no. 4 (2014): 394–405.

6. Elizabeth J. Bell, Pamela L. Lutsey, Beverly G. Windham, and Aaron R. Folsom, "Physical Activity and Cardiovascular Disease in African Americans in Atherosclerosis Risk in Communities," *Medicine & Science in Sports & Exercise* 45, no. 5 (2013): 901–7.

7. François Boudreau and Gaston Godin, "Participation in Regular Leisure-Time Physical Activity Among Individuals with Type 2 Diabetes Not Meeting Canadian Guidelines: The Influence of Intention, Perceived Behavioral Control, and Moral Norm," *International Journal of Behavioral Medicine* 21 (2014): 918–26.

8. Maria Horne and Stephanie Tierney, "What Are the Barriers and Facilitators to Exercise and Physical Activity Uptake and Adherence Among South Asian Older Adults: A Systematic Review of Qualitative Studies," *Preventive Medicine* 55 (2012): 276–84.

9. Markus Gerber, Serge Brand, Catherine Elliot et al., "Aerobic Exercise, Ball Sports, Dancing, and Weight Lifting as Moderators of the Relationship Between Stress and Depressive Symptoms: An Exploratory Cross-Sectional Study with Swiss University Students," *Perceptual & Motor Skills* 119, no. 3 (2014): 679–97.

10. Peter Schnohr, James H. O'Keefe, Jacob L. Marott, and Peter Lange, "Dose of Jogging and Long-Term Mortality," *Journal of the American College of Cardiology* 65, no. 5 (2015): 411–19.

REFERENCES AND RESOURCES

Magazines, Journals, and Newspapers

Bell, Elizabeth J., Pamela L. Lutsey, Beverly G. Windham, and Aaron R. Folsom. "Physical Activity and Cardiovascular Disease in African Americans in Atherosclerosis Risk Communities." *Medicine & Science in Sports & Exercise* 45, no. 5 (2013): 901–7.

Boudreau, François, and Gaston Godin. "Participation in Regular Leisure-Time Physical Activity Among Individuals with Type 2 Diabetes Not Meeting Canadian Guidelines: The Influence of Intention, Perceived Behavioral Control, and Moral Norm." *International Journal of Behavioral Medicine* 21 (2014): 918–26.

Dulfer, Karolijn, Nienke Duppen, Irene M. Kuipers et al. "Aerobic Exercise Influences Quality of Life of Children and Youngsters with Congenital Heart Disease: A Randomized Controlled Trial." *Journal of Adolescent Health* 55 (2014): 65–72.

Gerber, Markus, Michael Kellmann, Catherine Elliot et al. "Perceived Fitness Protects Against Stress-Based Mental Health Impairments Among Police Officers Who Report Good Sleep." *Journal of Occupational Health* 55 (2013): 376–84.

Gerber, Markus, Serge Brand, Catherine Elliot et al. "Aerobic Exercise, Ball Sports, Dancing, and Weight Lifting as Moderators of the Relationship Between Stress and Depressive Symptoms: An Exploratory Cross-Sectional Study with Swiss University Students." *Perceptual & Motor Skills* 119, no. 3 (2014): 679–97.

Horne, Maria, Uptake and Stephanie Tierney. "What Are the Barriers and Facilitators to Exercise and Physical Activity uptake and Adherence Among South Asian Older Adults: A Systematic Review of Qualitative Studies." *Preventive Medicine* 55 (2012): 276–84.

Kollarova, H., K. Azeem, H. Tomaskova et al. "Is Physical Activity a Protective Factor Against Pancreatic Cancer?" *Bratislava Medical Journal* 115, no. 8 (2014): 474–78.

Matthews, Charles E., Sarah S. Cohen, Jay H. Fowke et al. "Physical Activity, Sedentary Behavior, and Cause-Specific Mortality in Black and White Adults in the Southern Community Cohort Study." *American Journal of Epidemiology* 180, no. 4 (2014): 394–405.

McGale, Nadine, Siobhain McArdle, and Paul Gaffney. "Exploring the Effectiveness of an Integrated Exercise/CBT Intervention for Young Men's Mental Health." *British Journal of Health Psychology* 16 (2011): 457–71.

Schnohr, Peter, James H. O'Keefe, Jacob L. Marott, and Peter Lange. "Dose of Jogging and Long-Term Mortality." *Journal of the American College of Cardiology* 65, no. 5 (2015): 411–19.

Terry-McElrath, Yvonne M., and Patrick M. O'Malley. "Substance Use and Exercise Participation Among Young Adults: Parallel Trajectories in a National Cohort-Sequential Study." *Addiction* 106 (2011): 1855–65.

Yang, Xiaolin, Mirja Hirvensalo, Mirka Hintsanen et al. "Longitudinal Associations Between Changes in Physical Activity and Depressive Symptoms in Adulthood: The Young Finns Study." *International Journal of Behavioral Medicine* 21 (2014): 908–17.

Participate in Group Sports

OVERVIEW

While it is evident that many teens will never excel in sports, participating in a group sport as a teen serves a number of positive functions. Teens who play in group sports work with other teens to achieve a common goal. They learn how to interact effectively with others, an essential part of life. They practice leadership, communication, and build self-confidence, which will help guide them to future successes. Teens who take part in group sports are far more likely to eat a healthier diet and are less likely to be overweight.

Moreover, between the practices and the games, group sports require a good deal of time. Of course, in addition to the group sports, there are classes, homework, and maybe a part-time job. All those responsibilities keep teens very busy. Busy teens are not as likely to participate in less desirable activities, such as smoking and drinking. Coaches frequently forbid team members from smoking and drinking. Schools may require team members to maintain a certain grade point average and to be a good school citizen. Teens who do well in school and in sports have more self-esteem, and there is a better chance that they will want to attend college.

WHAT THE EXPERTS SAY

Participation in Club Sports Benefits Both Children and Teens

In a study published in 2015 in the *Journal of Science and Medicine in Sport*, researchers from Australia investigated the longitudinal effect of sports club (group sports) participation on fitness and body fat changes during childhood and adolescence. The cohort consisted of 134 Australian males and 155 Australian females between the ages of 8 and 16 years. The data were obtained at age 8, 9, 10, 11, 12, and 16 years from 2005 to 2013. The goal of the study was to compare the club sports participants to the nonparticipants across time. Participants who changed their sport participation status were eliminated from the analysis. At baseline, 79 percent of the males and 65 percent of the females participated in club sports. Unfortunately, over the course of the study there was a 47 percent attrition rate for the males and a 43 percent attrition rate for the females. By the time they were 16 years old, there was an 8 percent decline in sports participation among the males and a 6 percent decline among the females. Still, sports club participants were more physically active at all age groups. Both male and female sport club participants had a high level of fitness, and the females, but not the males, had less body fat. The researchers commented that "strategies aiming to maximize the benefits associated with sport participation are required and should be adapted to the specific gender, age-group and stage of development of the group."[1]

Participation in Group Sports May Be Helpful for Younger People with Attention Deficit/Hyperactivity Disorder

In a study published in 2014 in the journal *Adapted Physical Activity Quarterly*, researchers from the University of Alberta, Canada, wanted to learn more about the youth sport experiences of young adult males with attention deficit/hyperactivity disorder. The cohort consisted of six males, with a mean age of 22.7 years, who had attention deficit/hyperactivity disorder and played at least four different team sports from the ages of five to 18 years. Each participant completed two semistructured one-hour interviews with the lead researcher. The researchers learned that the participants' symptoms introduced some negative interpersonal and performance-related problems, such as being distracted by their surroundings, having difficulty following the instructions from the coaches, and making inappropriate comments. However, the participants agreed that taking part in the group sports supported social interactions, especially for those with the most pronounced social difficulties, and improved academic performance. The physical exercise also had stress-releasing benefits. The group sport experiences were best for those who had "supportive coaches, understanding teammates, and personal coping strategies." The researchers concluded that "it may be that by educating coaches and teammates and finding ways to help individuals with ADHD cope more effectively with their behavioral symptoms, we will be able to improve their experiences in sport, the longevity of their involvement, and the potential benefits that may accrue."[2]

A Football Program Appears to Have Psychological Benefits for Overweight Boys

In a study published in 2014 in the *Scandinavian Journal of Medicine & Science in Sports*, researchers based in Portugal examined the association between a five-month football instruction and practice intervention and the psychological status and body composition of overweight boys. The cohort consisted of 12 males between the ages of 8 and 12 years; all of the boys were overweight. The males participated in a structured five-month football program that consisted of four weekly 60- to 90-minute sessions. A control group included eight boys of the equivalent age from an obesity clinic located near the school attended by the intervention children. Both groups of children participated in two school-based physical education sessions of 45 to 90 minutes per week. By the end of the intervention, much to the surprise of the researchers, there were no differences in body fat and lean body mass between the two groups. As one might assume, the researchers hypothesized that the intervention group would have less body fat and leaner body mass. However, the intervention group showed improvements in all the indicators of psychological status, such as significantly better body image and self-esteem. The researchers commented that their "results were consistent with a previous study highlighting the importance of PA [physical activity] in enhancing the psychological health of overweight and obese children."[3]

Participation in After-School Group Sports May Foster Positive Youth Development

In a study published in 2013 in the journal *Research Quarterly for Exercise and Sport*, researchers from New York and Connecticut wanted to learn more about the black and Latino males in their early teens who participated in a Hartford, Connecticut, positive youth development program that focused on group sports. On any given day, between 6 and 12 boys between the ages of 10 and 13 years attended. During the study, researchers conducted semistructured individual interviews with eight daily program participants. The researchers learned that the teens joined the program primarily because of its emphasis on sports. And, they continued to attend the program because it was a safe, trouble-free place that "led to positive personal development." While participating in the activities, they increased their communication skills and learned to resolve conflict. Moreover, they realized that different choices have varying consequences and that goals may be achieved through specific actions. The researchers noted that "this youth-centered model personally benefited each of the study's participants."[4]

BARRIERS AND PROBLEMS

Adolescent Female Soccer Players Appear to Have High Rates of Injury

In a study published in 2014 in the *American Journal of Sports Medicine*, researchers from Denmark wanted to learn more about the actual injury incidence among adolescent female soccer players. They believed that previous studies, based on reports from coaches or medical staff, had significantly underestimated the rate of injury in this population. Unlike the other studies, the researchers obtained their data from self-reports via mobile telephone text messaging. The cohort consisted of 498 females between the ages of 15 to 18 years from 32 teams. During the February to June 2012 female soccer season, the players sustained a total of 434 soccer injuries, defined as "any new onset of pain or discomfort reported by the players." This represented an overall injury incidence of 15.3 per 1,000 hours of exposure. The incidence of severe injuries was 1.1 per 1,000 hours of exposure. The researchers noted that the incidence of soccer injuries in female players in Denmark is "very high." Severe injuries commonly occurred to the knee, ankle, groin, and lumbar spine. Frequent players have far fewer injuries than those with low soccer participation. Infrequent soccer players "may represent a population exhibiting unsafe behavior and a possible major cost to society in terms of medical expenses."[5]

Researchers Have Determined Specific Barriers to Female Teen Participation in Team Sports

In a study published in 2013 in the journal *BioMed Research International*, researchers from the United Kingdom wanted to learn more about barriers to female teen participation in team sports. The researchers began by underscoring the many physical and psychological benefits of participating in sports. To learn more, they asked 60 15- and 16-year-old females to complete questionnaires, and they conducted semistructured interviews with six females of the same age. All of the participants attended two high schools in the English Midlands. The researchers discovered four main reasons that the teens failed to participate in team sports. The first was internal factors such as the lack of confidence or feelings of embarrassment. A second reason was negative stereotypes about female athletes and the scarcity of female athletic role models. Third, the students had other hobbies or commitments that left little time for participation in team sports. And fourth, there was a perception that the teachers concentrated on the male teams and the females with the higher levels of sporting ability. The researchers noted a need to address these concerns so that more female teens would participate in team sports. For example, teachers who focus on male team sports should be encouraged to also direct their attention to female teams, and the media should feature more female athletes. "This needs to be maintained to allow girls more opportunities, role models, and motivation to participate in sport."[6]

High School Football Players Know Too Little About Concussions

In a study published in 2014 in *Journal of Athletic Training*, researchers from the University of Florida, Gainesville, noted that people with symptoms of a concussion who continue to participate in sports may place their health in serious danger. Yet, it is not well known how much sports players, specifically football players, know about concussion symptoms. In recent years, legislation in Florida has attempted to address this situation through parental consent forms. Was the legislation making a difference? The researchers surveyed a total of 334 varsity football players from 11 high schools in north-central Florida. Slightly more than half of the participants reported receiving concussion instruction from their parents; 60 percent received this from a formal source. A startling 25 percent had not received any concussion education. Almost all of the participants were aware that headache, dizziness, and confusion were potential signs of a concussion. But, they were generally unaware of other signs, such as nausea, vomiting, grogginess, difficulty concentrating, and personality and/or behavior changes. Only a small proportion knew that inappropriate care after a concussion may trigger very serious medical problems, such as brain hemorrhage, coma, or death. "Even with parents or guardians signing a consent form indicating they discussed concussion awareness with their child, 46 percent of athletes suggested they had not." The researchers commented that "action should be taken to better educate athletes and to ensure the proper recognition and management of concussions."[7]

NOTES

1. Rohan M. Telford, Richard D. Telford, Thomas Cochrane et al., "The Influence of Sport Club Participation on Physical Activity, Fitness and Body Fat During Childhood and Adolescence: The LOOK Longitudinal Study," *Journal of Science and Medicine in Sport*, published online May 14, 2015.

2. Homan Lee, Janice Causgrove Dunn, and Nicolas L. Holt, "Youth Sport Experiences of Individuals with Attention Deficit/Hyperactivity Disorder." *Adapted Physical Activity Quarterly* 31, no. 4 (2014): 343–61.

3. A. C. Seabra, A. F. Seabra, J. Brito et al., "Effects of a Five-Month Football Program on Perceived Psychological Status and Body Composition of Overweight Boys," *Scandinavian Journal of Medicine & Science in Sports* 24, Supplement 1 (2014): 10–16.

4. R. D. Fuller, V. E. Percy, J. E. Bruening, and R. J. Cotrufo, "Positive Youth Development: Minority Male Participation in a Sport-Based Afterschool Program in

an Urban Environment." *Research Quarterly for Exercise and Sport* 84, no. 4 (2013): 469–82.

5. Mikkel Bek, Clausen Mette Kreutzfeldt Zebis, Merete Møller et al., "High Injury Incidence in Adolescent Female Soccer," *American Journal of Sports Medicine* 42, no. 10 (2014): 2487–94.

6. Abigail R. Wetton, Rebecca Radley, Angela R. Jones, and Mark S. Pearce, "What Are the Barriers Which Discourage 15–16 Year-Old Girls from Participating in Team Sports and How Can We Overcome Them?" *BioMed Research International* Article ID 738705 (2013): 8 pages.

7. J. Cournoyer and B. L. Tripp, "Concussion Knowledge in High School Football Players," *Journal of Athletic Training* 49, no. 5 (2014): 654–58.

REFERENCES AND RESOURCES

Magazines, Journals, and Newspapers

Bradley, John, Francis Keane, and Susan Crawford. "School Sport and Academic Achievement." *Journal of School Health* 83, no. 1 (2013): 8–13.

Clausen, Mikkel Bek, Mette Kreutzfeldt Zebis, Merete Møller et al. "High Injury Incidence in Adolescent Female Soccer." *American Journal of Sports Medicine* 42, no. 10 (2014): 2487–94.

Cournoyer, J., and B. L. Tripp. "Concussion Knowledge in High School Football Players." *Journal of Athletic Training* 49, no. 5 (2014): 654–58.

Fuller, R. D., V. E. Percy, J. E. Bruening, and R. J. Cotrufo. "Positive Youth Development: Minority Male Participation in a Sport-Based Afterschool Program in an Urban Environment." *Research Quarterly for Exercise and Sport* 84, no. 4 (2013): 469–82.

Lee, Homan, Janice Causgrove Dunn, and Nicolas L. Holt. "Youth Sport Experiences of Individuals with Attention Deficit/Hyperactivity Disorder." *Adapted Physical Activity Quarterly* 31, no. 4 (2014): 343–61.

Miller, Elizabeth, Madhumita Das, Daniel J. Tancredi et al. "Evaluation of a Gender-Based Violence Prevention Program for Student Athletes in Mumbai, India." *Journal of Interpersonal Violence* 29, no. 4 (2014): 758–78.

Seabra, A. C., A. F. Seabra, J. Brito et al. "Effects of a Five-Month Football Program on Perceived Psychological Status and Body Composition of Overweight Boys." *Scandinavian Journal of Medicine & Science in Sports* 24, Supplement 1 (2014): 10–16.

Telford, Rohan M., Richard D. Telford, Thomas Cochrane et al. "The Influence of Sport Club Participation on Physical Activity, Fitness and Body Fat During Childhood and Adolescence: The LOOK Longitudinal Study." *Journal of Science and Medicine in Sport*, published online May 14, 2015.

Wetton, Abigail R., Rebecca Radley, Angela R. Jones, and Mark S. Pearce. "What Are the Barriers Which Discourage 15–16 Year-Old Girls from Participating in Team Sports and How Can We Overcome Them?" *BioMed Research International* Article ID 738705 (2013): 8 pages.

Web Site

The Nemours Foundation. www.kidshealth.org.

Walk or Bike Instead of Driving Whenever Possible

OVERVIEW

When one owns a car, it is always tempting to drive, even to nearby destinations. The car is readily available and, in most instances, makes traveling from one point to another relatively effortless. However, it is sometimes possible to leave the car at home and walk or bike to a destination. Walking and biking are simple and fun ways to promote health. Walking and biking burn calories, support cardiovascular well-being, and reduce anxiety and depression. There is even the possibility that walking and biking may lower the risk of developing Alzheimer's disease and dementia.

Walkers and bikers save money on their transportation costs. Purchasing and maintaining a car is expensive. Street parking in a city tends to be problematic; finding a permanent parking spot may add even more expense. Walking is essentially free. Biking does necessitate having a bike, but many new or used models may be purchased for relatively modest sums. Bikes may also be rented. In addition, walkers and bikers also have a positive impact on the environment. There is even a term for walking or biking to commute to school and/or work: active commuting.

WHAT THE EXPERTS SAY

Active Commuting Appears to Improve Cardiovascular Health

In a study published in 2013 in the *American Journal of Preventive Medicine*, researchers from London examined the association between active commuting to work and cardiovascular health. Data were obtained from Understanding Society, a nationally representative survey of residents of the United Kingdom. The cohort consisted of 20,458 individuals 16 years of age or older. Only 12 percent of those surveyed walked to work; an even smaller number, 3 percent, cycled to work. Yet, participants who used any form of active commuting were significantly less likely to be overweight or obese than those who used private transportation, such as cars. Walkers and cyclists were less likely to have diabetes, and walkers were less likely to have hypertension than those who had private transport. The researchers noted that active commuting and traveling "should be prioritized within national and local prevention strategies for obesity, diabetes, and cardiovascular disease."[1]

Active Commuting Appears to Improve Psychological Well-Being

In a study published in 2014 in *Preventive Medicine*, researchers from the United Kingdom wanted to learn more about the association between active commuting and psychological well-being. The cohort consisted of 17,985 adult commuters from the British Household Panel Survey. When compared to commuting in a car, the researchers found a significant association between overall psychological well-being and active commuting. In fact, "avoiding car driving may be beneficial to wellbeing." According to the researchers, these psychological benefits should be considered when evaluating the cost-benefit assessments that promote active commuting.[2]

Active Commuting from Youth to Adulthood May Lead to a More Physical Early Midlife

In a study published in 2014 in *Preventive Medicine*, researchers from Finland investigated the association between active commuting and physical activity from youth until early midlife. Using five self-reporting questionnaires administered between 1980 and 2007, the researchers followed 2,072 men and women from youth (9–18 years) into adulthood (30–45 years). The researchers found that active commuting was common in childhood and adolescence but declined after the age of 12. Yet, those who continued commuting actively from youth to adulthood were more likely to maintain physical activity. The researchers concluded that "regular AC [active commuting] may promote overall PA [physical activity] and fitness, which, in turn, increases the probability of being active in later life and of enhancing health."[3]

Many People Support Infrastructure Changes That May Increase Active Commuting

In a study published in 2015 in *Preventive Medicine*, researchers from Los Angeles wanted to determine if residents of Los Angeles County would back infrastructure changes that support walking and biking. Los Angeles County is well known for having residents who spend large amounts of time driving their cars. As a result, in the fall of 2013, the Los Angeles County Department of Public Health arranged for an independent California-based survey firm to conduct a 15-minute telephone survey with a random sample of 1,005 registered voters. Participants were asked a series of questions about their attitudes toward the construction of infrastructure that would facilitate walking, biking, and public transportation. Although few of the participants actually walked or biked, large numbers were supportive of infrastructure improvements. The highest number backed improvements that would support walking. "Overall, the study provides support for voter appreciation and interest in investing more in active communities."[4] If people perceive that they are able to walk and bike with increased safety, there is a greater probability that they will participate in active commuting, which is a healthier alternative for them and the community.

Active Commuting Is Associated with Improved Metabolic Health

In a study published in 2013 in the *Journal of Behavioral Nutrition and Physical Activity*, researchers based in Portugal examined the relationship between active commuting and metabolic risk factors in 229 pre-teens between the ages of 10 to 12 years. These students, who lived in Porto, Portugal, were asked how they usually traveled to and from school. Body measurements and blood testing were administered at the schools. The researchers found a significant beneficial association between walking to and from school and waist circumference and levels of HDL (good) cholesterol. The researchers noted that "these findings could be especially significant for obese children that usually have less PA [physical activity] opportunities implying that walking to school may be a simple and effective strategy, that can be implemented almost everywhere, to help control and reduce overweight."[5]

BARRIERS AND PROBLEMS

More Work Needs to Be Directed toward Increasing the Numbers of People Who Actively Commute

In a study published in 2014 in the *Health Promotion Journal of Australia*, researchers from Australia investigated active commuting in the greater metropolitan area of Sydney. According to the researchers, in Australia, the rates of walking or biking to work tend to be low. The researchers purchased data from the 2001, 2006, and 2011 Australian Census of Population and Housing from the Australian Bureau of Statistics. Then, they analyzed this data for three regional groupings—inner Sydney, outer Sydney, and the greater metropolitan region of Sydney. The researchers found that between 2001 and 2011 the proportion of people walking or biking to work in inner Sydney rose, but it fell in outer Sydney and the greater metropolitan area. However, when all three areas were combined, the increases in active commuting outweighed the decreases, "resulting in a small but significant increase in proportion of people actively traveling to work." The researchers concluded that there is a need for a multiagency approach to increasing the numbers of people who actively commute. This should begin with "marketing, transport strategies, and parking and road network strategies." But, it should also include input from agencies involved with roads infrastructure, public transport, and health promotion.[6]

Not All Employers Are Excited About Active Commuting

In a study published in 2015 in the *International Journal of Behavioral Nutrition and Physical Activity*, researchers from the United Kingdom wanted to learn more about how employers felt about the development of an employer-led scheme to promote active commuting. The researchers conducted interviews with 29 employers from 26 small, medium, and large workplaces. The employers' approaches to active commuting varied widely—"from active support through uncertainty and cynicism to resistance." Most of the employers appeared unclear as to how to support employees who wished to walk to and from work; they seemed to know more about supporting those who wished to bicycle. Some employers resisted the notion that they should be telling employees how to commute. And, they tended to emphasize that their primary role was to support the health of the business. The researchers concluded that "it is clear that employers need more evidence of the effectiveness of such schemes, and the costs and benefits to employers as well as employees."[7]

NOTES

1. Anthony A. Laverty, Jennifer S. Mindell, Elizabeth A. Webb, and Christopher Millett, "Active Travel to Work and Cardiovascular Risk Factors in the United Kingdom," *American Journal of Preventive Medicine* 45, no. 3 (2013): 282–88.

2. Martin Adam, Yevgeniy Goryakin, and Marc Suhrcke, "Does Active Commuting Improve Psychological Wellbeing? Longitudinal Evidence from Eighteen Waves of the British Household Panel Survey," *Preventive Medicine* 69 (2014): 296–303.

3. Xiaolin Yang, Risto Telama, Mirja Hirvensalo et al., "Active Commuting from Youth to Adulthood As a Predictor of Physical Activity in Early Midlife: The Young Finns Study," *Preventive Medicine* 59 (2014): 5–11.

4. Lauren N. Gase, Noel C. Barrigan, Paul A. Simon et al., "Public Awareness of and Support for Infrastructure Changes Designed to Increase Walking and Biking in Los Angeles County," *Preventive Medicine* 72 (2015): 70–75.

5. A. N. Pizarro, J. C. Ribeiro, E. A. Marques et al., "Is Walking to School Associated with Improved Metabolic Health?" *International Journal of Behavioral Nutrition and Physical Activity* 10 (2013): 12+.

6. Alexis Zander, Chris Rissel, Kris Rogers, and Adrian Bauman, "Active Travel to Work in NSW: Trends Over Time and the Effect of Social Advantage," *Health Promotion Journal of Australia* 25 (2014): 167–73.

7. Suzanne Audrey and Sunita Procter, "Employers' Views of Promoting Walking to Work: A Qualitative Study," *International Journal of Behavioral Nutrition and Physical Activity* 12 (2015): 12+.

REFERENCES AND RESOURCES

Magazines, Journals, and Newspapers

Audrey, Suzanne, and Sunita Procter. "Employers' Views of Promoting Walking to Work: A Qualitative Study." *International Journal of Behavioral Nutrition and Physical Activity* 12 (2015): 12+.

Gase, Lauren N., Noel C. Barragan, Paul A. Simon et al. "Public Awareness of and Support for Infrastructure Changes Designed to Increase Walking and Biking in Los Angeles County." *Preventive Medicine* 72 (2015): 70–75.

Hume, Clare, Anna Timperio, Jo Salmon et al. "Walking and Cycling to School." *American Journal of Preventive Medicine* 36, no. 3 (2009): 195–200.

Laverty, Anthony A., Jennifer S. Mindell, Elizabeth A. Webb, and Christopher Millett. "Active Travel to Work and Cardiovascular Risk Factors in the United Kingdom." *American Journal of Preventive Medicine* 45, no. 3 (2013): 282–88.

Martin, Adam, Yevgenity Goryakin, and Marc Suhrcke. "Does Active Commuting Improve Psychological Wellbeing? Longitudinal Evidence from Eighteen Waves of the British Household Panel Survey." *Preventive Medicine* 69 (2014): 296–303.

Oluyomi, Abiodun O., Chanam Lee, Eileen Nehme et al. "Parental Safety Concerns and Active School Commute: Correlates Across Multiple Domains in the Home-to-School Journey." *International Journal of Behavioral Nutrition and Physical Activity* 11 (2014): 32+.

Pizarro, A. N., J. C. Ribeiro, E. A. Marques et al. "Is Walking to School Associated with Improved Metabolic Health?" *International Journal of Behavioral Nutrition and Physical Activity* 10 (2013): 12+.

Smith, Liz, Sarah H. Norgate, Tom Cherrett et al. "Walking School Buses as a Form of Active Transportation for Children—A Review of the Evidence." *Journal of School Health* 85, no. 3 (2015): 197–210.

St-Louis, Evelyne, Kevin Manaugh, Dea van Lierop, and Ahmed El-Geneidy. "The Happy Commuter: A Comparison of Commuter Satisfaction Across Modes." *Transportation Research Part F* 26 (2014): 160–70.

Sugiyama, Takemi, Ding Ding, and Neville Owen. "Commuting By Car." *American Journal of Preventive Medicine* 44, no. 2 (2013): 169–73.

Yang, Xiaolin, Risto Telama, Mirja Hirvensalo et al. "Active Commuting from Youth to Adulthood As a Predictor of Physical Activity in Early Midlife: The Young Finns Study," *Preventive Medicine* 59 (2014): 5–11.

Zander, Alexis, Chris Rissel, Kris Rogers, and Adrian Bauman. "Active Travel to Work in NSW: Trends Over Time and the Effect of Social Advantage." *Health Promotion Journal of Australia* 25 (2014): 167–73.

Web Site

The Nemours Foundation. www.kidshealth.org.

Medical Care and Avoiding Medical Issues

Don't Use Antibiotics Unless Necessary

OVERVIEW

Until the discovery of antibiotics, countless numbers of people of all ages were seriously harmed or killed by infectious bacteria. It was not uncommon for small, local bacterial infections to evolve into systemic illnesses that ravaged the entire body. Sometimes, serious medical problems, such as bacterial pneumonia, became a rapid death sentence. The untimely passing of children, teens, and young adults from problems related to infectious diseases was a fairly common occurrence.

Then, in the 1920s, Alexander Fleming, a British scientist who was working in a laboratory at St. Mary's Hospital in London, discovered that a naturally growing substance could attack and trigger the elimination of certain bacteria. Fleming found that when *Staphylococcus aureus*, a common bacterium, was placed in the same petri dish as mold, the bacterium was damaged or destroyed. The mold made a substance, which Fleming called penicillin, that could wipe out bacteria.

Soon, other researchers were also conducting experiments on penicillin in both animals and humans. It was evident that penicillin was saving lives and improving the outcomes of many illnesses. Not surprisingly, drug companies began to develop other antibiotics. Today, there are dozens of different antibiotics. It has been estimated that at least 150 million prescriptions for antibiotics are written each year.[1] The number is probably much higher. Some of the more common antibiotics are azithromycin, amoxicillin, amoxicillin/clavulinic acid (augmentin), ciprofloxacin, and cephalexin.

Nevertheless, it is well known that many illnesses may be treated without antibiotics. In a 2014 article in the *New Statesman*, an English physician noted that about 35 million antibiotic prescriptions are issued each year in England. These are primarily for respiratory infections such as, "coughs, colds, sore throats, sinusitis, [and] earache." This is extremely problematic. "Studies have repeatedly shown that in these scenarios, antibiotics do little or no good." With or without the antibiotics, these illnesses will run their natural course. Moreover, "there is good evidence that antibiotic use interrupts the development of a robust immune response." That makes people more susceptible to future infections.[2] Overuse of antibiotics can also lead to strains of bacteria that have become resistant to existing antibiotics. As a result, certain infections with these antibiotic-resistant strains of bacteria become extremely difficult to treat. Many experts fear that antibiotic resistance will become a major public health problem in the next decades if steps to reduce antibiotic use are not undertaken.

WHAT THE EXPERTS SAY

Reductions in Antibiotic Use Are Possible

In a study published in 2014 in the *Journal of Antimicrobial Chemotherapy*, researchers from the United Kingdom wanted to learn if they could reduce the duration of antibiotic therapy in patients with lower respiratory infections. According to these researchers, it is not uncommon for people with lower respiratory infections to be treated with antibiotics for "prolonged" periods of time. For one year, the researchers followed over 500 patients with lower respiratory tract infections. During the first six months, the researcher observed how the patients used their antibiotics; during the second six months, patients were placed on a new prescribing protocol. In the new protocol, there were automatic stop dates, time limits on prescriptions, and support from pharmacists. Throughout the study, the researchers monitored antibiotic side effects, length of hospital stays, and patient deaths. The results were notable. When the patients followed the new protocol, they used 18.1 percent fewer antibiotics, and they had a 39.3 percent reduction in antibiotic-related side effects. The researchers concluded that "a simple intervention can significantly reduce antibiotic duration and antibiotic-related side effects."[3]

There May Be an Association between Treating Farm Animals with Antibiotics and Obesity in Children, Teens, and Adults

In a study published in 2012 in the journal *Nature*, researchers from New York City and Rockville, Maryland, wrote that farmers have used low doses of antibiotics for more than 50 years to promote the growth of animals. As a result, they could not help but wonder if antibiotics were contributing to high rates of obesity in children, teens, and adults. Surely, it was at least possible that the same antibiotics that increased the weight of animals could also increase the weight of humans. The researchers tested their hypothesis in young mice that they exposed to four different types of antibiotics, given in subtherapeutic doses in drinking water. Of course, some mice were given no antibiotics; they served as the control mice. After seven weeks, the researchers observed that all of the mice on antibiotics had total fat mass levels that were significantly higher than the control mice. The researchers concluded that the "administration of subtherapeutic antibiotic therapy increased adiposity [body fat] in young mice and increased hormone levels related to metabolism."[4]

Antibiotics Also Kill Beneficial Bacteria

In an article published in 2011 in *Nature*, Martin Blaser, MD, chair of the Department of Medicine, New York University Langone Medical Center in New York City, noted that not all bacteria are bad, especially those in the gastrointestinal tract. And, even a short course of antibiotics can drastically reduce the number of bacteria in the gut. This, in turn, may trigger a difficult-to-cure case of diarrhea or a worse medical problem. Sometimes the friendly bacteria never fully recover. "Evidence is accumulating that our welcome residents [friendly bacteria] do not, in fact, recover completely." Why is that so important? According to Dr. Blaser, by the time the average child has matured into an 18-year-old teen, he or she has received 10 to 20 courses of antibiotics.[5]

There May Be an Association between the Use of Antibiotics and the Development of Celiac Disease

In a population case-controlled study published in 2013 in *BMC Gastroenterology*, researchers based in Sweden examined the association between exposure to antibiotics and the development of celiac disease, a common autoimmune disorder in which products containing gluten must be eliminated from the diet. In order to examine the relationship between the use of systemic antibiotics and the subsequent development of celiac disease, the researchers obtained histopathology data on 2,933 people with celiac disease. They also reviewed antibiotic use in 2,118 people with inflammation and 620 people with normal mucosa but positive celiac disease serology. All of the participants were matched for age and sex with 28,262 controls. The researchers noted that they "hypothesized a positive association between antibiotic use and CD." And, they did indeed find a positive relationship between antibiotic use and the subsequent development of celiac disease. Moreover, "antibiotic exposure was also linked to small-intestinal inflammation and to normal mucosa with positive CD serology, both of which may represent early CD." How does this happen? The researchers suggested that antibiotics may alter the gut microbiota.[6]

There May Be an Association between Antibiotic Treatment during Infancy and Body Mass Index in Boys

In an international, cross-sectional study published in 2014 in the *International Journal of Obesity*, researchers from New Zealand investigated whether the exposure to antibiotics during the first year of life increased childhood body mass index. The cohort consisted of 74,946 children from 18 countries who were between five and eight years old. Parents or guardians contributed information on their antibiotic usage during the first 12 months of life as well as their current body mass index. The researchers learned that the use of antibiotics during the first year of life ranged dramatically; while it was 76 percent in Thailand, it was a much lower 22 percent in Taiwan. And, they found an association between early-life antibiotic use and body mass index in boys but not girls. This relationship existed until the boys were at least 8 years old. Why would there be a difference between boys and girls? The researchers noted that their findings "might be explained by sex-specific differences in intestinal adaptation to early-life antibiotic exposure or to how antibiotic drugs are metabolised."[7]

There May Be an Association between Exposure to Antibiotics during Infancy and Early-Life Body Mass

In a study that was published in 2013 in the *International Journal of Obesity*, researchers from several New York University departments wanted to learn if the exposure of infants to antibiotics affected their early-life body mass. The cohort consisted of 11,532 children from the Avon Longitudinal Study of Parents and Children. The researchers found that nearly one-third of these children received antibiotics between the time they were born and six months of age. On the other hand, by the age of two years, 25.7 percent of the children had not taken any antibiotics. The researchers learned that exposure to antibiotics early in life was associated with increases in body mass. For example, "at 38 months, children who had been exposed to antibiotics during the earliest period had significantly higher standardized BMI scores, and were 22 percent more likely to be overweight than children who had not been exposed."[8]

BARRIERS AND PROBLEMS

While There Is Greater Awareness of the Overuse of Antibiotics, They Are Still Being Used Too Often

In a study published in 2014 in *Antimicrobial Agents and Chemotherapy*, researchers from the University of Alabama at Birmingham examined the use of antibiotics in emergency departments to treat acute respiratory tract infections, such as sinusitis, otitis media, and tonsillitis. The researchers analyzed 2001 to 2010 data from the National Ambulatory Care Survey; the cohort consisted of 126 million emergency department visits for acute respiratory tract infections. Despite the fact that many of these medical problems were viral, in 61 percent of the cases, antibiotics were prescribed. Children under the age of five years received the fewest antibiotic prescriptions; adults who were 65 years and older received the most. The researchers concluded that "although significant progress has been made toward reduction of antibiotic utilization for pediatric patients with ARTI [acute respiratory tract infections], the proportion of adult ARTI patients receiving antibiotics in U.S. EDs [emergency departments] is inappropriately high. Institution of measures to reduce inappropriate antibiotic use in the ED setting is warranted."[9]

In a study published in 2011 in the journal *Pediatrics*, researchers from Utah, California, and Pennsylvania wanted to learn more about the antibiotic prescribing practices in ambulatory pediatrics. The researchers used 2006 to 2008 data from the National Ambulatory Medical Care Survey and the National Hospital Ambulatory Medical Care Survey, which are nationally representative samples of ambulatory care visits in the United States. During this time period, there were 64,753 sampled visits in these surveys. The researchers determined that antibiotics were prescribed in 21 percent of the pediatric ambulatory visits. In 23 percent of these visits, the patients had respiratory conditions "for which antibiotics were not clearly indicated." Moreover, the medical providers frequently prescribed "broad-spectrum antibiotics, which are often inappropriate. The researchers commented that this inappropriate use of broad-spectrum antibiotics "raises serious concerns about the overuse of broad-spectrum antibiotics, particularly for patients for whom antibiotics therapy is not indicated at all." The overuse of broad-spectrum antibiotics is problematic; "these agents are prescribed unnecessarily, have high cost, and promote bacterial resistance."[10]

Antibiotic Prescribing for Common Pediatric Infections Varies from Practice to Practice

In a retrospective study published in 2015 in the *Journal of the Pediatric Infectious Diseases Society*, researchers from different locations in Pennsylvania noted that the most common reason for prescribing antibiotics is to treat outpatient respiratory tract infections. As a result, the researchers wanted to learn more about outpatient antibiotic prescribing practices. The cohort consisted of 25 distinct but diverse pediatric practices with 222 clinicians. The practices varied markedly in racial characteristics and payer types. Data were obtained from January 1 until December 31, 2009. The researchers found that a total of 28 percent of acute visits resulted in antibiotic prescriptions. But, the prescribing practices ranged from 18 percent to 36 percent of acute visits. Certain practices appeared to be more likely to prescribe antibiotics than other practices. "Compared with a child seeking care at a low-antibiotic use practice, a similar child visiting a high use practice is twice as likely to receive an antibiotic prescription at any acute visit." The researchers concluded that "antibiotic prescribing for common pediatric infections varied substantially across practices."[11]

NOTES

1. American Academy of Pediatrics, healthychildren.org.

2. Phil Whitaker, "If We Don't Treat Antibiotics with Respect, Hoping to Avoid Resistance Will Be Futile," *New Statesman*, January 10, 2014: 67.

3. Colin Murray, Arlene Shaw, Matthew Lloyd et al., "A Multidisciplinary Intervention to Reduce Antibiotic Duration in Lower Respiratory Tract Infections," *Journal of Antimicrobial Chemotherapy* 69, no. 2 (2012): 515–18.

4. Ilseung Cho, Shingo Yamanishi, Laura Cox et al., "Antibiotics in Early Life Alter the Murine Colonic Microbiome and Adiposity," *Nature* 488 (2012): 621–26.

5. Martin Blaser, "Stop the Killing of Beneficial Bacteria," *Nature* 476 (2011): 393–94.

6. Karl Mårild, Weimin Ye, Benjamin Lebwohl et al., "Antibiotic Exposure and the Development of Coeliac Disease: A Nationwide Case-Control Study," *BMC Gastroenterology* 13 (2013): 109+.

7. R. Murphy, A. W. Stewart, I. Braithwaite et al., "Antibiotic Treatment During Infancy and Increased Body Mass Index in Boys: An International Cross-Sectional Study," *International Journal of Obesity* 38 (2014): 1115–19.

8. L. Trasande, J. Blustein, M. Liu et al., "Infant Antibiotic Exposures and Early-Life Body Mass," *International Journal of Obesity* 37 (2013): 16–23.

9. J. P. Donnelly, John W. Baddley, and H. E. Wang, "Antibiotic Utilization for Acute Respiratory Tract Infections in U. S. Emergency Departments," *Antimicrobial Agents and Chemotherapy* 58, no. 3 (2014): 1451–57.

10. Adam L. Hersh, Daniel J. Shapiro, Andrew T. Pavia, and Samir S. Shah, "Antibiotic Prescribing in Ambulatory Pediatrics in the United States," *Pediatrics* 128, no. 6 (2011): 1053–61.

11. Jeffrey S. Gerber, Priya A. Prasad, A. Russell Localio et al., "Variation in Antibiotic Prescribing Across a Pediatric Primary Care Network," *Journal of the Pediatric Infectious Diseases Society* 4, no. 4 (2015): 297–304.

REFERENCES AND RESOURCES

Magazines, Journals, and Newspapers

Blaser, Martin. "Stop the Killing of Beneficial Bacteria." *Nature* 476 (2011): 393–94.

Cho, Ilseung, Shingo Yamanishi, Laura Cox et al. "Antibiotics in Early Life Alter the Murine Colonic Microbiome and Adiposity." *Nature* 488 (2012): 621–26.

Donnelly, J. P., J. W. Baddley, and H. E. Wang. "Antibiotic Utilization for Acute Respiratory Infections in U. S. Emergency Departments." *Antimicrobial Agents and Chemotherapy* 58, no. 3 (2014): 1451–57.

Gerber, Jeffrey S., Priya A. Prasad, A. Russell Localio et al. "Variation in Antibiotic Prescribing Across a Pediatric Primary Care Network." *Journal of the Pediatric Infectious Diseases Society* 4, no. 4 (2015): 297–304.

Hersh, Adam L., Daniel J. Shapiro, Andrew T. Pavia, and Samir S. Shah. "Antibiotic Prescribing in Ambulatory Pediatrics in the United States." *Pediatrics* 128, no. 6 (2011): 1053–61.

Mårild, Karl, Weimin Ye, Benjamin Lebwohl et al. "Antibiotic Exposure and the Development of Coeliac Disease: A Nationwide Case-Control Study." *BMC Gastroenterology* 13 (2013): 109+.

Murphy, R., A. W. Stewart, I. Braithwaite et al. "Antibiotic Treatment During Infancy and Increased Body Mass Index in Boys: An International Cross-Sectional Study." *International Journal of Obesity* 38 (2014): 1115–19.

Murry, Colin, Arlene Shaw, Matthew Lloyd et al. "A Multidisciplinary Intervention to Reduce Antibiotic Duration in Lower Respiratory Trace Infections." *Journal of Antimicrobial Chemotherapy* 69, no. 2 (2012): 515

Trasande, L., J. Blustein, M. Liu et al. "Infant Antibiotic Exposures and Early-Life Body Mass." *International Journal of Obesity* 37 (2013): 16–23.

Whitaker, Phil. "If We Don't Treat Antibiotics with Respect, Hoping to Avoid Resistance Will Be Futile." *New Statesman*, January 10, 2014: 67.

Web Sites

Alliance for the Prudent Use of Antibiotics. www.tufts.edu/med/apua.
American Academy of Pediatrics. Healthychildren.org.

Get Vaccinated for Conditions That Affect Teens

OVERVIEW

While the vast majority of childhood vaccinations are scheduled during the first several years of life, some vaccinations are, ideally, administered during the preteen and teen years. These include the Tdap and meningococcal vaccines. In the case of the human papillomavirus, it should be administered at the ages of 11 and 12 years. And, of course, teens and young adults need a yearly influenza (flu) vaccine.

The Tdap vaccine is similar to Td vaccine, which was given every 10 years for tetanus and diphtheria. However, Tdap now also offers protection from pertussis or whooping cough. Over time, immunity from pertussis diminishes. Thus, the disease is no longer uncommon in older children and adults. And, it is the older children and adults who have the potential to pass along their illness to infants who are not yet protected by immunization. These young children may become seriously ill and require hospitalization. The elderly are also at increased risk.

Meningococcal vaccine protects against most of the bacteria that can cause meningococcal diseases, such as sepsis and meningitis. It is recommended that the first dose be administered between the ages of 11 and 12 years, and the second dose be administered at age 16 years.

Like everyone else, teens are at risk for the flu, a miserable viral illness that has respiratory symptoms, body aches, and an elevated body temperature. Unless someone has an allergy to some component of the influenza vaccine, all children over the age of six months should have a flu vaccine each year, preferably in the fall.

WHAT THE EXPERTS SAY

Direct Messaging to Parents Appears to Improve Adolescent Immunization Compliance

In a study published in 2015 in the *Journal of Adolescent Health*, researchers from Ohio wanted to learn more about the impact of messaging via automated text, prerecorded voice messages, and/or postcards sent in the mail on adolescent vaccination compliance. Did contacting the parents by whichever of these methods were available make a difference? The parents/guardians of 3,393 teens, between the ages of 11 and 18 years, in need of at least one vaccination, were contacted by these methods. A total of 7,094 messages were sent. After the first message was sent, 865 teens received at least one vaccine. Within 24 weeks of messaging, 1,324 vaccinations occurred in 959 visits. "Average visits generated $204 gross reimbursement for $1.77 in messaging expenses per vaccine given." Though the populations surveyed were diverse, the interventions were useful in all the groups. The researchers concluded that "automated texts, voice messages, and postcards had a significant positive effect on vaccination rates in adolescents needing vaccination and required minimal financial expenditure."[1]

In a study that was also published in 2015 in the *Journal of Adolescent Health*, researchers from San Diego and La Jolla, California, used data from the San Diego Immunization Registry to assess the effectiveness and cost efficacy of vaccination reminder messages sent via postal mail, text messaging, and/or emails. Parents of 5,050 adolescents, between the ages of 11 and 17 years, whose records at the San Diego Immunization Registry indicated that they lacked one or more vaccines, were contacted by telephone. The parents who consented to further communication were then asked how they would like to be contacted in the future. The vast majority wanted to be sent postcards. But, because that form of reminder has been previously studied, the number was limited. In the end, 963 were sent emails, 552 were sent text messages, and 282 were sent postal mailings. Subjects who declined to participate were placed in the primary control group. A second control group consisted of teens who met the criteria for inclusion but were not contacted by phone. Three follow-up reminders were sent to participants who did not update their vaccinations. The researchers found that the participants who received any type of reminder were more likely to update their vaccinations than those who only received the initial enrollment call. By the end of the study, 32.1 percent of the text message recipients, 23.0 percent of the postcard recipients, and 20.8 percent of the email recipients were up-to-date on their vaccinations. Those figures stood in contrast to the 12.4 percent of the enrollment call recipients who were up-to-date. Only 9.7 percent of the nonintervention teens were up-to-date. The researchers concluded that "text messaging and email as reminder methods for receiving vaccinations should be considered for use to boost vaccination completion among adolescents."[2]

Parents of Adolescents Tend to Support School-Based Vaccinations

In a study published in 2015 in the *Journal of Community Health*, researchers from Atlanta, Georgia, noted that school-based vaccination clinics increase access to teen immunizations. But, they wanted to learn more about what the parents of middle and high school students thought about these clinics. The researchers conducted telephone and Web-based surveys of parents of students enrolled in six middle schools and five high schools in one county in Georgia. Though the researchers reached out to thousands, in the end they had completed survey materials from 686 people. The researchers determined that parents were most willing to have their teens vaccinated for Tdap and influenza. (Tdap vaccination is now required in Georgia for all teens entering sixth grade.) And, although they were least willing to have their teen vaccinated for HPV, "a high proportion of parents who intended to vaccinate their adolescent against HPV would allow them to receive a vaccine at school." Generally, the majority of parents were accepting of these clinics. "Perceived severity of illness and intention to get their adolescent vaccinated were the most consistent correlates of parental SLVC [school-located vaccination clinics] acceptance for all vaccines."[3]

Provider Recommendations Make a Difference

In a study published in 2015 in *Women's Health Issues*, researchers from Boston compared factors associate with the vaccination of meningococcal vaccine and HPV vaccine in adolescent teens in the United States. Data were obtained from the public files of the National Immunization Survey-Teen for the years 2008 to 2012, which contained parental/guardian input on 48,527 girls between the ages of 13 and 17 years. The researchers found that providers who recommended both vaccinations had higher rates of compliance. In fact, provider recommendation "was the most important factor in receipt of both vaccines." However, white girls were 10 percent more likely than black or Hispanic girls to report that their provider recommended vaccination. Yet, the white girls did not have higher rates of vaccination. According to the researchers, this suggested that the parents of the white girls had higher rates of refusal. The researchers commented that because the rates of meningococcal vaccination are 20 percent higher than HPV vaccination, "improving provider recommendation for co-administration of HPV and meningococcal vaccines would reduce missed opportunities for initiating the HPV vaccine series."[4]

BARRIERS AND PROBLEMS

School-Based Influenza Vaccinations May Improve Rates of Immunization, But Large Numbers of Parents Do Not Want Their Children to Be Included

In a study published in 2014 in *Academic Pediatrics*, researchers based in Colorado wanted to learn more about school-based influenza vaccination programs. So, they offered a survey from April 2010 to June 2010 to 1,000 parents of randomly selected, primarily low-income children at 20 elementary schools. Seventy percent of the parents responded. Of these, 81 percent indicated that they were comfortable with school-based vaccinations. However, many believed that it was better to be vaccinated at the office of the child's physician. Twenty-five percent did not want to provide health insurance information, which would be required for billing. Parents with a high school education or less or Hispanic ethnicity were more likely to support the program. Parents who had concerns about the safety of the influenza vaccine and who did not want their children vaccinated without their presence were less likely to support the program. When asked where was the "best place" for their child to receive the influenza vaccine next year, 47 percent said the doctor's office and 47 percent said the school. The remaining parents suggested other locations. The researchers noted that "parental concerns about not being present for vaccination and about the safety and efficacy of the vaccine will need to be addressed."[5]

Parents Vary in Their Support of School-Based Vaccinations; Those Who Are More Economically Challenged Appear to Be More Supportive

In a study published in 2012 in *Journal of Adolescent Health*, researchers from Colorado and Georgia wanted to learn more about parental attitudes about school-based vaccinations for adolescents. From July 2009 to September 2009, the researchers mailed 806 surveys to the parents of incoming sixth graders in three urban/suburban middle schools in Aurora, Colorado. Five hundred parents (62 percent) responded. They reported that 82 percent of their teens had a regular site for obtaining healthcare, but 17 percent were uninsured. Overall, 71 percent of the parents indicated that they would give consent to have their teen vaccinated at school. However, while 72 percent would give permission for a Tdap vaccination, only 53 percent would give permission for their girls to be vaccinated for HPV. Single parents of uninsured children and children who received free and reduced lunches "were significantly more willing to consent for vaccinations at school." The researchers suggested that it may be more useful to focus school-based vaccination programs in schools in lower-income areas where there are more underserved teens. Furthermore, "targeting schools with a high percentage of uninsured and low-income teens for school-located vaccination program may be particularly effective in increasing vaccination rates in these adolescents who are often difficult to reach."[6]

Some States Need to Increase Their Efforts to Improve Immunization Rates

In a study published in 2014 in the OSMA *Journal* (*Oklahoma State Medical Association Journal*), researchers based in Oklahoma compared the adolescent vaccination rates in Oklahoma to rates in the entire United States. The researchers obtained their data from the 2010–2012 National Immunization Survey of Teens, which includes input from about 20,000 parents or legal guardians of teens between the ages of 13 and 17 years. Of these, between 300 and 360 lived in

Oklahoma. The researchers found that the rates of Tdap and meningococcal vaccination "are consistently lower in Oklahoma compared to the US." For example, Tdap rates in the United States increased from 69 percent in 2010 to 85 percent in 2012. In Oklahoma, the rate in 2010 was 55 percent; and in 2012, the rate was 77 percent. According to the researchers, healthcare providers in Oklahoma are less likely to mention vaccinations. That is why these providers must be encouraged to "recommend vaccines for adolescents they care for in an effort to improve our immunization rates." The researchers also suggested all members of medical practices, not just the clinicians, express positive comments about vaccines and discuss the benefits of vaccinations.[7]

NOTES

1. David S. Bar-Shain, Margaret M. Stager, Anne P. Runkle et al., "Direct Messaging to Parents/Guardians to Improve Adolescent Immunization," *Journal of Adolescent Health* 56 (2015): S21–S26.

2. Jessica Morris, Wendy Wang, Lawrence Wang et al., "Comparison of Reminder Methods in Selected Adolescents with Records in an Immunization Registry," *Journal of Adolescent Health* 56 (2015): S27–S32.

3. Lisa M. Gargano, Paul Weiss, Natasha L. Underwood et al., "School-Located Vaccination Clinics for Adolescents: Correlates of Acceptance Among Parents," *Journal of Community Health* 40, no. 4 (2015): 660–69.

4. Rebecca B. Perkins, Mengyun Lin, Rebecca A. Silliman et al., "Why Are U. S. Girls Getting Meningococcal but Not Human Papilloma Virus Vaccines? Comparison of Factors Associated with Human Papilloma Virus and Meningococcal Vaccination Among Adolescent Girls 2008 to 2012," *Women's Health Issues* 25, no. 2 (2015): 97–104.

5. Allison Kempe, Matthew F. Daley, Jennifer Pyrzanowski et al., "School-Located Influenza Vaccination with Third-Party Billing: What Do Parents Think? *Academic Pediatrics* 14, no. 3 (2014): 241–48.

6. Karen Kelminson, Alison Saville, Laura Seewald et al., "Parental Views of School-Located Delivery of Adolescent Vaccines," *Journal of Adolescent Health* 51 (2012): 190–96.

7. Monique M. Naifeh, James R. Roberts, Benyamin Margolis et al., "Adolescent Vaccination in Oklahoma: A Work in Progress," *OSMA Journal* (2014): 510–16.

REFERENCES AND RESOURCES

Magazines, Journals, and Newspapers

Bar-Shain, David S., Margaret M. Stager, Anne P. Runkle et al. "Direct Messaging to Parents/Guardians Improve Adolescent Immunization." *Journal of Adolescent Health* 56 (2015): S21–S26.

Gargano, Lisa M., Paul Weiss, Natasha L. Underwood et al. "School-Located Vaccination Clinics for Adolescents: Correlates of Acceptance Among Parents." *Journal of Community Health* 40, no. 4 (2015): 660–69.

Gilkey, Melissa B., Annie-Laurie McRee, and Noel T. Brewer. "Forgone Vaccination During Childhood and Adolescence: Findings of a Statewide Survey of Parents." *Preventive Medicine* 56 (2013): 202–6.

Kelminson, Karen, Alison Saville, Laura Seewald et al. "Parental Views of School-Located Delivery of Adolescent Vaccines." *Journal of Adolescent Health* 51 (2012): 190–96.

Kempe, Allison, Matthew F. Daley, Jennifer Pyrzanowski et al. "School-Located Influenza Vaccination with Third-Party Billing: What Do Parents Think?" *Academic Pediatrics* 14, no. 3 (2014): 241–48.

Morris, Jessica, Wendy Wang, Lawrence Wang et al. "Comparison of Reminder Methods in Selected Adolescents with Records in an Immunization Registry." *Journal of Adolescent Health* 56 (2015): S27–S32.

Naifeh, Monique M., James R. Roberts, Benyamin Margolis et al. "Adolescent Vaccination in Oklahoma: A Work in Progress." *OSMA Journal* (2014): 510–16.

Perkins, Rebecca B., Mengyun Lin, Rebecca A. Silliman et al. "Why Are U. S. Girls Getting Meningococcal but Not Human Papilloma Virus Vaccines? Comparison of Factors Associated with Human Papilloma Virus and Meningococcal Vaccination Among Adolescent Girls 2008 to 2012." *Women's Health Issues* 25, no. 2 (2015): 97–104.

Rambout, Lisa, Mariam Tashkandi, Laura Hopkins, and Andrea C. Tricco. "Self-Reported Barriers and Facilitators to Preventive Human Papillomavirus Vaccination Among Adolescent Girls and Young Women: A Systematic Review." *Preventive Medicine* 58 (2014): 22–32.

Web Site

Centers for Disease Control and Prevention. www.cdc.gov.

Maintain Good Bone Density

OVERVIEW

During the childhood and adolescent years, it is very important to build and maintain bones. In fact, the bones that adults have are in many ways a function of the bones that were built and maintained during the first few decades of life. By age 18, females have acquired up to 90 percent of their peak bone mass; in males, that occurs by age 20. The goal is to have strong bones that will lower the risk of developing the bone loss medical problems known as osteopenia, or the more serious bone loss problem known as osteoporosis. Osteopenia and osteoporosis increase the risk of stress fractures and other types of fractures, especially hip fractures. Hip fractures are serious and may be life-altering or life-threatening.

Building and maintaining strong bones should be an integral part of living a healthy lifestyle. First and foremost, it is important to eat a diet filled with vitamin- and nutrient-enriched foods, especially calcium-enriched foods such as yogurt, cheese, milk, collard greens, and spinach. Since calcium and vitamin D work together to support bone health, foods with vitamin D, such as shrimp, egg yolks, sardines, and tuna are an important part of a healthy diet. Vitamin D is frequently added to cereals and orange juice. Sometimes vitamin D levels may be hard to maintain. Consider discussing vitamin D supplementation with a medical provider. Vitamin K is another bone builder. It is found in kale, broccoli, Swiss chard, and spinach. And, potassium neutralizes acid that may remove calcium from the body. So, include potassium-rich foods such as sweet potatoes, white potatoes, yogurt, and bananas.

Exercise needs to become a priority. It actually helps build bones and reduces bone loss. The most effective exercises are the weight-bearing ones such as running, walking, jumping rope, skiing, and stair climbing. Resistance training is similarly useful. And, add still another reason not to smoke: smokers have a harder time absorbing calcium and building bone mass.[1]

WHAT THE EXPERTS SAY

Resistance Training Improves Skeletal Growth in Female Teens

In a study published in 2014 in the journal *Osteoporosis International*, researchers from Madison, Wisconsin, examined the effect of a middle-school-based resistance-training program on the skeletal growth of perimenarcheal females. Forty-five sixth grade females, who were 11 and 12 years old, participated in a seven-month resistance training program as part of their regular physical education classes, held two or three times each week. Every few weeks, the exercise difficulty was increased. The researchers noted that the intervention required a minimal amount of equipment and was easily taught to the new instructors. Meanwhile, the researchers had 23 controls from students in a matched neighboring school. Scans analyzed levels of bone density. The researchers learned that the resistance intervention produced bone gains in the girls. The less mature girls benefited most at the hip, and the more mature girls benefited most at the spine. The researchers concluded that "this program provides an attractive, easily-generalized, public health intervention to minimize the significant morbidity associated with osteoporosis."[2]

Physical Activity Supports Strong Bones

In an article published in 2013 in BMC *Musculoskeletal Disorders*, researchers based in Brazil reviewed 19 studies on the association between physical activity and bone mineral density in young adults. Fourteen of these studies were performed in Europe. Only six studies had more than 200 subjects. Fifteen of the studies focused on the lumbar spine. The researchers found that younger people who participated in "high peak strain" sports, such as team sports, experienced improvements in bone density. That is why, according to the researchers, the promotion of sports in schools is so crucial. The researchers commented that "physical activity may play an important role on reducing the risk of osteoporosis in women."[3]

In a seven-year prospective, longitudinal study published in 2010 in the *Journal of Bone and Mineral Research*, researchers from Finland and Memphis,

Tennessee, examined the association between leisure-time physical activity and bone mineral content and bone mineral density. At baseline, the cohort consisted of 202 Finnish females who were 10 to 13 years old. They were divided into four groups—consistently low physical activity, consistently high physical activity, change from low to high physical activity, and change from high to low physical activity. The teens were followed for seven years. The researchers found that the females with a consistently higher level of physical activity had higher bone gain at various bone sites. They concluded that "maximizing bone accrual during childhood and adolescence is critical for optimizing peak bone mass."[4]

Among Teens, Calcium Intake Makes a Difference

In a 12-month study published in 2014 in the *British Journal of Nutrition*, researchers from China wanted to learn more about the association between calcium supplementation and bone density in teens. The researchers recruited 220 teens between the ages of 12 and 14 years. There were almost equal numbers of males and females. The subjects were randomly placed in one of three groups—low calcium, middle calcium, and high calcium. The total supplemental calcium levels were 300, 600, and 900 mg/day for the three different groups, respectively. One hundred and ninety-eight subjects completed the study. The calcium supplementation appeared to have "moderate" effects on the bones of the teens. The researchers commented that their findings "revealed that Ca [calcium] supplementation caused a clinically important decrease in the risk of osteoporosis and fractures."[5]

BARRIERS AND PROBLEMS

Teens with the Eating Disorder Anorexia Nervosa May Compromise Their Bone Health

In an article published in 2014 in the journal HORMONES, researchers from Greece discussed some of the bone problems associated with the psychiatric eating disorder known as anorexia nervosa. The researchers noted that people with anorexia have extremely low levels of body fat, and females tend to experience the loss of menstruation. Bone problems in teens and young adults with anorexia are not uncommon. These include impaired linear growth, reductions in bone mineral density, changes in bone turnover, and microarchitectural alterations, and they may lead to an increased risk for bone fractures. In addition, the researchers added that it is difficult to treat bones in patients with anorexia. While there is a need to return to a normal weight, most often that is an exceedingly difficult undertaking, "due to a high propensity for relapse into disordered eating behavior." The researchers concluded that anorexia clearly has detrimental effects on bones, especially during the teen years when bones should be building strength. "Complete recovery from bone disease is not universal and the increase of fracture risk is prevalent even years after treatment of the disease."[6]

Low-Dose Oral Contraceptives Are Associated with Lower Bone Mineral Content

In a study published in 2015 in *BMC Endocrine Disorders*, researchers from Brazil wanted to learn more about the association between intake of low-dose combined oral contraceptives and bone mass density and bone mass content. The cohort consisted of 67 female teens, between the ages of 12 and 19 years, and the study took place over a one-year period of time. Forty-one of the teens used oral contraceptives; 26 did not. Bone density evaluations were conducted at baseline and after one year. Thirty-five users of oral contraceptives completed the study; all of the nonusers finished the study. The researchers determined that the females who used oral contraceptives had lower levels of bone mass acquisition than the nonusers. Since many teens take oral contraceptives to prevent unplanned pregnancies, "new studies are required to establish which estrogenic and progestagenic components and their ideal doses would be safe and adequate for appropriate bone mass acquisition in this age group to favor complete development of the bone mineral capital, a protective factor against osteopenia and/or osteoporosis in later life."[7]

Vitamin D Deficiency Is Very Common

In a cross-sectional study published in 2012 in the online journal *PLoS ONE*, researchers from Helsinki, Finland, noted that vitamin D insufficiency in children may effect calcium absorption, bone mineralization, and bone mass attainment, which may have long-term skeletal consequences. Did Finnish children have adequate amounts of serum vitamin D? To learn more, the researchers established a cohort of 195 Finnish children and teens between the ages of 7 and 19 years. Sixty-two percent were females and 38 percent were males. The vast majority of the teens were physically active. A variety of tests were administered, including measurements of serum vitamin D and evaluations of bone mineral density. The researchers determined that 71 percent of the subjects had insufficient levels of vitamin D. That means that only 29 percent of the children and teens had sufficient vitamin D status. According to the researchers, "vitamin D insufficiency is alarmingly prevalent." The researchers commented that their findings indicated an "urgent need to increase vitamin D intake to optimize bone health in children."[8]

People with Excess Abdominal Fat Tend to Have Lower Bone Density

In a study published in 2015 in the *American Journal of Clinical Nutrition*, researchers based in Ann Arbor, Michigan, wanted to learn more about the association between excess abdominal fat, known as visceral adiposity, and bone density. The cohort consisted of 8,833 thoracic or abdominal tomography scans from 7,230 patients at the University of Michigan Health System. Slightly over half were from men. At the time of the scans, the patients were between 18 and 65 years.

The researchers found that excess abdominal fat was associated with lower bone density. "These findings are important considering that obesity is often touted as a protective factor for bone health." Since about 35 percent of the United States population is obese, the negative association between excess abdominal fat and bone health may have important public health implications.[9]

NOTES

1. National Institute of Arthritis and Musculoskeletal and Skin Diseases, www.niams.nih.gov.

2. Brittney Bernardoni, Jill Thein-Nissenbaum, Joshua Fast et al., "A School-Based Resistance Intervention Improves Skeletal Growth in Adolescent Females," *Osteoporosis International* 25, no. 3 (2014): 1025–32.

3. Renata M. Bielemann, Jeovany Martinez-Mesa, and Denise Petrucci Gigante, "Physical Activity During Life Course and Bone Mass: A Systematic Review of Methods and Findings from Cohort Studies with Young Adults," BMC *Musculoskeletal Disorders* 14 (2013): 77+.

4. Eszter Völgyi, Arja Lyytikäinen, Frances A. Tylavsky et al., "Long-Term Leisure-Time Physical Activity Has a Positive Effect on Bone Mass Gain in Girls," *Journal of Bone and Mineral Research* 25, no. 5 (2010): 1034–41.

5. Xiao-ming Ma, Zhen-wu Huang, Xiao-guang Yang, and Yi-xiang Su, "Calcium Supplementation and Bone Mineral Accretion in Chinese Adolescents Aged 12–14 Years: A 12-Month, Dose-Response, Randomised Intervention Trial," *British Journal of Nutrition* 112 (2014): 1510–20.

6. Anastasia D. Dede, George P. Lyritis, and Symeon Tournis, "Bone Disease in Anorexia Nervosa," *HORMONES* 13, no. 1 (2014): 38–56.

7. Talita Poi Biason, Tamara Beres Lederer Goldberg, Cilmery Suemi Kurokawa et al., "Low-Dose Combined Oral Contraceptive Use Is Associated with Lower Bone Mineral Content Variation in Adolescents Over a One-Year Period," *BMC Endocrine Disorders* 15 (2015): 15+.

8. M. Pekkinen, H. Viljakainen, E. Saarnio et al., "Vitamin D Is a Major Determinant of Bone Mineral Density at School Age," *PLoS ONE* 7, no. 7 (2012): e40090.

9. Peng Zhang, Mark Peterson, Grace L. Su, and Stewart C. Wang, "Visceral Adiposity Is Negatively Associated with Bone Density and Muscle Attenuation," *American Journal of Clinical Nutrition* 101 (2015): 337–43.

REFERENCES AND RESOURCES

Magazines, Journals, and Newspapers

Alyahya, Khulood, Warren T. K. Lee, Zaidan Al-Mazidi et al. "Risk Factors of Low Vitamin D Status in Adolescent Females in Kuwait: Implications for High Peak Bone Mass Attainment." *Archives of Osteoporosis* 9 (2014): 178+.

Behringer, Michael, Sebastian Gruetzner, Molly McCourt, and Joachim Mester. "Effects of Weight-Bearing Activities on Bone Mineral Content and Density in Children and Adolescents: A Meta-Analysis." *Journal of Bone and Mineral Research* 29, no. 2 (2014): 467–78.

Bernardoni, Brittney, Jill Thein-Nissenbaum, Joshua Fast et al. "A School-Based Resistance Intervention Improves Skeletal Growth in Adolescent Females." *Osteoporosis International* 25, no. 3 (2014): 1025–32.

Biason, Talita Poli, Tamara Beres Lederer Goldberg, Cilmery Suemi Kurokawa et al. "Low-Dose Combined Oral Contraceptive Use Is Associated with Lower Bone Mineral Content Variation in Adolescents Over a One-Year Period." *BMC Endocrine Disorders* 15 (2015): 15+.

Bielemann, Renata M., Jeovany Martinez-Mesa, and Denise Petrucci Gigante. "Physical Activity During Life Course and Bone Mass: A Systematic Review of Methods and Findings from Cohort Studies with Young Adults." *BMC Musculoskeletal Disorders* 14 (2013): 77+.

Dede, Anastasia D., George P. Lyritis, and Symeon Tournis. "Bone Disease in Anorexia Nervosa." *HORMONES* 13, no. 1 (2014): 38–56.

Pekkinen, M., H. Viljakainen, E. Saarnio et al. "Vitamin D Is a Major Determinant of Bone Mineral Density at School Age." *PLoS ONE* 7 no. 7 (2012): e40090.

Völgyi, Eszter, Arja Lyytikäinen, Frances A. Tylavsky et al. "Long-Term Leisure-Time Physical Activity Has a Positive Effect on Bone Mass Gains in Girls." *Journal of Bone and Mineral Research* 25, no. 5 (2010): 1034–41.

Winther, Anne, Luai Awad Ahmed, Anne-Sofie Furberg et al. "Leisure Time Computer Use and Adolescent Bone Health—Findings from the Tromsø Study, *Fit Futures*: A Cross-Sectional Study." *BMJ Open* 5 (2015): e006665.

Xiao-ming, Ma, Zhen-wu Huang, Xiao-guang Yang, and Yi-xiang Su. "Calcium Supplementation and Bone Mineral Accretion in Chinese Adolescents Aged 12–14 Years: A 12-Month, Dose-Response, Randomised Intervention Trial." *British Journal of Nutrition* 112, no. 9 (2014): 1510–20.

Zhang, Peng, Mark Peterson, Grace L. Su, and Stewart C. Wang. "Visceral Adiposity Is Negatively Associated with Bone Density and Muscle Attenuation." *American Journal of Clinical Nutrition* 101 (2015): 337–43.

Zouch, Mohamed, Anis Zribi, Christian Alexandre et al. "Soccer Increases Bone Mass in Prepubescent Boys During Growth: A 3-Year Longitudinal Study." *Journal of Clinical Densitometry* 18, no. 2 (2015): 179–86.

Web Site

National Institute of Arthritis and Musculoskeletal and Skin Diseases. www.niams.nih.gov.

Practice Excellent Home Dental Care

OVERVIEW

Oral health impacts the health and well-being of the entire body. If you have a problem with your oral health, such as an infection, it may spread to other parts of the body. No longer a localized problem, the infection may require more aggressive treatment, even hospitalization. In addition, problems in your body, such as nutritional deficiencies, may first appear as oral lesions.

Of course, it is important to have regular visits with your dentist and hygienist. But, it is equally essential to practice excellent home dental care. Though teens lead very busy lives, it is crucial that they make time for brushing their teeth a minimum of two times per day and flossing a minimum of once per day. For teens who are wearing dental braces or other orthodontic devices, brushing and flossing may be a little more challenging. Ask your dental provider to recommend products that will improve your ability to brush and floss effectively. Often, teens and others are able to obtain samples from dental professionals. If possible, it is a good idea to keep a small toothbrush and small tube of toothpaste in your locker at school. This is especially important for teens who eat larger amounts of sugary foods and sugary snacks. It is best not to eat these foods, but many teens do.

WHAT THE EXPERTS SAY

Text Messages Tend to Improve Oral Hygiene in Orthodontic Patients

In a prospective, randomized study published in 2014 in *Angle Orthodontist*, researchers from Richmond, Virginia, wanted to learn if text message reminders would improve oral hygiene compliance among patients. Forty-two patients, with a mean age of 14.2 years, were given detailed oral hygiene instructions and assigned to one of two groups. In one group, parents received one weekly oral hygiene text message. In the second group, no one received oral hygiene text messages. The text messages reminded the parents that their teens should brush their teeth for three minutes after every meal or at least three times each day. Then it noted that "cleaning your teeth will help to keep them healthy and beautiful." On average, subjects remained in the groups for almost 11 months. Oral compliance was assessed using a number of different clinical factors, such as bleeding index and modified gingival index. The researchers found the children of the parents receiving the oral hygiene text messages had significantly better hygiene than the other participants. The researchers noted that the technology to add this service to a dental practice is already readily available. While they are now generally used to remind patients about upcoming appointments, these messages could be easily modified to serve other functions. The researchers noted that "providing such a service will maintain good communication between the orthodontist and the patient and shows that the orthodontist is concerned about each patient's well-being."[1]

Difficult Economic Times Do Not Necessarily Mean Inadequate Dental Care

In a study published in 2014 in *Community Dentistry and Oral Epidemiology*, researchers from Iceland and Alexandria, Virginia, wanted to learn more about the effects of economic recession on dental health behaviors. Like many other countries throughout the world, in 2008, Iceland experienced an economic collapse. Using a cohort of 4,100 residents of Iceland, the researchers examined the demographics, dental behaviors, and dental checkup frequency of the respondents. Participants were first contacted from October to December 2007; they were contacted a second time from November to December 2009. The researchers found "no strong evidence for drastic changes in dental health behaviors" from 2007 to 2009. While there were significant increases in people, especially men, flossing every day, there were no significant increases in the proportion of people brushing daily. According to these researchers, their findings did "not indicate an overall change in dental health behaviors."[2]

Fluoride May Be an Integral Component of Dental Home Care for Some Children and Teens

In an article published in 2014 in *Compendium of Continuing Education in Dentistry*, dentists from several locations in the United States noted that the home dental care of some children and teens should include fluoride. According to these researchers, some children, teens, and parents may not have the time or ability to provide adequate flossing and brushing. Moreover, poor dietary choices may further place the teeth and gums at increased risk. Preadolescents and teens with dental braces often do not take the added time needed to clean their teeth. According to the authors, these are the children and teens who may benefit from an in home fluoride program. And, it is important that dentists explain to patients and their parents the need to adhere to the at home protocol. "The protocols take into consideration safety (to minimize ingestion of the material), costs, practicality, efficacy, frequency of intervention, and types of fluoride products to be used."[3]

Oscillating-Rotating Power Brushes Appear to Remove More Plaque Than Sonic Brushes

In a randomized, examiner-blind, four-week study published in 2014 in the *American Journal of Dentistry*, researchers from Ohio and Germany compared the plaque-removing ability of an oscillating-rotating power brush to a sonic brush. The cohort consisted of 131 subjects; 65 were assigned to the oscillating-rotating group and 66 were in the sonic group. Over the course of the trial, both brushes significantly reduced plaque. However, the oscillating-rotating brush removed significantly more plaque. "Compared to the sonic power brush, the adjusted mean plaque reduction scores for the oscillating-rotating power brush were more than five times greater for whole mouth and approximal areas."[4]

Use of a Disclosing Agent Appears to Improve Patient Compliance with Plaque Control

In a randomized, prospective study published in 2014 in *Journal of Oral Research and Review*, researchers from India wondered if the use of a disclosing agent would help individuals have better control of the plaque on their teeth. Disclosing agents are preparations that contain coloring that highlights bacterial plaque. The cohort consisted of 100 dental patients between the ages of 18 and 50 years who suffered from chronic gingivitis. Fifty of the patients were instructed to use the disclosing agent for 21 days; the 50 patients in the second group did not use a disclosing agent. At the end of the trial, the researchers assessed the plaque status of all the subjects. They found that the subjects using disclosing agents had significantly lower plaque scores than the other subjects. By using the disclosing agent, patients were able to detect the presence of plaque and focus on removing it. "It is imperative to remove plaque in [a] timely manner in order to limit the progression of periodontal disease process and further calculus formation."[5]

Lower-Priced Toothpaste Appears to Work as Well as High-Priced Alternatives

In a randomized, double-blind trial published in 2014 in the *European Journal of Dentistry*, researchers from India wanted to compare the antiplaque efficacy of lower-priced and higher-priced commercially available toothpastes. For four weeks, 65 patients with dental plaque and gingivitis were assigned to use either a lower-cost or a higher-cost toothpaste. Plaque and gingival assessments were made at baseline and at the end of the trial. The researchers found that both groups had significant reductions in plaque and gingival scores. The researchers concluded that "low cost dentifrice is equally effective to the high cost dentifrice in reducing plaque and gingival inflammation."[6]

BARRIERS AND PROBLEMS

People Wearing Fixed Orthodontic Appliances Have Higher Amounts of Plaque on Their Teeth

In a study published in 2011 in the *American Journal of Orthodontics and Dentofacial Orthopedics*, researchers from Ohio, Germany, and the United Kingdom wanted to learn more about the build-up of plaque on the teeth of people with fixed orthodontic appliances. The cohort consisted of 32 males and 20 females with fixed orthodontic appliances undergoing treatment in Mainz, Germany. All the participants were at least 12 years old. The researchers found plaque levels ranging from 5.1 percent to 85.3 percent of the analyzed tooth areas. Approximately 37 percent of the patients had plaque levels over 50 percent of the dentition, while only 10 percent had plaque levels below 15 percent of tooth coverage. Most often, the plaque could be found along the gum line and around the orthodontic brackets and wires. "Plaque values measured in orthodontic populations are much higher than levels in nonorthodontic patients." While it may be a daunting task, in order to prevent caries or periodontal disease, it is important to lower these elevated levels of plaque with regular professional care and excellent home dental care. The researchers concluded that "improved hygiene, chemotherapeutic regimens, and compliance facilitators are necessary in these patients."[7]

Dental Anxiety Appears to Negatively Impact Oral Hygiene

In a study published in 2015 in the journal *Oral Health & Preventive Dentistry*, researchers from Poland wanted to learn more about the oral health habits of people who experience dental anxiety, a disorder in which people have excessive amounts of anxiety associated with their dental visits. The researchers noted that in Poland it has been estimated that 40 percent of patients have dental anxiety. The cohort consisted of 117 consecutive dental patients between the ages of 18 and 77 years; their mean age was 36.57 years. All the participants completed questionnaires and had oral examinations by a dentist. The researchers found that increased dental anxiety was associated with higher levels of dental calculus (hardened dental plaque). So, dental anxiety appears to play a role in people failing to provide the best care for their teeth and oral health. This, in turn, has been associated with a "lower quality of life." The researchers emphasized the need to develop psychosocial interventions "which may help patients deal with their dental anxiety."[8]

Mexican American Teens and Adults May Have Special Barriers to Adequate Home Dental Care

In a study published in 2015 in the *Journal of Public Health Dentistry*, researchers from Indianapolis, Indiana, wanted to identify specific dental hygiene beliefs and behaviors held by Mexican American adults and teens. The researchers conducted semistructured interviews with 16 adults between the ages of 33 and 52 years and 17 teens between the ages of 14 and 19 years. The most common reason cited for inadequate dental care was expense. But, there were also problems navigating the dental care system and finding someone to provide childcare while they went for appointments. In addition, there was skepticism that the amount of care recommended was actually required. However, parents were more likely to provide dental care for children than they were for themselves. What was perhaps most interesting was the finding that no participant remembered being given any training in dental hygiene in the dental office. Yet, 76 percent of the participants indicated that they brushed their teeth at least once per day, and almost everyone used toothpaste. Adults frequently used mouth rinses. "It was often implied that appropriate tooth brushing regimes would be an effective way to altogether avoid needing dental care." Still, flossing patterns varied; some doubted the value of flossing, especially since it caused their gums to bleed.[9] In reality, the gum bleeding was in all probability related to insufficient and/or inadequate dental hygiene.

NOTES

1. Matthew Eppright, Bhavna Shroff, Al M. Best et al., "Influence of Active Reminders on Oral Hygiene Compliance in Orthodontic Patients," *Angle Orthodontist* 84, no. 2 (2014): 208–13.

2. C. B. McClure and S. R. Saemundsson, "Effects of National Economic Crisis on Dental Habits and Checkup Behaviors—A Prospective Cohort Study," *Community Dentistry and Oral Epidemiology* 42, no. 2 (2014): 106–12.

3. T. P. Croll and J. H. Berg, "Use of Fluoride Products for Young Patients at High Risk of Dental Caries," *Compendium of Continuing Education in Dentistry* 35, no. 8 (2014): 602–6.

4. Barbara Büchel, Markus Reise, Malgorzata Klukowska et al., "A 4-Week Clinical Comparison of an Oscillating-Rotating Power Brush Versus a Marketed Sonic Brush in Reducing Dental Plaque," *American Journal of Dentistry* 27, no. 1 (2014): 56–60.

5. Mayuri Bhikaji Nepale, Siddhartha Varma, Girish Suragimath et al., "A Prospective Case-Control Study to Assess and Compare the Role of Disclosing Agent in Improving the Patient Compliance in Plaque Control," *Journal of Oral Research and Review* 6, no. 2 (2014): 45–48.

6. Rahul Ganavadiya, B. R. Chandra Shekar, Pankaj Goel et al., "Comparison of Anti-Plaque Efficacy Between a Low and High Cost Dentifrice: A Short Term Randomized Double-Blind Trial," *European Journal of Dentistry* 8, no. 3 (2014): 381–88.

7. M. Koukowska, A. Bader, C. Erbe et al., "Plaque Levels of Patients with Fixed Orthodontic Appliances Measured by Digital Plaque Image Analysis," *American Journal of Orthodontics and Dentofacial Orthopedics* 139, no. 5 (2011): e463–e470.

8. Urszula Kanaffa-Kilijańska, Urszula Kaczmarek, Barbara Kilijańska, and Dorota Frydecka, "Oral Health Condition and Hygiene Habits Among Adult Patients with Respect to Their Level of Dental Anxiety," *Oral Health & Preventive Dentistry* 12, no. 3 (2014): 233–39.

9. Gerardo Maupome, Odette Aguirre-Zero, and Chi Westerhold, "Qualitative Description of Dental Hygiene Practices Within Oral Health and Dental Care Perspectives of Mexican-American Adults and Teenagers," *Journal of Public Health Dentistry* 75, no. 2 (2015): 93–100.

REFERENCES AND RESOURCES

Magazines, Journals, and Newspapers

Büchel, Barbara, Markus Reise, Malgorzata Klukowska et al. "A 4-Week Clinical Comparison of an Oscillating-Rotating Power Brush Versus a Marketed Sonic Brush in Reducing Dental Plaque." *American Journal of Dentistry* 27, no. 1 (2014): 56–60.

Croll, T. P., and J. H. Berg. "Use of Fluoride Products for Young Patients at High Risk of Dental Caries." *Compendium of Continuing Education in Dentistry* 35, no. 8 (2014): 602–6.

Eppright, Matthew, Bhavna Shroff, Al M. Best et al. "Influence of Active Reminders on Oral Hygiene Compliance in Orthodontic Patients." *Angle Orthodontist* 84, no. 2 (2014): 208–13.

Ganavadiya, Rahul, B. R. Chandra Shekar, Pankaj Goel at al. "Comparison of Anti-Plaque Efficacy Between a Low and High Cost Dentifrice: A Short Term Randomized Double-Blind Trial." *European Journal of Dentistry* 8, no. 3 (2014): 381–88.

Geisinger, M. L., N. C. Geurs, J. L. Bain et al. "Oral Health Education and Therapy Reduces Gingivitis During Pregnancy." *Journal of Clinical Periodontology* 41, no. 2 (2014): 141–48.

Jordan, R. A., H. M. Hong, A. Lucaciu, and S. Zimmer. "Efficacy of Straight Versus Angled Interdental Brushes on Interproximal Tooth Cleaning: A Randomized Controlled Trial." *International Journal of Dental Hygiene* 12 (2014): 152–57.

Kanaffa-Kilijańska, Urszula, Urszula Kaczmarek, Barbara Kilijańska, and Dorota Frydecka. "Oral Health Condition and Hygiene Habits Among Adult Patients with Respect to Their Level of Dental Anxiety." *Oral Health & Preventive Dentistry* 12, no. 3 (2014): 233–39.

Koukowska, M., A. Bader, C. Erbe et al. "Plaque Levels of Patients with Fixed Orthodontic Appliances Measured by Digital Plaque Image Analysis." *American Journal of Orthodontics and Dentofacial Orthopedics* 139, no. 5 (2011): e463–e470.

Maupome, Gerardo, Odette Aguirre-Zero, and Chi Westerhold. "Qualitative Description of Dental Hygiene Practice Within Oral Health and Dental Care Perspectives of Mexican-American Adults and Teenagers." *Journal of Public Health Dentistry* 75, no. 2 (2015): 93–100.

McClure, C. B., and S. R. Saemundsson. "Effects of a National Economic Crisis on Dental Habits and Checkup Behaviors—A Prospective Cohort Study." *Community Dentistry and Oral Epidemiology* 42, no. 2 (2014): 106–12.

Nepale, Mayuri Bhikaji, Siddhartha Varma, Girish Suragimath et al. "A Prospective Case-Control Study to Assess and Compare the Role of Disclosing Agent in Improving the Patient Compliance in Plaque Control." *Journal of Oral Research and Review* 6, no. 2 (2014): 45–48.

Web Site

American Dental Association. www.ada.org.

Prevent Vitamin D Deficiency

OVERVIEW

Vitamin D is an oil-soluble vitamin that plays a number of important roles in the body. Probably the most important functions of vitamin D are to absorb dietary calcium and phosphorus from the intestines and to suppress the release of parathyroid hormone, a hormone that causes bone reabsorption. These processes help maintain normal levels of calcium and phosphorus in the blood, which, in turn, promotes bone health.

Triggered by sunlight, vitamin D is made in the skin. People who spend little time outside or who use sunscreen diligently tend to not make a sufficient amount of vitamin D. People who live in colder climates or in areas where sunlight is a rarer event tend to have low levels of serum vitamin D. In addition, people with darker skin tones need more sunlight to make adequate amounts of vitamin D.

Vitamin D is found in certain foods, such as fatty fish, red meat, liver, cod liver oil, and eggs. In the United States, milk is often fortified with vitamin D. An 8-ounce glass of milk has about 100 IU of vitamin D. But, large numbers of people of all ages fail to make enough from the sun and/or consume enough vitamin D in their diet. For teens and young adults, who are still building the bones they will need for a lifetime, the lack of sufficient vitamin D needs to be addressed.

Vitamin D deficiency may be diagnosed through a simple blood test called 25 hydroxyvitamin D or 25(OH)D. Serum concentrations above 50 nmol/L are considered normal. In general, teens should take in about 600 IU per day. Potential vitamin D supplementation is a good topic to address with medical providers.[1]

WHAT THE EXPERTS SAY

Vitamin D Deficiency Appears to Be Independently Associated with the Extent of Coronary Artery Disease

In a study published in 2014 in the *European Journal of Clinical Investigation*, researchers from Italy evaluated the association between levels of vitamin D and the extent of coronary artery disease in patients undergoing coronary angiography, a medical test that uses dyes and special x-rays to see inside coronary arteries. Of the 1,484 patients in the cohort, a stunning 70.4 percent had low levels of vitamin D. Those with the lowest levels of vitamin D appeared to have the most coronary artery disease. "The association between low vitamin D levels and CAD reached a statistical significance." Patients with very low levels of vitamin D should be considered at increased risk for cardiovascular disease. The researchers concluded that there should be more research on this topic. "Additional studies are needed to evaluate the potential benefits of vitamin D supplementation on the prevention of CAD and its progression."[2]

Low Vitamin D Appears to Be Associated with Hypertension in Obese Children and Teens

In a retrospective, cross-sectional study published in 2015 in the *Journal of Paediatrics and Child Health*, researchers from Australia and Turkey investigated the cardiometabolic risk factors in a children and teens who received outpatient pediatric obesity services in Melbourne, Australia, between 2008 and 2011.

Slightly more than half the cohort was male, and the mean age was 12.1 years. Vitamin D data were available on 229 patients between the ages of 2 and 18 years. Forty-five percent of the cohort had deficient levels of vitamin D (<50 nmo/L). Interestingly, there was an association between the degree of obesity and levels of vitamin D. The more obese youth had lower levels of vitamin D. Youth with lower levels of vitamin D were also at increased risk for hypertension or elevated blood pressure. Why is this important? "Hypertension is the most common component of metabolic syndrome and contributes substantially to atherosclerosis." The researchers suggested that obese youth may well prove to be good candidates of vitamin D supplementation.[3]

There May Be an Association between Low Levels of Vitamin D and Obesity and the Risk for Type 2 Diabetes

In a study published in 2012 in the *Journal of Clinical Endocrinology & Metabolism*, researchers based in Dallas, Texas, determined the prevalence of vitamin D deficiency in children referred to an obesity clinic in north Texas and compared that prevalence to similar non-overweight children. They also examined associations between levels of vitamin D and type 2 diabetes. The cohort consisted of 411 obese children between the ages of 6 and 16 years and 89 non-overweight children, with the same age range. All the data were collected in 2009 and 2010. When compared to the normal weight children, the researchers found that the obese children were far more likely to have lower levels of vitamin D. Moreover, lower levels of Vitamin D were associated with risk factors for type 2 diabetes, such as insulin resistance, in obese children. "Thus, low 25(OH)D levels may play a role in the pathophysiology of impaired glucose tolerance in obese children."[4]

Fortification of Staple Foods with Vitamin D Increases the Consumption of Vitamin D among Groups at Risk of Deficiency

In a study published in 2015 in the *American Journal of Clinical Nutrition*, researchers from the United Kingdom noted that certain groups of people, such as children between the ages of 18 and 36 months, females between the ages of 15 and 49 years, and adults 65 years and older, are at increased risk for vitamin D deficiency. In the United Kingdom, it has been estimated that one-fifth of the population has poor vitamin D status. As a result, researchers identified wheat and milk as two foods that may be good candidates for vitamin D fortification; they are the most widely consumed foods within the population. To simulate the impact of fortification, the researchers used consumption data from the U.K. National Diet and Nutrition Survey Rolling Programme, which estimates individual dietary intake in the general U.K. population. The researchers determined that the most effective and useful fortification was 10 micrograms per 100 grams of wheat flour. "The simulation of the fortification of wheat flour at this concentration was more effective than that of the fortification of milk . . . or the fortification of milk and flour combined."[5]

There Seems to Be an Association between Vitamin D and Autism Spectrum Disorder

In a study published in 2015 in the journal *European Child & Adolescent Psychiatry*, researchers from China and the Netherlands wanted to learn if vitamin D played a role in the etiology of autism spectrum disorder. (Autism spectrum disorder is a brain disorder characterized by deficits in social interaction, verbal and nonverbal communication, and restricted and repetitive behaviors.) The researchers conducted a meta-analysis that included 11 studies with 870 children with some type of autism spectrum disorder and 782 healthy controls. All the children were between the ages of 2 and 16 years. The researchers found that compared to the controls, the people with autism spectrum disorders had significantly lower levels of vitamin D. And, they suggested that lower levels of vitamin D may place people at increased risk for autism spectrum disorders.[6]

In fact, in an article published in 2015 in the journal *Pediatrics*, researchers from China and the Netherlands described the case of a 32-month-old boy from China with autism spectrum disorder and vitamin D deficiency. He appeared to have a number of autism symptoms. "No urge for social interaction, no response to facial expression or to other people, no social interactional smiling, not following instructions from his parents, no response when somebody calls his name, avoidance of eye contact and physical contact, strange gestures." The toddler also had temper tantrums, attacked other children, and hurt himself when he banged his head against objects. Upon testing, his medical providers found that he had very low levels of serum vitamin D. As a result, he received both IV and oral vitamin D supplementation. After two months, the parents reported noticeable improvements in behavior. The child responded when his name was called and was no longer preoccupied with running in circles. Self-injury had almost stopped, and he allowed his parents to hold him in their arms. Because no other medical abnormalities were found other than vitamin D deficiency, "the marked improvement in the relatively brief period of treatment that was observed in this case appears to be related to vitamin D supplementation."[7]

BARRIERS AND PROBLEMS

People Who Practice Sun-Protective Behaviors May Have Lower Levels of Vitamin D

In a cross-sectional study published in 2012 in the journal *Cancer Causes & Control*, researchers from Redwood City, Palo Alto, and San Francisco, California,

examined the association between sun-protective practices and levels of vitamin
D in the blood. The researchers used data from the US National Health and
Nutrition Examination Survey 2003–2006 that contained information obtained
from adults between the ages of 18 and 60 years. The researchers analyzed questionnaire responses about sun-protective behaviors such as staying in the shade,
wearing long sleeves, wearing a hat, and using sunscreen. Their data also included vitamin D levels of 5,367 participants. The researchers learned that the
people who remained in the shade and wore long sleeves had significantly lower
levels of vitamin D. This was particularly true for the white participants. "White
individuals who protect themselves from the sun by seeking shade or wearing
long sleeves may require higher oral intake of vitamin D than the currently recommended 200–400 IU."[8]

Vitamin D Deficiency Is Very Common, Even among Apparently Healthy People

In a study published in 2015 in the online journal *PLoS ONE*, researchers based
in Saudi Arabia wanted to learn more about the rates of vitamin D deficiency
among Arab adolescent and adult males and females. The cohort consisted of
1,187 males and 1,038 females between the ages of 13 and 17 years and 368 men
and 462 women between the ages of 18 and 50 years. Sizeable numbers of these
seemingly healthy people had some level of vitamin D deficiency. Almost half of
the female teens and almost one-fifth of the male teens had a deficiency. Almost
two-fifths of the women and one-fifth of the men were deficient. In addition to
the high prevalence of vitamin D deficiency, the researchers found an association
between low vitamin D levels in male teens and cardiometabolic risk factors.
According to the researchers, this finding "indicated a sex and age-related disad-
vantage for boys with low vitamin D status and challenges the extra-skeletal protection of vitamin D correction in adolescent females."[9]

Children and Teens with Normal Levels of Vitamin D Do Not Appear to Benefit from Vitamin D Supplementation

In a study published in 2011 in the journal *BMJ*, researchers from Australia
examined the effectiveness of vitamin D supplementation for improving bone mineral density in children and adolescents. They conducted a meta-analysis of six relevant studies with 343 participants receiving placebos and 541 participants receiving
vitamin D. To be eligible for inclusion, trials had to be randomized and placebo
controlled and to last for at least three months. The children and teens ranged in age
from 8 to 17 years. The researchers learned that it is unlikely that children or teens
with normal levels of vitamin D benefit from supplementation. However, the researchers commented that it is possible that children and teens deficient in vitamin
D might experience "clinically useful improvements, particularly in lumbar spine

bone mineral density and total body bone mineral count" from supplementation. But, this needs to be confirmed in future studies.[10]

NOTES

1. Vitamin D Council, www.vitmindcouncil.org.

2. Monica Verdoia, Alon Schaffer, Chiara Sartori et al., "Vitamin D Deficiency Is Independently Associated with the Extent of Coronary Artery Disease," *European Journal of Clinical Investigation* 44, no. 7 (2014): 634–42.

3. Kung-Ting Kao, Nobia Abidi, Sanjeeva Ranasinha et al., "Low Vitamin D Is Associated with Hypertension in Paediatric Obesity," *Journal of Paediatrics and Child Health* 51, no. 12 (2015): 1207–13.

4. Micah L. Olson, Naim M. Maalouf, Jon D. Oden et al., "Vitamin D Deficiency in Obese Children and Its Relationship to Glucose Homeostasis," *Journal of Clinical Endocrinology & Metabolism* 97, no. 1 (2012): 279–85.

5. R. E. Allen, A. D. Dangour, A. E. Tedstone, and Z. Chalabi, "Does Fortification of Staple Foods Improve Vitamin D Intakes and Status of Groups At Risk of Deficiency? A United Kingdom Modeling Study," *American Journal of Clinical Nutrition* 102, no. 2 (2015): 338–44.

6. T. Wang, L. Shan, L. Du et al., 2015. "Serum Concentration of 25-Hydroxyvitamin D in Autism Spectrum Disorder: A Systematic Review and Meta-Analysis," *European Child & Adolescent Psychiatry* 25, no. 4 (April 2016): 341–50.

7. Feiyong Jia, Bing Wang, Ling Shan et al., "Core Symptoms of Autism Improved After Vitamin D Supplementation," *Pediatrics* 135, no. 1 (2015): e196–e198.

8. Eleni Linos, Elizabeth Keiser, Matthew Kanzler et al., "Sun Protective Behaviors and Vitamin D Levels in the US Population: NHANES 2003–2006," *Cancer Causes & Control* 23, no. 1 (2012): 133–40.

9. Nasser M. Al-Daghri, Yousef Al-Saleh, Naji Aljohani et al., "Vitamin D Deficiency and Cardiometabolic Risks: A Juxtaposition of Arab Adolescents and Adults," *PLoS ONE* 10, no. 7 (2015): e0131315.

10. T. Winzenberg, S. Powell, K. A. Shaw, and G. Jones, "Effects of Vitamin D Supplementation on Bone Density in Healthy Children: Systematic Review and Meta-Analysis," *BMJ* 342 (2011): c7254.

REFERENCES AND RESOURCES

Magazines, Journals, and Newspapers

Al-Daghri, Nasser M., Yousef Al-Saleh, Naji Aljohani et al. "Vitamin D Deficiency and Cardiometabolic Risks: A Juxtaposition of Arab Adolescents and Adults." *PLoS ONE* 10, no. 7 (2015): e0131315.

Allen, R. E., A. D. Dangour, A. E. Tedstone, and Z. Chalabi. August 2015. "Does Fortification of Staple Foods Improve Vitamin D Intakes and Status of Groups at Risk of Deficiency? A United Kingdom Modeling Study." *American Journal of Clinical Nutrition* 102, no. 2 (2015): 338–44.

Ataie-Jafari, Asal, Mostafa Qorbani, Ramin Heshmat et al. "The Association of Vitamin D Deficiency with Psychiatric Distress and Violence Behaviors in Iranian

Adolescents: The CASPIAN-III Study." *Journal of Diabetes & Metabolic Disorders* 14 (2015): 62+.

Jia, Feiyong, Bing Wang, Ling Shan et al. "Core Symptoms of Autism Improved After Vitamin D Supplementation." *Pediatrics* 135, no. 1 (2015): e196–e198.

Kao, Kung-Ting, Nobia Abidi, Sanjeeva Ranasinha et al. "Low Vitamin D Is Associated with Hypertension in Paediatric Obesity." *Journal of Paediatrics and Child Health* 51, no. 12 (2015): 1207–13.

Linos, Eleni, Elizabeth Keiser, Matthew Kanzler et al. "Sun Protective Behaviors and Vitamin D Levels in the US Population: NHANES 2003–2006." *Cancer Causes & Control* 23, no. 1 (2012): 133–40.

Olson, Micah L., Naim M. Maalouf, Jon D. Oden et al. "Vitamin D Deficiency in Obese Children and Its Relationship to Glucose Homeostasis." *Journal of Clinical Endocrinology & Metabolism* 97, no. 1 (2012): 279–85.

Pilz, Stefan, Martin Gaksch, Katharina Kienreich et al. "Effects of Vitamin D on Blood Pressure and Cardiovascular Risk Factors: A Randomized Controlled Trial." *Hypertension* 65 (2015): 1195–201.

Verdoia, Monica, Alon Schaffer, Chiara Sartori et al. "Vitamin D Deficiency Is Independently Associated with the Extent of Coronary Artery Disease." *European Journal of Clinical Investigation* 44, no. 7 (2014): 634–42.

Wang, T., L. Shan, L. Du et al. "Serum Concentration of 25-Hydroxyvitamin D in Autism Spectrum Disorder: A Systematic Review and Meta-Analysis." *European Child & Adolescent Psychiatry* 25, no. 4 (April 2016): 341–50.

Winzenberg, T., S. Powell, K. A. Shaw, and G. Jones. "Effects of Vitamin D Supplementation on Bone Density in Healthy Children: Systematic Review and Meta-Analysis." *BMJ* 342 (2011): c7254.

Web Site

Vitamin D Council. www.vitamindcouncil.org.

Protect Your Hearing

OVERVIEW

The statistics of the National Institute on Deafness and Other Communication Disorders on hearing impairment in the United States are sobering. Based on standard hearing examinations, one in every eight people aged 12 years or older has hearing loss in both ears. That represents about 30 million people or 13 percent of the population.[1] And, those numbers seem to be growing, especially for adolescents.

Why are teens at such an increased risk for hearing loss? Large numbers of teens spend endless hours exposed to loud noises as they listen to music, attend concerts, use power equipment, and/or mow the lawn. An occasional exposure for a limited period of time likely causes little harm; but the continuous exposure places teens and others at increased risk for hearing loss. Probably the best solution for background noise that you are unable to control is to wear noise-cancelling headphones. If you have flown in a plane, you have seen people wearing them. They greatly reduce exposure to outside noise in a plane. But, they are useful in other settings. While these headphones are not inexpensive, they can play a role in preventing hearing loss. You may purchase headphones at electronic stores; a good store should have an excellent selection.

There are also problems associated with teens and young adults who raise the sound of personal music players. In response, the American Speech-Language-Hearing Association launched a campaign called "Listen to Your Buds." (Buds are the portion of the personal music players that fit into the ears. They are speakers in your ears.) The campaign is trying to "educate children and parents about practicing safe listening habits when using personal listening devices, in order to avoid possible noise-inducing hearing loss in the future."[2] It is always best to lower the volume of your music and limit the amount of time you spend with buds in your ears.

It is possible that you already have hearing loss from excessive noise, a condition known as noise-induced hearing loss. Symptoms of this disorder are ringing, buzzing, or roaring in the ears after hearing loud noise, and the distortion of sounds.[3] If you are experiencing these symptoms, make an appointment with your healthcare provider. You will then be referred to the correct professional for future care and treatment.

WHAT THE EXPERTS SAY

Children Are Able to Learn Healthier Personal Listening Device Behavior

In a pilot study published in 2013 in the journal *Noise & Health*, researchers from South Africa and Australia wanted to learn if a noise-induced hearing loss prevention program, known as Cheers for Ears, was effective in changing the self-reported listening behaviors of Australian students between 9 and 13 years. All the students participated in two interactive sessions, which were held six weeks apart, and a total of 318 students were selected to be surveyed. At baseline, 91.8 percent of the surveyed students owned or had access to a personal listening device. And, the vast majority, 79.1 percent, could control the volume on their devices. The researchers found that after the sessions, the students reduced the volume of their listening devices. Three months after the program ended, the students were again surveyed. The researchers found that their behavior changes "were stable and sustained." And, they noted that the program "is effective in increasing knowledge on the harmful effects of noise and therefore, it may prevent future noise-induced hearing loss."[4]

In a study published in 2011 in the journal *The Laryngoscope*, researchers from Canada assessed the efficacy of a hearing conservation program (Sound Sense™) in elementary school children. The cohort consisted of sixth grade students, between the ages of 9 and 13 years, from 16 Vancouver School Board schools. The schools were randomized to be either an intervention school or a control group school. Students completed an initial questionnaire, a second questionnaire two weeks after the intervention, and a third questionnaire six months later. The surveys, which were administered by the teachers during regular school hours, asked about personal music playing habits, exposure to noise during daily activities, and about the use of earplugs. The students in the control schools completed questionnaires but had no intervention. The researchers learned that at baseline 43 of the 775 students had some degree of hearing loss. The use of a personal listening devise was reported by 515 of the 771 students. When compared to the children in the control, the researchers found that the children who participated in the intervention had significant improvements in use of earplugs. The children in the intervention group also reduced their use of personal music devices. The researchers concluded that the Sound Sense™ program "improved earplug use practices in elementary school children in the short and long term." Moreover, "the development, implementation and evaluation of a community-based health promotion project around hearing loss can serve as a tremendous opportunity for students to develop their knowledge and skills in health advocacy."[5]

Interventions to Prevent Hearing Loss Made at Younger Ages May Prevent More Serious Problems

In a randomized, controlled trial published in 2012 in the journal *Occupational & Environmental Medicine*, researchers from Wisconsin and Canada had an opportunity to follow 392 young workers for up to 16 years and to determine if the measures taken to prevent hearing loss when people were still in high school were effective over a long period of time. When the teens were first evaluated, they were 12 to 16 years old, with a mean age of 14.5 years. During their most recent evaluation, they were aged 29 to 33 years. While most of the participants originally worked in agriculture, over time they entered other occupations. The participants completed questionnaires that asked about their exposure to high levels of occupational and recreational noise, as well as their use of hearing protection devices. The researchers found that hearing loss was more evident in the men than the women. As a result, they limited their final analysis to men. They found a high variation in the use of protective devices—ranging from 3.85 to 67.3 percent. Still, the devices "appeared to offer some protection to participants." The researchers suggested that hearing conservation programs "should focus on a broader range of exposures, whether in occupational or non-occupational settings."[6]

BARRIERS AND PROBLEMS

Hearing Loss Interventions May Only Work for a Relatively Short Period of Time

In a study published in 2011 in the journal *Pediatrics*, researchers from Wisconsin, Minnesota, and Canada examined the long-term effects of a well-designed hearing conservation intervention. The researchers wanted to learn if the intervention reduced the amount of hearing loss and sufficiently supported the sustained use of hearing protective devices. Between 1992 and 1996, 34 rural Wisconsin schools with vocational agriculture programs were recruited. The students in 17 of these schools, who were all in grades 7 through 9, were randomly assigned to receive a comprehensive, three-year hearing conservation intervention or no intervention. Noise exposure questionnaires were completed at the beginning and ending of the intervention. From 2009 to 2010, the researchers made "extensive efforts" to contact all 690 of the students who had completed the original trial. The researchers were able to recruit 392 participants from the original trial—200 were in the intervention group and 192 were in the control group. Of these, 355 completed a questionnaire and had clinical hearing tests conducted by trained audiologists. The researchers found that among the participants exposed to agricultural noise, the members of the intervention group were significantly more likely to use hearing protection than those in the control group. The members of the intervention group were also more likely to use hearing protection when they used firearms. But, in other areas of their lives, the members of both groups used about the same amount of protection. The researchers found no significant difference between the groups with respect to objective measures of noise-induced hearing loss (NIHL). The researchers concluded that their "findings suggest that this comprehensive, well-designed, well-executed intervention aimed at educating rural high school students about hearing conservation was of limited effectiveness in preventing early NIHL."[7]

Most Teens Appear to Need More Information About Hearing Health

In a descriptive study published in 2012 in the journal *Language, Speech, and Hearing Services in Schools*, researchers from Santa Barbara, California, and Auburn, Alabama, wanted to learn more about what high school students knew about hearing health and the impact of using personal listening devices. In December 2009, an 83-item questionnaire was administered to students at a California high school. One hundred and thirty-one completed the survey, which was a response rate of 56 percent. Most of the students thought they used their iPods safely. Only a small percentage noted that the volume was too loud. And, many increased the volume when they listened to favorite songs, when there was background noise, and/or when they exercised. It became evident that the students expressed incorrect information on some areas of hearing health. For example, most of the teens did not realize that using cotton in the ears does not provide protection from hearing loss caused by loud noises. Perhaps one of the most disturbing findings was that more than one-third of the students said that the scientific findings that using high volume on their iPods damaged hearing would not cause them to change their behaviors. The researchers concluded that "most of the students needed education . . . about hearing health, the warning signs of hearing loss, and how to prevent hearing loss."[8]

In a study published in 2013 in the *International Journal of Audiology*, researchers from Australia noted that occupational noise tended to be fairly predictable. So, work environments may already have plans in place to protect hearing. On the other hand, noise in leisure environments may be variable, and protecting oneself from such noise is dependent on "personal regulation," the ability of each individual to take action to protect his or her hearing. The researchers wanted to learn more about the ability of people to take this action. The cohort consisted of 1,000 Australian males and females between the ages of 18 and 35 years. They all completed an online questionnaire, which asked about participation in noisy leisure activities and what the participants did to protect their hearing. While most of the participants reported good current hearing health, more than one-fifth showed the early signs of damage. About half took some measures to reduce their exposure to noise. However, this preventive action was found not to be related to hearing loss symptoms or "perceived personal risk" of damage from noise. Instead, these measures were taken because of the participants' "beliefs about the risk posed by leisure noise, hearing health awareness, and the importance of hearing." The researchers underscored the need for more education about the risks leisure time activities may pose to hearing. "Placing a stronger emphasis on educating young adults about the risk for hearing loss from their leisure activities, and personalizing this risk to make it relevant to their own participation is likely to be an important motivator."[9]

Undergraduate Music Students May Have a Greatly Increased Risk of Hearing Loss

In a study published in 2010 in the journal *Medical Problems of Performing Artists*, a researcher from the United Kingdom wanted to know more about the hearing problems associated with undergraduate students who were enrolled in popular music courses. The researcher hypothesized that these students would have "a higher than average noise exposure hazard." The cohort consisted of 100 students, with a mean age of 22.6 years, enrolled in nine undergraduate courses. In a 30-point questionnaire, the 92 males and 8 females were surveyed about their musical habits, both within and outside the university setting. When the researcher compared exposure to noise during supervised time, such as lectures and tutorials, to exposure to noise during unsupervised activities, such as rehearsals and recordings, the differences were dramatic. "Unsupervised activities were more likely to exceed noise recommendations, particularly as they were generally based on practical, noise-making activities." If hearing protection is not used during these unsupervised times, there appeared to be "a significant hazard to the hearing of music students." This was most apparent in the students studying music performance. "Although there was a high reported level of education on noise exposure, many students were still choosing to use loud sound levels and opting not to use hearing protection."[10]

NOTES

1. National Institute on Deafness and Other Communication Disorders, http://www.nidcd.nih.gov.
2. American Speech-Language-Hearing Association, www.asha.org.
3. The Nemours Foundation, http://kidshealth.org.
4. D. S. Taljaard, N. F. Leischman, and R. H. Eikelboom, "Personal Listening Devises and the Prevention of Noise Induced Hearing Loss in Children. The Cheers for Ears Pilot Program," *Noise & Health* 15, no. 65 (2013): 261–68.
5. Anastasia Neufeld, Brian D. Westerberg, Shahin Nabi et al., "Prospective, Randomized Controlled Assessment of the Short- and Long-Term Efficacy of a Hearing Conservation Education Program in Canadian Elementary School Children," *The Laryngoscope* 121 (2011): 176–81.
6. Barbara Marlenga, Richard L. Berg, James G. Linneman et al., "Determinants of Early-Stage Hearing Loss Among a Cohort of Young Workers with 16-Year Follow-Up," *Occupational & Environmental Medicine* 69 (2012): 479–84.
7. Barbara Marlenga, James G. Linneman, William Pickett et al., "Randomized Trial of a Hearing Conservation Intervention for Rural Students: Long-Term Outcomes," *Pediatrics* 128, no. 5 (2011): e1139–e1146.
8. Jeffrey L. Danhauer, Carole E. Johnson, Aislinn F. Dunne et al., "Survey of High School Students' Perceptions About Their iPod Use, Knowledge of Hearing Health, and Need for Education," *Language, Speech, and Hearing Services in Schools* 43 (2012): 14–35.
9. Megan Gilliver, Elizabeth Francis Beach, and Warwick Williams, "Noise with Attitude: Influences on Young People's Decisions to Protect their Hearing," *International Journal of Audiology* 52 (2013): S26–S32.
10. Christopher Barlow, "Potential Hazard of Hearing Damage to Students in Undergraduate Popular Music Courses," *Medical Problems of Performing Artists* 25 (2010): 175–82.

REFERENCES AND RESOURCES

Magazines, Journals, and Newspapers

Auchter, Melissa, and Colleen G. Le Prell. "Hearing Loss Prevention Education Using Adopt-a-Band Changes in Self-Reported Earplug Use in Two High School Marching Bands." *American Journal of Audiology* 23 (2014): 211–26.
Barlow, Christopher. "Potential Hazard of Hearing Damage to Students in Undergraduate Popular Music Courses." *Medical Problems of Performing Artists* 25 (2010): 175–82.

Danhauer, Jeffrey L., Carole E. Johnson, Aislinn F. Dunne et al. "Survey of High School Students' Perceptions About Their iPod Use, Knowledge of Hearing Health, and Need for Education." *Language, Speech, and Hearing Services in Schools* 43 (2012): 14–35.

Gilliver, Megan, Elizabeth Francis Beach, and Warwick Williams. "Noise with Attitude: Influences on Young People's Decisions to Protect their Hearing." *International Journal of Audiology* 52 (2013): S26–S32.

Marlenga, Barbara, James G. Linneman, William Pickett et al. "Randomized Trial of a Hearing Conservation Intervention for Rural Students: Long-Term Outcomes." *Pediatrics* 128, no. 5 (2011): e1139–e1146.

Marlenga, Barbara, Richard L. Berg, James G. Linneman et al. "Determinants of Early-State Hearing Loss Among a Cohort of Young Workers with 16-Year Follow-Up." *Occupational & Environmental Medicine* 69 (2012): 479–84.

Neufeld, Anastasia, Brian D. Westerberg, Shahin Nabi et al. "Prospective, Randomized Controlled Assessment of the Short- and Long-Term Efficacy of a Hearing Conservation Education Program in Canadian Elementary School Children." *The Laryngoscope* 121 (2011): 176–81.

Rosemberg, Marie-Anne S., Marjorie C. McCullagh, and Megan Nordstrom. "Farm and Rural Adolescents' Perspective on Hearing Conservation: Reports from a Focus Group Study." *Noise & Health* 17, no. 76 (2015): 134–40.

Taljaard, D. S., N. F. Leischman, and R. H. Eikelboom. "Personal Listening Devices and the Prevention of Noise Induced Hearing Loss in Children. The Cheers for Ears Pilot Program." *Noise & Health* 15, no. 65 (2013): 261–68.

Web Sites

American Speech-Language-Hearing Association. www.asha.org.

National Institute on Deafness and Other Communication Disorders. http://www.nidcd.nih.gov.

The Nemours Foundation. http://kidshealth.org.

Take Care of Your Feet

OVERVIEW

It is easy to take feet for granted. In one way or another, they are involved in just about all daily activities. Yet, while teens and young adults often spend lots of time caring for their skin, teeth, hair, and other parts of their bodies, they devote little if any time to their feet. It is important to remember that foot health is an integral component of overall health and wellness. Female teens may polish the nails on their feet, but that does not really support healthy feet.

According to the Michigan Podiatric Medical Association, though most people tend to address foot issues later in life, it is important to begin a good foot care routine during the teen years. Such a routine includes washing feet every day with soap and water. After the feet have been washed, they should be dried. If not, fungus may easily begin to grow, especially between the toes. In fact, wet socks may also foster the growth of fungus. Wet socks should be changed as soon as possible. It is a good idea to store a dry pair of socks in a school locker. Toenails should not be allowed to grow beyond the toes; toenails should be trimmed every few weeks with a toenail clipper. Supportive and properly fitted shoes should be worn. Shoes that lack basic support and fit poorly may be a source of foot pain and injury.[1]

Like adults, teens are at risk for a number of foot problems. One of the most common concerns is feet that have an unpleasant smell. This is caused by bacteria that live on the feet and in shoes. Washing your feet with soap every day, wearing a clean pair of socks, and alternating shoes should correct this problem. Removing insoles from shoes and sponge washing them with a little soap and water may also be helpful. Plantar warts, also known as verruca, are caused by a virus that enters the skin through a small crack. To survive on floors, the virus requires a warm and wet environment, such as a communal changing room or sports center. As it thickens, a plantar wart may become painful. If a plantar wart does not resolve by itself, it may be treated by a medical provider. Ingrown toenails are another common medical problem. These occur when a small amount of nail grows forward and digs into the skin. They may become infected and be painful. Again, you may need the care of a medical provider who will use special clippers, and, perhaps, a local anesthetic, to resolve the issue. Another frequent medical problem among teens is foot pain. This is often related to rapid foot growth and the need for larger and more supportive shoes, which may or may not be fashionable. In females, foot pain may be associated with wearing high-heeled shoes. Foot pain that persists should be discussed with a medical provider.[2]

WHAT THE EXPERTS SAY

Running on Grass Reduces In-Shoe Pressures on Feet

In a study published in 2012 in the *Journal of Sports Sciences*, researchers from Brazil noted that recreational running has become quite popular throughout the world, and with this practice has come related lower limb injuries. The researchers wanted to investigate the ability of the varying running surfaces—asphalt, concrete, rubber, and natural grass—to reduce the incidence of these injuries. The cohort consisted of 47 adult recreational runners between the ages of 18 and 50 years, with a mean age of 35.1 years for men and 38.9 years for women. For inclusion in the study, the participants were required to run at least 20 km weekly (about 12 1/2 miles) for at least one year, and they had to be experienced running in long-distance competitions and on different surfaces. During the study, participants ran 40 minutes on all four different surfaces. The researchers initially hypothesized that there would be lower pressure on the grass and rubber surfaces. Surprisingly, the rubber acted like the more rigid concrete and asphalt surfaces. The researchers suggested that this result may have occurred because the rubber was five years old. Running on grass appeared to be the most favorable option for the feet. Still, there may be problems with grass. "The non-uniformity of natural grass, due to such factors as holes and tree roots, and also the higher energy expenditure by the runner are disadvantages that should be taken into account when considering a training surface." On the other hand, "if a runner controls his/her amount and intensity of practice, running on grass may reduce the total stress on the musculoskeletal system."[3]

Shock-Absorbing Insoles May Help Protect Feet

In a prospective, randomized study published in 2014 in the *Journal of Orthopaedic and Sports Physical Therapy*, researchers from Denmark and Spain compared the ability of shock-absorbing insoles and regular insoles to reduce the amount of pain experienced by young soccer players on artificial turf. The cohort consisted of 75 adolescent players who were divided into two groups. An initial baseline assessment was conducted. Then, for three weeks, the teens in one group used the shock-absorbing insoles and the teens in the other used regular insoles. Assessments were made at the end of the three weeks of training and at a six-week follow-up. The researchers found that the shock-absorbing insoles reduced the amount of pain experienced by the players. They noted that the use of shock-absorbing insoles "may play a protective role in pressure sensitivity and pain prevention." Likewise, these insoles "caused larger decreases in pressure pain sensitivity and pain intensity compared with usual insoles."[4]

Sanitizing Athletic Shoes May Help Prevent Foot Infections and Reduce Unpleasant Odors

In a crossover study published in 2015 in the *Journal of Athletic Training*, researchers based in Italy evaluated the efficacy of a sanitizing technique for reducing the bacterial and fungal contamination of footwear. According to the researchers, people tend to wash their feet with some regularity, but they devote little attention to the inside areas of their shoes. The cohort consisted of 27 male athletes and four coaches, with a total of 62 shoes. The researchers began their experimental protocol by using swabs to take samples from the interior sections of all of the shoes. Then the participants were supplied with a sanitizing product and told to use it on dry shoes before they were worn. Second samples of the shoes were taken after about four weeks. The researchers found that the shoe sanitizing product resulted in a "general reduction in the microbial population." The researchers commented that "the sanitizing technique significantly reduced the bacterial presence in athletes' shoes."[5]

BARRIERS AND PROBLEMS

High Heels May Impair Static Balance

In a cross-sectional study published in 2012 in the journal *Human Movement Science*, researchers from Brazil assessed the effect of high-heeled shoes (seven centimeters) on the static balance of young adult women. (Static balance is the ability to maintain one's balance when not moving.) The cohort consisted of 53 women between the ages of 18 and 30 years who regularly wore high-heeled shoes. None of the women had experienced any "orthopedic or neurologic alterations." Static balance assessments were made when the women were barefoot and when they were wearing high-heeled shoes, and when their eyes were open and their eyes were closed. All the assessments were conducted on a single day. The women who were barefoot with their eyes open had the best static balance, and the women wearing the high-heeled shoes who had their eyes closed had the most problems with static balance. The researchers commented that in their findings, "the use of high-heeled shoes had a negative influence over balance in the women evaluated . . ., which was accentuated when visual information was removed."[6]

Female Teens Do Not Necessarily Consider Foot Health When Selecting Shoes

In an investigation published in 2013 in the *Journal of Health Psychology*, researchers from the United Kingdom wanted to learn more about the role that foot health plays in the shoe choices of female teens. The cohort consisted of 162 female students with a mean age of 17 years. The students completed questionnaires about their thoughts and emotions concerning their footwear purchases made during the previous six months. During that time, they collectively purchased a total of 458 pairs of shoes. The high-heeled shoes, which were purchased for occasions and parties, made the teens the happiest. In fact, the height of the heel was a statistically significant choice. Flat shoes, which were worn for everyday and school, were not associated with positive or negative emotions. Casual shoes, such as wool boots, were often worn on weekends. The researchers commented that footwear was a factor in fashion and self-image for female teens. But, foot functions and foot health did not appear to influence the choice of footwear. Moreover, "foot measurements were not seen as an important consideration for footwear purchases."[7]

Wearing Flip-Flop Style Shoes Appears to Alter Human Gait

In a study published in 2010 in the *Journal of the American Podiatric Medical Association*, researchers from Auburn University in Alabama noted that flip-flop style shoes have become a common footwear option. As a result, they wanted to learn more about the effect flip-flops have on human gait. The cohort consisted of 37 women and 19 men, who were all college students with a mean age of 20.85 years. The students were videotaped wearing flip-flops and athletic style sneakers. The researchers found that flip-flops did indeed alter human gait. While wearing their flip-flops, the students took shorter steps and their heels hit the ground with less vertical force than they did with sneakers. In addition, while wearing flip-flops, the students did not raise their toes as much during the leg's swing phase, which resulted in a larger ankle angle and a shorter stride length. This was possibly because they tended to grip the flip-flops with their toes. The researchers commented that their findings suggested that "flip-flops have an effect on several kinetic and kinematic variables compared with sneakers."[8]

NOTES

1. Michigan Podiatric Medical Association, www.mpma.org.

2. The College of Podiatry, www.scpod.org.

3. V. Tessutti, A.P. Ribeiro, F. Trombini-Souza, and I. C. Sacco, "Attenuation of Foot Pressure During Running on Four Different Surfaces: Asphalt, Concrete, Rubber, and Natural Grass," *Journal of Sports Sciences* 30, no. 14 (2012): 1545–50.

4. Pascal Madeleine, Brian P. Hoej, César Fernández de las Peñas et al., "Pressure Pain Sensitivity Changes After Use of Shock-Absorbing Insoles Among Young Soccer Players Training on Artificial Turf: A Randomized Controlled Trial," *Journal of Orthopaedic and Sports Physical Therapy* 44, no. 8 (2014): 587–94.

5. G. Messina, S. Burgassi, C. Russo et al., "Is It Possible to Sanitize Athletes' Shoes?" *Journal of Athlete Training* 50, no. 2 (2015): 126–32.

6. Susana Baceete Gerber, Rafael Vital Costa, Luanda André Colange Grecco et al., "Interference of High-Heeled Shoes in Static Balance Among Young Women," *Human Movement Science* 31 (2012): 1247–52.

7. H. Branthwaite, N. Chockaingam, S. Grogan, and M. Jones, "Footwear Choices Made by Young Women and Their Potential Impact on Foot Health," *Journal of Health Psychology* 18, no. 11 (2013): 1422–31.

8. Justin F. Shroyer and Wendi H. Weimar, "Comparative Analysis of Human Gait While Wearing Thong-Style Flip-Flops Versus Sneakers," *Journal of the American Podiatric Medical Association* 100, no. 4 (2010): 251–57.

REFERENCES AND RESOURCES

Magazines, Journals, and Newspapers

Branthwaite, H., N. Chockalingam, S. Grogan, and M. Jones. "Footwear Choices Made by Young Women and Their Potential Impact on Foot Health." *Journal of Health Psychology* 18, no. 11 (2013): 1422–31.

Gerber, Susana Baceete, Rafael Vital Costa, Luanda André Colange Grecco et al. "Interference of High-Heeled Shoes in Static Balance Among Young Women." *Human Movement Science* 31 (2012): 1247–52.

Hoffman, Martin D., and Eswar Krishnan. "Health and Exercise-Related Medical Issues Among 1,212 Ultramarathon Runners: Baseline Findings from the Ultrarunners Longitudinal TRAcking (ULTRA) Study." *PLoS ONE* 9, no. 1 (2014): e83867.

Hollander, K., D. Riebe, S. Campe et al. "Effects of Footwear on Treadmill Running Biomechanics in Preadolescent Children." *Gait & Posture* 40, no. 2 (2014): 381–81.

Madeleine, Pascal, Brian P. Hoej, César Fernández de las Peñas et al. "Pressure Pain Sensitivity Changes After Use of Shock-Absorbing Insoles Among Young Soccer Players Training on Artificial Turf: A Randomized Controlled Trial." *Journal of Orthopaedic and Sports Physical Therapy* 44, no. 8 (2014): 587–94.

Messina, G., S. Burgassi, C. Russo et al. "Is It Possible to Sanitize Athletes' Shoes?" *Journal of Athlete Training* 50, no. 2 (2015): 126–32.

Robinson, L. E., M. E. Rudisill, W. H. Weimar et al. "Footwear and Locomotor Skill Performance in Preschoolers." *Perceptual and Motor Skills* 113, no. 2 (2011): 534–38.

Shroyer, Justin F., and Wendi H. Weimar. "Comparative Analysis of Human Gait While Wearing Thong-Style Flip-Flops Versus Sneakers." *Journal of the American Podiatric Medical Association* 100, no. 4 (2010): 251–57.

Silva, Anniele Martins, Gisela Rocha de Siqueira, and Giselia Alves P. da Silva. "Implications of High-Heeled Shoes on Body Posture of Adolescents." *Revista Paulista de Pediatria* 31, no. 2 (2013): 265–71.

Simon, J., E. Hall, and C. Docherty. "Prevalence of Chronic Ankle Instability and Associated Symptoms in University Dance Majors: An Exploratory Study." *Journal of Dance Medicine & Science* 18, no. 4 (2014): 178–84.

Tessutti, V., A. P. Ribeiro, F. Trombini-Souza, and I. C. Sacco. "Attenuation of Foot Pressure During Running on Four Different Surfaces: Asphalt, Concrete, Rubber, and Natural Grass." *Journal of Sports Sciences* 30, no. 14 (2012): 1545–50.

Web Sites

Michigan Podiatric Medical Association. www.mpma.org.
The College of Podiatry. www.scpod.org.

Safety

Don't Text While Driving

OVERVIEW

We have all seen other drivers texting while they are driving. We may have even texted while driving. Texting while driving is a type of distracted driving. According to the Centers for Disease Control and Prevention, distracted driving is "driving while doing another activity that takes your attention away from driving." There are three main types of distraction. In the first, your eyes are not looking at the road. In the second, your hands are off the wheel. And, in the third, your mind is thinking of something other than driving. Texting combines all three of these types. While texting, one must focus on the text; the head is focused on the text for at least a few seconds. Younger, less experienced drivers under the age of 20 have the highest rate of distraction-related fatal crashes. That makes texting especially dangerous.[1]

Every year, thousands of people in the United States are killed in distracted driver crashes and hundreds of thousands are injured. In 2011, 17 percent of all crashes involved a distracted driver. A Centers for Disease Control and Prevention study found that 31 percent of U.S. drivers between the ages of 18 and 64 years reported that they had read or sent text messages or email messages while driving at least once within 30 days of the survey. That's almost a third of all drivers.[2]

Many states have enacted laws against texting while driving. And, there are a few federal laws, such as the September 17, 2010, law issued by the Federal Railroad Administration, that banned the use of cell phones and electronic devices by employees while they are working. The next month, on October 27, 2010, the Federal Motor Carrier Safety Administration prohibited commercial vehicle drivers from texting while driving.[3] In April 2014, the National Highway Safety Administration launched its first national advertising campaign to combat distracted drivers. Multiple media advertisements were designed to coincide with a "nationwide law enforcement crackdown in states with distracted driving bans." Before starting the car engine, all drivers need to turn off their phones, and place them out of reach. And, older drivers should set an example for younger drives. Parents should make a point of talking to their teens about responsible driving.[4]

WHAT THE EXPERTS SAY

Distracted Driving Is Dangerous Driving

In an article published in 2015 in the *Journal of Trauma and Acute Care Surgery*, researchers from several locations in the United States and Nairobi, Kenya, assembled 19 evidence-based review articles on distracted driving. The researchers directed their attention to articles published between 2000 and 2013, a time period when it became increasingly evident that large numbers of people were texting and driving. In addition, they noted that the National Highway Traffic Safety Administration has declared that motor vehicle crashes are the number one cause of death and disability among teens. "Inexperience and distracted driving are common contributing factors for the teen driver involved in collisions." As a result, the researchers issued several recommendations for drivers. First, drivers should minimize all in-vehicle distractions. Second, drivers should not use any messaging device. And, finally, in addition to not using any messaging systems, younger drivers should avoid using cell phones. The researchers concluded that "competent driving involves dedicated attention to road conditions using all senses; dangerously, both the novice and the distracted drivers fail to appreciate their responsibility. Elimination of distraction is key to preventing further mortality."[5]

Driving Context Influences the Drivers' Decision to Engage in Visual-Manual Phone Tasks

In a study published in 2015 in the *Journal of Safety Research*, researchers from Sweden investigated the association between the driving context and the drivers' decision to engage in visual-manual phone tasks, such as texting and dialing. Using several devices, everyday data were collected from 100 Volvo cars over a one-year period of time. The cars were driven in real traffic with their normal drivers. Video recordings of 1,432 car trips were used for the analysis. The researchers learned that visual-manual phone tasks were generally initiated when the car was stopped; these tasks were less likely to occur when the car was at a higher speed or a passenger was present. Drivers were more likely to complete these tasks when there were clear weather conditions, lower traffic density, and when they were driving on rural roads, motorways, or highways. When drivers had higher-demand driving maneuvers, such as sharp turns and roundabouts, they would delay using their phones until the maneuver was completed. Thus, the researchers noted that the use of phones does not occur at random. Drivers are deciding when and how to use their devices. Moreover, "this adaptive behavior of task timing clearly suggests that drivers are aware of the increased risk of VM [visual-motor] phone tasks while driving."[6]

Though Aware of the Dangers, College Students Continue to Drive While They Are Texting

In a study published in 2011 in the journal *Accident Analysis and Prevention*, a researcher from Middletown, Pennsylvania, wanted to quantify the amount of text messaging and other types of distracted driving practiced by college students. The cohort consisted of 91 college students (60 females and 31 males); they drove a mean of 6.08 days per week. A stunning 91 percent of the students reported that they have used text messaging while driving. They sent text messages even if other people, including children, were in the car. In addition, the students reported that they drove above the speed limit and drifted into other lanes while text messaging. Almost 40 percent of the students have driven while eating and text messaging. At the same time, the researcher noted that "most people in this study believed that texting while driving is dangerous, distracting, and should be illegal." The researcher concluded that there is a need for stronger anti-texting laws and more rigorous enforcement of these laws. And, she concluded her article with a poignant statement: "The irony is not lost in that texting while driving may lead to devastating consequences for one's self and for others, including never seeing again the people to whom one has an ostensibly obsessive desire to stay connected."[7]

BARRIERS AND PROBLEMS

Texting with Google Glass Is Still Distracted Driving

In a study published in 2014 in the journal *Human Factors*, researchers from Florida and Ohio wanted to learn more about the distraction potential of texting with Google Glass, a "mobile wearable platform capable of receiving and sending short-message-service and other messaging formats," while driving. Google Glass enables people to send text messages using voice transcription as well as head commands. Was texting with Google Glass safer than texting with a phone, as some have claimed? During the trial, about 40 participants drove in a simulator while they texted about arithmetic problems via Google Glass or a smartphone. While this was taking place, the drivers had to deal with the car in front of them braking suddenly. When compared to driving without any distractions, the researchers found that messaging using either Google Glass or a smartphone impaired driving. The researchers noted that Google Glass messages "served to moderate but did not eliminate distracting cognitive demands."[8]

While Texting Is a Serious Distraction, There Are Many Others

In a study published in 2015 in the journal *Traffic Injury Prevention*, researchers from the United Kingdom, Spain, and Turkey wanted to learn more about the prevalence of observable driving distractions. As a result, two independent researchers collected data at four randomly selected locations in the United Kingdom. Of the 10,984 drivers who were seen, 16.8 percent were engaged in "a secondary task." The most common distraction was talking to passengers (8.8 percent). This was followed by smoking (1.9 percent) and by talking on a hands-free mobile phone (1.7 percent). One percent of the drivers were seen talking on a hand-held phone, and texting was observed in less than one percent. Middle-aged and older drivers were less likely to engage in these behaviors than younger drivers. The researchers concluded that their study offered "further evidence of the relatively high rate of distracted driving in the UK."[9]

Alabama Teen Drivers and Their Passengers Reported Multiple Types of Risky Behaviors in Cars, Including Frequent Texting

In a study published in 2014 in *Southern Medical Journal*, researchers from Alabama investigated the types of risky behaviors practiced by teen drivers and their passengers in Jefferson County, Alabama. According to these researchers, Alabama ranked fourth in the United States for teen crash fatalities. The cohort consisted of 1,399 teens, between the ages of 15 and 18 years, who completed surveys in 2009 and 2010. Fifty-two percent of the participants were males; 64 percent were white; and, 29 percent were African American. When the teens were asked about their behaviors during the previous 30 days, 41 percent reported texting and 11 percent reported driving after drinking. Sixty-seven percent of the teens said that they had been in a car in which the driver was texting. The researchers noted that their findings were "alarming." And, they concluded that, "a concerning number of teens are not receiving safe driving educational messages from parents, doctors, or driver's education classes." According to these researchers, there is a need for stronger driving laws and more education for both parents and teens.[10]

Texting While Driving Has Become a "Cultural Artifact" in the United States

In a study published in 2015 in *Cyberpsychology, Behavior, and Social Networking*, a researcher from Tennessee examined social factors that lead people to text while driving. The cohort consisted of adults aged 18 years and older who were surveyed by the Pew Research Center for the 2010 Spring Change Assessment.

The researcher learned that more than 27 percent of adults in the United States text while driving and more than 60 percent report talking on their mobiles while driving. People who use the Internet on their mobiles are more likely to text while driving; people who talk on their mobiles while driving are more likely to text while driving than those who do not. Interestingly, people who ride with drivers who text are more likely to text, and people who ride with others who use their mobiles in a dangerous way are more likely to text while driving.

People who use their mobiles when they are bored are more likely to text while driving; men are more likely than women to text while driving. The researcher commented that his findings "provide substantial evidence that a variety of complex social factors impact the likelihood of texting while driving." And, though texting while driving is illegal in many states and people are generally aware that it is inherently unsafe, it "has become normalized." The researchers offered a few suggestions for reducing this practice. Awareness campaigns could stress the dangers of texting while driving and the role that peer pressure appears to play in the decision to text while driving. Cars could be built with reminders not to text, similar to the seatbelt reminders that they now have. And, third, technologies should be developed that enable drivers to use voice prompts to text. "Automobile companies must continue to integrate hands-free technologies for mobile multiplexing into vehicles innovatively and ergonomically."[11]

NOTES

1. Centers for Disease Control and Prevention, www.cdc.gov.
2. Ibid.
3. Ibid.
4. National Highway Traffic Safety Administration, www.nhtsa.gov.
5. Luis E. Llerena, Kathy V. Aronow, Jana Macleod et al., "An Evidence-Based Review: Distracted Driver," *Journal of Trauma and Acute Care Surgery* 78, no. 1 (2015): 147–52.
6. E. Tivesten and M. Dozza, "Driving Context Influences Drivers' Decision to Engage in Visual-Manual Phone Tasks: Evidence from a Naturalistic Driving Study," *Journal of Safety Research* 53 (2015): 87–96.
7. Marissa A. Harrison, "College Students' Prevalence and Perceptions of Text Messaging While Driving," *Accident Analysis and Prevention* 43 (2011): 1516–20.
8. B. D. Sawyer, V. S. Finomore, A. A. Calvo, and P. A. Hancock, "Google Glass: A Driver Distraction Cause or Cure?" *Human Factors* 56, no. 7 (2014): 1307–21.
9. M. J. Sullman, F. Prat, and D. K. Tasci, "A Roadside Study of Observable Driver Distractions," *Traffic Injury Prevention* 16, no. 6 (2015): 552–57.
10. E. Irons, M. Nichols, W. D. King et al., "Teen Driving Behaviors in a Rural Southern State," *Southern Medical Journal* 107, no. 12 (2014): 735–38.
11. Steven J. Seiler, "Hand on the Wheel, Mind on the Mobile: An Analysis of Social Factors Contributing to Texting While Driving," *Cyberpsychology, Behavior, and Social Networking* 18, no. 2 (2015): 72–78.

REFERENCES AND RESOURCES

Magazines, Journals, and Newspapers

Barr, Jr., Gavin C., Kathleen E. Kane, Robert D. Barraco et al. "Gender Differences in Perceptions and Self-Reported Driving Behaviors Among Teenagers." *Journal of Emergency Medicine* 48, no. 3 (2015): 366–70.
Harrison, Marissa A. "College Students' Prevalence and Perceptions of Text Messaging While Driving." *Accident Analysis and Prevention* 43 (2011): 1516–20.

Hill, Linda, Jill Rybar, Tara Styer et al. "Prevalence of and Attitudes About Distracted Driving in College Students." *Traffic Injury Prevention* 16, no. 4 (2015): 362–67.

Irons, E., M. Nichols, W. D. King et al. "Teen Driving Behaviors in a Rural Southern State." *Southern Medical Journal* 107, no. 12 (2014): 735–38.

Llerena, Luis E., Kathy V. Aronow, Jana Macleod et al. "An Evidence-Based Review: Distracted Driver." *Journal of Trauma and Acute Care Surgery* 78, no.1 (2015): 147–52.

Sawyer, B. D., V. S. Finomore, A. A. Calvo, and P. A. Hancock. "Google Glass: A Driver Distraction Cause or Cure?" *Human Factors* 56, no. 7 (2014): 1307–21.

Seiler, Steven J. "Hand on the Wheel, Mind on the Mobile. An Analysis of Social Factors Contributing to Texting While Driving." *Cyberpsychology, Behavior, and Social Networking* 18, no. 2 (2015): 72–78.

Sullman, M. J., F. Prat, and D. K. Tasci. "A Roadside Study of Observable Driver Distractions." *Traffic Injury Prevention* 16, no. 6 (2015): 552–57.

Tivesten, E., and M. Dozza. "Driving Context Influences Drivers' Decision to Engage in Visual-Manual Phone Tasks: Evidence from a Naturalistic Driving Study." *Journal of Safety Research* 53 (2015): 87–96.

Web Sites

Centers for Disease Control and Prevention. www.cdc.gov.

National Highway Traffic Safety Administration. www.nhtsa.gov.

Learn Ways to Prevent Violence

OVERVIEW

Anyone who watches local or national news knows that violence is a fairly common occurrence. And, violence is not confined to the big cities. While it is a part of daily life in cities, violent acts also take place in the suburbs and small towns. Moreover, teens are not spared this violence. According to the Palo Alto Medical Foundation, almost 16 million teens have witnessed some form of violent assault. About one in eight people murdered in the United States each year is younger than 18 years old. Generally, violent acts occur between people who know each other; stranger violence is far less common. And, homes that have guns place family members at increased risk for gun violence against a family member.[1]

Teens who are raised in homes with violence are more likely to be violent. Even if parents do not discuss violence, they are teaching by example. Parents need to demonstrate how to solve problems without resorting to violence. Parents should model nonphysical solutions to problems. It is also important to eliminate exposure to violent programming. In fact, all types of screen time should be limited, especially on school days.

Between school, after-school activities, part-time jobs, and other responsibilities, teens spend much of their day away from home. As a result, they must learn to avoid potentially dangerous and violent situations. If they become overwhelmed with anger and feel they might become violent, teens need to learn to step back and take a time out to regain control. Teens should understand that it is okay to turn to a third party to help resolve a potentially violent situation.

In an article published in 2013 in the journal *Adolescent Medicine: State of the Art Reviews*, researchers from New York City outlined some of the behaviors that characterize adolescent victims and perpetrators of violence. A common theme in victims and perpetrators is maltreatment. Adolescents who visit Internet chat rooms, meet unknown individuals, and are later sexually assaulted have often been a victim of sexual assault earlier in childhood. Teens who are perpetrators of violence tend to have a history of childhood physical abuse and ongoing exposure to violence in their homes. When medical providers recognize that a child is being mistreated, they may take action to stop the situation before the child grows into a teen victim or perpetrator. "Identification and provision of services to families involved in domestic violence situations can help children establish positive adult roles with peers and future partners."[2]

WHAT THE EXPERTS SAY

Athletic Coaches May Teach Violence Prevention

In a study published in 2015 in the *Journal of Interpersonal Violence*, researchers from several different locations in the United States noted that there is a program, Coaching Boys into Men (CBIM), that trains coaches to deliver violence prevention messages to male athletes. The researchers wondered if it was really working. Was the program teaching nonviolence and having an impact? To determine the answer, the researchers asked 176 coaches in 16 high schools in Northern California to complete baseline surveys. Coaches were then randomly assigned to receive the CBIM materials (intervention group) or to continue to coach as usual (control group). While 59 coaches were lost to follow-up, the remaining coaches completed postseason surveys that assessed their attitudes and confidence in delivering the program. A smaller group of 36 intervention coaches participated in semistructured face-to-face interviews that addressed "program acceptability, feasibility, and impact." When compared to the control coaches, the intervention coaches demonstrated more confidence in intervening when they saw abusive behaviors in their athletes. They also had more bystander intervention and more violence-related discussions with athletes and other coaches. The coaches reported that the program was easy to implement and a valuable addition to athletics. The researchers commented that "this brief curriculum appears to impact both coach confidence to enact behavior change and actual positive behavior changes."[3]

Many Teens Think Their Schools Are Unsafe

In a study published in 2015 in the *Journal of School Health*, researchers from New York City wanted to determine the prevalence of aggressive and violent behaviors in the schools that teens in the United States attend. When they analyzed multiple years of data from 84,734 participants in the Youth Risk Behavior Surveillance System, the researchers found that many teens feel unsafe in their schools. They bring weapons to school and engage in physical fights at school. Minority teens are more affected by the violence than nonminority teens. Hispanic males and females have the highest rates of feeling unsafe in school, 8.5 percent and 9.6 percent respectively. Hispanic and black teens were more likely to report that they had recently been threatened in school. Males are more likely than females to carry weapons to school. The researchers noted that many schools and communities are addressing issues of school safety. However, they are not uniformly effective. According to the researchers, in order to improve the violence that occurs in schools, "schools must have the support and resources to facilitate a caring environment that encourages connectedness, academic engagement, and positive relationships among youth and with school staff."[4]

Childhood Exposure to Violence Impacts Adult Physical Health

In a cross-sectional study published in 2015 in the *Journal of Family and Community Medicine*, researchers from Seattle, Washington, and Baghdad, Iraq, wanted to estimate the effect of childhood experiences, at age 15 years or younger, on the physical health of adults in Baghdad. The study was conducted from January 2013 to January 2014 on 1,000 people, between the ages of 18 and 59 years, living in Baghdad, the capital of Iraq. Slightly less than half of the respondents reported that they witnessed a parent or household member being yelled at, screamed at, sworn at, insulted, or humiliated in their home. A third of the respondents reported seeing or hearing a parent or household member being slapped, kicked, punched, or beaten. Almost half of the respondents have observed someone being beaten, and almost 20 percent have been threatened with a knife or gun. And, about half of the respondents lived in a violent environment in their childhood. Meanwhile, more than one-third of the respondents had gastrointestinal diseases and symptoms, and more than one-fifth had cardiovascular diseases. The researchers found that the respondents exposed to a high level of community violence and household dysfunction and abuse had a dramatically increased risk of a chronic physical disease. At the same time, higher levels of family bonding were associated with a lower risk of chronic physical disease. The researchers concluded that "adverse childhood experiences increase the risk of a chronic physical illness in adult life." But, "family bonding appears an important protective factor against physical diseases."[5]

BARRIERS AND PROBLEMS

School Programs Have the Potential to Reduce Some Aspects of Violence, But the Results Appear to Be Variable, and Too Many Programs Seem to Be Ineffective

In a longitudinal study published in 2013 in the *Journal of Adolescent Health*, researchers from Illinois, Arizona, and Washington evaluated the ability of a middle school program, known as Second Step: Student Success Through Prevention (SS-SSTP), to reduce violent acts among sixth-grade students. The violent acts included peer aggression, peer victimization, homophobic name calling, and sexual violence perpetration. The researchers randomly assigned 18 matched pairs of 36 middle schools in Illinois and Kansas to receive the SS-SSTP program or serve as controls. The program included 15 lessons on social emotional learning skills such as empathy, communication, bully prevention, and problem-solving skills. All of the sixth graders in both the intervention and control groups, a total of 3,616 students, completed questionnaires on various aspects of violence. The researchers learned that students in the intervention schools were 42 percent less likely to report physical aggression than students in the control schools. The researchers emphasized that "the magnitude of this finding should not be minimized." In 2009, almost one-third of all students in the United States in grades 9 through 12 reported that they had engaged in physical fighting in the previous 12 months. On the other hand, the intervention did not appear to have an effect on verbal/relational bully perpetration peer victimization, homophobic teasing, and sexual violence.[6]

In a study published in 2014 in *Child Abuse & Neglect*, researchers from New Hampshire and Tennessee investigated the percentages of children who are exposed to violence prevention programs as well as the potential benefits of these programs. Their data were obtained from the National Survey of Children's Exposure to Violence II, which consisted of 4,503 children between the ages of one month to 17 years in 2011. For their study, the researchers used a subset of 3,391 children between the ages of 5 and 17 years. The researchers found that 65 percent of the children had been exposed to a violence prevention program; 55 percent had been exposed during the previous year. Seventy-one percent of the respondents rated the programs as very or somewhat helpful. Children between the ages of 5 and 9 years who had been exposed to higher quality prevention programs had lower levels of peer victimization and perpetration. But, this association did not exist for older youth or youth exposed to lower quality programs. Children exposed to higher quality programs who had experienced peer victimization or conventional crime victimization were more likely to disclose what happened to authorities. Disclosure is a key component. It allows parents and authorities to intervene. So, good programs have clear benefits. But, it is also evident that there are programs in need of serious improvement. Apparently, "too few programs currently include efficacious components."[7]

It May Be Difficult to Predict Which Violence Prevention Programs Will Be Effective

In a study published in 2013 in the *Journal of Adolescent Health*, researchers from San Antonio, Texas, examined the violence protection effects of two different school-based programs in an economically disadvantaged and predominantly Latino school district. One program, El Joven Noble, was a "culturally tailored character development program." It was the intervention program. The other offering, Teen Medical Academy, was a health career promotion program that focused on common medical conditions. It was the control. Both programs consisted of a series of 18 45-minute sessions that were conducted twice a week. The participants self-reported acts of nonphysical aggression, physical violence, and intimate partner violence during the previous 30 day at baseline and at three months and nine months. At baseline, when El Joven Noble had 96 students and the Teen Medical Academy had 127 students, there were no significant differences between the students in the groups. After nine months in the programs, there were uneven results. The high school students who participated in the Teen Medical Academy reported fewer acts of aggression and violence. As a result, positive results were observed in the control but not the intervention program. The researchers concluded that "participating in a health career promotion program may be an effective youth violence strategy for high-risk high school students in Latino communities."[8]

NOTES

1. Palo Alto Medical Foundation, www.pamf.org.

2. Lori Legano and Margaret McHugh, "Adolescents as Victims and Perpetrators of Violence," *Adolescent Medicine: State of the Art Reviews* 24, no. 1 (2013): 155–66.

3. Maria Catrina D. Jaime, Heather L. McCauley, Daniel J. Tancredi et al., "Athletic Coaches as Violence Prevention Advocates," *Journal of Interpersonal Violence* 30, no. 7 (2015): 1090– 1111.

4. Sonali Rajan, Rachel Namdar, and Kely V. Ruggles, "Aggressive and Violent Behaviors in the School Environment Among a Nationally Representative Sample of Adolescent Youth," *Journal of School Health* 85, no. 7 (2015): 446–57.

5. Ameel F. Al-Shawi and Riyadh K. Lafta, "Effect of Adverse Childhood Experiences on Physical Health in Adulthood: Results of a Study Conducted in Baghdad City," *Journal of Family and Community Medicine* 22, no. 2 (2015): 78–84.

6. Dorothy L. Espelage, Sabina Low, Joshua R. Polanin, and Eric C. Brown, "The Impact of a Middle School Program to Reduce Aggression, Victimization, and Sexual Violence," *Journal of Adolescent Health* 53 (2013): 180–86.

7. David Finkelhor, Jennifer Vanderminden, Heather Turner et al., "Youth Exposure to Violence Prevention Programs in a National Sample," *Child Abuse & Neglect* 38 (2014): 677–86.

8. Manuel Ángel Oscós-Sánchez, Janna Lesser, and L. Dolores Oscós-Flores, "High School Students in a Health Career Promotion Program Report Fewer Acts of Aggression and Violence," *Journal of Adolescent Health* 52 (2013): 96–101.

REFERENCES AND RESOURCES

Magazines, Journals, and Newspapers

Al-Shawi, Ameel F., and Riyadh K. Lafta. "Effect of Adverse Childhood Experiences on Physical Health in Adulthood: Results of a Study Conducted in Baghdad City." *Journal of Family and Community Medicine* 22, no. 2 (2015): 78–84.

Chapman, R. L., L. Buckley, B. Reveruzzi, and M. Sheehan. "Injury Prevention Among Friends: The Benefits of School Connectedness." *Journal of Adolescence* 37 (2014): 937–44.

Espelage, Dorothy L., Sabina Low, Joshua R. Polanin, and Eric C. Brown. "The Impact of a Middle School Program to Reduce Aggression, Victimization, and Sexual Violence." *Journal of Adolescent Health* 53 (2013): 180–86.

Finkelhor, David, Jennifer Vanderminden, Heather Turner et al. "Youth Exposure to Violence Prevention Programs in a National Sample." *Child Abuse & Neglect* 38 (2014): 677–86.

Jaime, Maria Catrina D., Heather L. McCauley, Daniel J. Tancredi et al. "Athletic Coaches as Violence Prevention Advocates." *Journal of Interpersonal Violence* 30, no. 7 (2015): 1090–1111.

Legano, Lori, and Margaret McHugh. "Adolescents as Victims and Perpetrators of Violence." *Adolescent Medicine: State of the Art Reviews* 24, no. 1 (2013): 155–66.

Mikton, C., H. Maguire, and T. Shakespeare. "A Systematic Review of the Effectiveness of Interventions to Prevent and Respond to Violence Against Persons with Disabilities." *Journal of Interpersonal Violence* 29, no. 17 (2014): 3207–26.

Oscós-Sánchez, Manuel Ángel, Janna Lesser, and L. Dolores Oscós-Flores. "High School Students in a Health Career Promotion Program Report Fewer Acts of Aggression and Violence." *Journal of Adolescent Health* 52 (2013): 96–101.

Rajan, Sonali, Rachel Namdar, and Kelly V. Ruggles. "Aggressive and Violent Behaviors in the School Environment Among a Nationally Representative Sample of Adolescent Youth." *Journal of School Health* 85, no. 7 (2015): 446–57.

Sharp, Adam, Lisa A. Prosser, Maureen Walton et al. "Cost Analysis of Youth Violence Prevention." *Pediatrics* 133, no. 3 (2014): 448–53.

Web Site

Palo Alto Medical Foundation. www.pamf.org.

Prevent Sports Injuries

OVERVIEW

It is generally agreed that participating in sports during the teen years supports overall health. Teens who regularly take part in sports tend to be thinner and eat a healthier diet. They are less likely to smoke, drink alcohol, and use illegal drugs. But, participating in sports also increases the risk of injury. And, sports injuries are not uncommon occurrences. In fact, they happen fairly often. According to Stanford Children's Health, in the United States, each year, about 30 million children and teens participate in some form of organized sports. At the same time more than 3.5 million of these teens sustain some type of injury, most often a sprain or strain, that occurs during a person-to-person contact or collision. Almost one-third of all injuries that occur in childhood are sports related.[1]

The American Academy of Orthopaedic Surgeons noted that there are two main types of teen sports injuries—acute injuries and overuse injuries. Acute injuries are the result of a sudden trauma, such as a collision with something or someone on the playing field. Overuse injuries occur over a period of time; an athlete keeps injuring the part or parts of the body. The body is repeatedly reinjured without having time to heal. Overuse injuries may affect muscles, ligaments, tendons, bones, and growth plates. For example, swimmers have a tendency for overuse injuries to their shoulders, and gymnasts may easily have overuse injuries to their wrists and elbows. Stress fractures are a common overuse injury in teens and young adults. When the body does not make sufficient bone to replace the breakdown of older bone, the bone is weakened and a stress fracture may occur.[2] Stress fractures are known for being exquisitely painful. So, it is important to find ways to help prevent some of these injuries.

WHAT THE EXPERTS SAY

Neuromuscular Warm-Ups May Reduce Lower Limb Injury

In a study published in 2012 in BMC *Medicine*, researchers from the United Kingdom noted that lower limb injuries in sports are quite common and are the cause of "large economic as well as personal burdens." As a result, they wanted to learn more about the use of neuromuscular warm-up strategies and injury prevention. Typically, these are movements that include stretching, strengthening, balance exercises, agility drills, and landing techniques. The researchers found nine relevant studies; six were randomized controlled trials and three were controlled clinical trials. Two studies had male and female participants; the other studies had only females. On average the studies included 1,500 participants. The age range of the participants was 13 to 26 years. The studies evaluated injuries from a variety of sports, such as football, basketball, and volleyball, and they determined that several of the neuromuscular warm-up strategies are useful in the prevention of lower limb injuries. But, these warm-up strategies need to be completed at all the training sessions for more than three consecutive months. The researchers commented that more studies are needed to identify which "neuromuscular warm-up strategy components are most beneficial and the mechanisms behind their effectiveness."[3]

Some School-Based Sports Injury Prevention Programs Appear to Be Highly Effective

In a study published in 2010 in the journal *Archives of Pediatrics & Adolescent Medicine*, researchers from the Netherlands investigated the effects of an eight-month school-based injury prevention program on the incidence and severity of physical activity injury. The cohort consisted of 2,210 children between the ages of 10 and 12 years from 40 primary schools throughout the Netherlands. The students in 20 schools were in the intervention group; the students in the other 20 schools were in the control group. The program included monthly newsletters, classroom posters, a Web site with an abundance of interactive material, and five-minute exercises at the beginning and ending of all physical education classes. Because they are the most common, the intervention focused primarily on preventing lower-extremity injuries. A total of 100 injuries in the intervention group and 104 injuries in the control group were registered. The intervention appeared to have a stronger effect in the less active students. The researchers commented that they "found a substantial and relevant reduction in physical activity injuries, especially in children in the low active group, because of the intervention."[4]

Mouthguards Provide Protection from Orofacial Injuries

In an article published in 2014 in *Sports Medicine*, two dentists from Turkey underscored the need for dentists to teach athletes, coaches, and patients about the importance of wearing mouthguards to prevent orofacial injuries. Injury to permanent teeth is not unusual; estimates range from 2.6 percent to 50 percent. Dental traumas most often happen between the ages of 6 and 12 years. But, they may occur at any age, especially for those engaged in contact sports and sports with higher rates of injury. "The prevalence of orofacial injuries varies depending on the type of sport played, the degree of contact, and the age, sex, and geographic location of the subject studied." The dentists noted that the primary means to prevent orofacial injury during sports is to wear protective devices such as mouthguards. Mouthguards "dissipate the energy of a traumatic blow," which prevents direct force to dental structures. There are three main types of mouthguards. The most common type of mouthguard, known as a mouth-formed guard or "boil-and-bite" mouthguard, is made from thermoplastic material. These mouthguards are molded into the individual's mouth using fingers, tongue, and bite pressure. There are also custom-fabricated mouthguards, which are made from a dental model of the patient's mouth, and stock mouthguards that are purchased over the counter. Since stock mouthguards may interfere with speaking and breathing, they are normally not recommended by dental professionals. The dentists concluded that "athletes, coaches, dentists, pediatricians, and other professionals should promote the use of mouth protection devices in children and adolescents to minimize the risk of sport-related injuries during professional or amateur sports activities."[5]

BARRIERS AND PROBLEMS

The Transmission of Injury Prevention Information between Players, Parents, and Coaches May Be Less Than Ideal

In a study published in 2013 in the *Scandinavian Journal of Medicine & Science in Sports*, researchers from Canada wanted to learn more about the transmission of information between players, parents, and coaches on female soccer knee injuries and how they may be prevented. During the 2007 indoor soccer season, a descriptive survey was administered to players, parents, and coaches from the Edmonton Minor Soccer Association. Information was obtained from people involved in both competitive (about 30 percent) and recreational (about 70 percent) teams. Over half of the people, a total of 773, responded to the survey. The average player was 14.2 years and had played soccer for an average of seven years. Seventy-one percent of the respondents were aware of a risk for knee injury. Parents and coaches were more likely than players to consider knee injuries to be preventable. However, they failed to identify prevention strategies. Almost 64 percent of the respondents reported that they had not received any information on knee injuries. The researchers noted that "substantial knowledge gaps regarding knee injury prevention and effective preventative strategies were identified." And, they concluded that given the high number of knee injuries in female teen soccer, "there is an urgent need for knowledge translation of prevention strategies to decrease both incidence and long-term consequences of knee injuries."[6]

Teens May Not Always Follow Sports Injury Prevention Programs

In a study published in 2014 in the *British Journal of Sports Medicine*, researchers from Sweden noted that neuromuscular training has been shown to reduce the rates of injury of the anterior cruciate ligaments, which are located in the knees. But, are the teens adhering to the training protocols? The researchers sent questionnaires to football (soccer) associations and coaches who participated in a previous related study (n=303) and coaches who did not participate in the initial study but were coaching female teen football teams during the 2012 season (n=496). The vast majority of the coaches appeared to be well versed in the injury prevention training. Yet, they often trained less than the recommended frequency or they modified aspects of the program. Though a high number of coaches initially adopted the program, there was a "low fidelity" with the program and the "lack of formal policies for its implementation." As a result, an altered program may not be as useful as the original was.[7]

There May Be Insufficient Readily Available Information on the Importance of Using an Injury Prevention Device, Such as a Mouthguard

In a study published in 2013 in the *Journal of Advanced Prosthodontics*, researchers from Korea examined the underuse of mouthguards by Korean Taekwondo athletes. (Taekwondo is an aggressive form of karate.) The cohort consisted of 152 athletes who participated in the Korea National Taekwondo team selection event for the 2010 Guangzhou Asian Games. They completed questionnaires, which asked a variety of questions about their use of mouthguards. Although the participants acknowledged that mouthguards prevented injury, the researchers found a relatively low level of mouthguard use. They noted that mouthguards made it more difficult to breathe and speak, and they caused jaw muscle fatigue. The participants suggested that they had inadequate information on mouthguards. When they did use mouthguards, it was most often the boil-and-bite type. Rarely did they use custom-made mouthguards, which would have been more comfortable. The researchers suggested that dentists provide more information to their patients on the importance of using mouthguards, especially custom-made mouthguards, which fit very well.[8]

NOTES

1. Stanford Children's Health, www.stanfordchildrens.org.

2. American Academy of Orthopaedic Surgeons, http://orthoinfo.aaos.org.

3. Katherine Herman, Christian Barton, Peter Malliaras, and Dylan Morrissey, "The Effectiveness of Neuromuscular Warm-Up Strategies, That Require No Additional Equipment, for Preventing Lower Limb Injuries During Sports Participation: A Systematic Review," *BMC Medicine* 10 (2012): 75+.

4. Dorine C. M. Collard, Evert A. L. M. Verhagen, Mai J. M. Chinapaw et al., "Effectiveness of a School-Based Physical Activity Injury Prevention Program," *Archives of Pediatrics & Adolescent Medicine* 164, no. 2 (2010): 145–50.

5. Elif Bahar Tuna and Emre Ozel, "Factors Affecting Sports-Related Orofacial Injuries and the Importance of Mouthguards," *Sports Medicine* 44 (2014): 777–83.

6. B. Orr, C. Brown, J. Hemsing et al., "Female Soccer Knee Injury: Observed Knowledge Gaps in Injury Prevention Among Players/Parents/Coaches and Current Evidence (the KNOW Study)," *Scandinavian Journal of Medicine & Science in Sports* 23 (2013): 271–80.

7. Hanna Lindblom, Markus Waldén, Siw Carlfjord, and Martin Hägglund, "Implementation of a Neuromuscular training Programme in Female Adolescent Football: 3-Tear Follow-Up Study After a Randomised Controlled Trial," *British Journal of Sports Medicine* 48 (2014): 1425–30.

8. J. W. Lee, C. K. Heo, S. J. Kim et al. "Mouthguard Use in Korean Taekwondo Athletes —Awareness and Attitude," *Journal of Advanced Prosthodontics* 5, no. 2 (2013): 147–52.

REFERENCES AND RESOURCES

Magazines, Journals, and Newspapers

Collard, Dorine C. M., Evert A. L. M. Verhagen, Mai J. M. Chinapaw et al. "Effectiveness of a School-Based Physical Activity Injury Prevention Program." *Archives of Pediatrics & Adolescent Medicine* 164, no. 2 (2010): 145–50.

Herman, Katherine, Christian Barton, Peter Malliaras, and Dylan Morrissey. "The Effectiveness of Neuromuscular Warm-Up Strategies, That Require No Additional Equipment, for Preventing Lower Limb Injuries During Sports Participation: A Systematic Review." *BMC Medicine* 10 (2012): 75+.

Lee, J. W., C. K. Heo, S. J. Kim et al. May "Mouthguard Use in Korean Taekwondo Athletes —Awareness and Attitude." *Journal of Advanced Prosthodontics* 5, no. 2 (2013): 147–52.

Lindblom, Hanna, Markus Waldén, Siw Carljord, and Martin Hägglund. "Implementation of a Neuromuscular Training Programme in Female Adolescent Football: 3-Year Follow-Up Study After a Randomised Controlled Trial." *British Journal of Sports Medicine* 48 (2014): 1425–30.

Orr, B., C. Brown, J. Hemsing et al. "Female Soccer Knee Injury: Observed Knowledge Gaps in Injury Prevention Among Players/Parents/Coaches and Current Evidence (the KNOW Study)." *Scandinavian Journal of Medicine & Science in Sports* 23 (2013): 271–80.

Padua, Darin A., Lindsay J. DiStefano, Stephen W. Marshall et al. ""Retention of Movement Pattern Changes After a Lower Extremity Injury Prevention Program Is Affected by Program Duration." *American Journal of Sports Medicine* 40, no. 2 (2012): 300–306.

Ting, D. K., and R. J. Brison. "Injuries in Recreational Curling Include Head Injuries and May Be Prevented by Using Proper Footwear." *Health Promotion and Chronic Disease Prevention in Canada* 35, no. 2 (2015): 29–34.

Tranaeus, Ulrika, Urban Johnson, Andreas Ivarsson et al. "Sports Injury Prevention in Swedish Elite Floorball Players: Evaluation of Two Consecutive Floorball Seasons." *Knee Surgery, Sports Traumatology, Arthroscopy* 23 (2015): 899–905.

Tuna, E. B., and E. Ozel. "Factors Affecting Sport-Related Orofacial Injuries and the Importance of Mouthguards." *Sports Medicine* 44 (2014): 777–83.

Web Sites

American Academy of Orthopaedic Surgeons. http://orthoinfo.aaos.org.
Stanford Children's Health. www.standfordchildrens.org.

Use Protective Gear

OVERVIEW

While it is true that participating in exercise, group sports, and other physical activities have a number of benefits, it also true that such participation places you at increased risk for injury. For example, while cycling, it is easy to hit a patch of sand, lose balance, and topple. According to the U.S. Centers for Disease Control (CDC), almost 30 million children and teens participate in youth sports in the United States.[1] Yet, these high numbers have led to increases in injuries. Each year, teens in high school have an estimated 2 million injuries, with 500,000 doctor visits and 30,000 hospitalizations. Meanwhile, each year, more than 3.5 million kids under the age of 14 years receive some type of medical treatment for a sports injury.[2]

Though the prevention of as many injuries as possible is always the goal, the prevention of concussions, which occur when the brain knocks against the skull's bony surface, is of prime importance. Most of the time, especially when the concussion is relatively mild, healing is fairly rapid. But, according to the Nemours Foundation, every year "more than 400,000 kids are sent to the emergency department for serious brain injuries."[3] Though these may well occur in car crashes, they may also be the result of playing a variety of different sports. Concussions vary in the degree of severity. It is not unusual for a concussion to result in a loss of consciousness for seconds, minutes, or longer. Common concussion symptoms include feeling groggy, dazed, and very confused. A medical provider should check anyone with a head injury.

One of the ways to lower these high rates of injury is to use protective gear, such as helmets, mouthguards, and pads. Probably the most important piece of protective gear is the helmet. Of course, there are different types of helmets. So, a helmet used for riding a bike is unlike a helmet used for playing football. It is important to use the correct helmet for the sport you are playing. A helmet for a different sport may not provide the protection you need. Purchase a helmet at a sporting goods store where the sales representatives are well trained. A helmet should be snug and not tilt backward or forward.

Many sports require eye protection. Look for eye protection made from polycarbonate. All types of eye protection should fit securely. Teens who wear prescription eyeglasses probably need prescription polycarbonate glasses or goggles. If you play a contact sport, such as hockey, football, basketball, it is important to protect your teeth, mouth, and tongue. For this, you need mouthguards. Although these may be obtained from your dentist, quality mouthguards may be purchased at better sporting goods stores. If you are wearing a retainer, as part of your orthodontic treatment, remove it before exercising.

People who are at increased risk for wrist, knee, and elbow injuries, such as those who ride scooters and skateboards, need to use wrist, knee, and elbow guards. These guards help prevent fractures and other injuries. Pads are recommended for many different types of contact sports. There are pads for the elbows, wrists, knees, and other parts of the body. Guys who play contact sports may require a protective cup, and guys who run may wish to use an athletic supporter.[4]

WHAT THE EXPERTS SAY

Protective Gear May Prevent Severe and Debilitating Water Sports Injuries

In a study published in 2013 in the *Journal of Pediatric Surgery*, researchers from Alabama, Washington, New York City, and Canada noted that children may suffer severe and debilitating injury from watercraft-associated trauma. The cohort consisted of 15 children, between the ages of 7 and 15 years, involved in 14 accidents who were admitted to the trauma service of Children's of Alabama (hospital) between September 1999 and August 2009. Most often, the injuries occurred while the children were riding inflatable tubes pulled by the boat. In these instances, the children lost control over their speed or direction of the pull. But, there were also other types of accidents. Though all the patients in this cohort lived, two required partial lower extremity amputations. None of the patients was reported to be wearing any protective gear. As a result of their investigation, the researchers recommended the mandatory use of protective gear, such as helmets, special clothing, life vests, and easily visible flotation devices, for children participating in water sports activities. And, they stressed a need for more awareness about safety measures to prevent these serious injuries.[5]

Using Hip Pads Prevents Injury in Recreational Snowboarders

In a study published in 2012 in the *British Journal of Sports Medicine*, researchers from Japan wanted to learn if hip pads reduced some of the injuries that happened to recreational snowboarders. The cohort consisted of 5,561 injured snowboarders who were admitted to a Japanese hospital during four snowboarding seasons. Distal radial fracture (broken wrist) and head injury were the two most common injuries. Other frequent injuries included clavicle fracture, humerus fracture, glenohumeral dislocation (shoulder dislocation), spinal burst, compression fractures, and elbow dislocation. The researchers found that the use of hip pads reduced the overall risk of these injuries. The researchers commented that the "reduction in the overall risk of common snowboarding injuries is necessary to make snowboarding safer." And, hip pads were the only "effective protective gear to reduce the overall risk of common injuries."[6]

Protective Gear Reduces Flag Football Injuries

In a study published in 2014 in the journal *Knee Surgery, Sports Traumatology, Arthroscopy*, researchers from Israel, Norway, and Belgium noted that playing American flag football often results in injuries to the fingers, face, knees, shoulders, and ankles. So, they decided to conduct a one-season trial to determine ways to lower the incidence and reduce the severity of injuries. The cohort consisted of American and Canadian precollege males and females (724 males and

114 females). The researchers created four different intervention measures. First, players were not permitted to wear pants with open side pockets. Second, before the first game, all the participants were given mouthguards, with instructions on how to use them. Third, players who had a history of at least two sprains were given ankle braces. And, fourth, every participant received an information brochure. To record all time-loss injuries, a questionnaire was administered. The most important finding was that the rule against open pockets resulted in significant reductions in finger and thumb injuries. Although the mouthguards were self-fitting and came with instructions, most of the players used them improperly. In fact, large numbers of players thought the mouthguards and ankle braces were not necessary. And, most players did not take the time to read the information brochure. The researchers suggested that, in the future, mouthguards should be "individually prepared for the players during the distribution process." And, in order to reduce the incidence of injuries, there is a need for improved education about the importance of the safety measures.[7]

Protective Gear Prevents Boxing Injuries

In a study published in 2010 in *Deutsches Ärzteblatt International*, researchers from Germany noted that boxing has been associated with a number of medical problems, including concussions and dementia. As a result, they conducted a comprehensive review of several studies on the acute, subacute, and chronic neuropsychiatric consequences of boxing to determine if the use of protective gear, such as a head guard and heavily cushioned gloves, could prevent some of these serious medical problems. The researchers found that protective gear has dramatically reduced the risk associated with amateur boxing. However, there appears to be a lack of interest in protective gear for professional boxing. Apparently, such gear has the potential to decrease the "thrill, which does appeal to many supporters."[8]

Using Helmets Prevents Injuries in Children Participating in Nonmotorized Wheeled Activities

In a study published in 2014 in *Chronic Diseases and Injuries in Canada*, researchers from British Columbia and Ontario, Canada, wanted to learn more about injuries and helmet use among children operating nonmotorized wheeled vehicles such as bikes. Data for the years 2004 to 2009 were obtained from the Canadian Hospitals Injury Reporting and Prevention Program. The researchers found that the vast majority (72.8 percent) of the 28,618 children between the ages of 1 and 16 years were injured while cycling. Boys were more likely than girls to be injured. Falls were the most common injury, and 8.3 percent of the children had head injuries. Regardless of age or sex, when compared to the children not wearing helmets, the children wearing helmets were less likely to have a head injury. Moreover, when compared with children who were allowed to return home, children who were admitted to the hospital were significantly less likely to be wearing a helmet. The researchers also found an association between helmet laws and helmet use. In areas where helmet use was required by law, the children more often wore helmets. The researchers commented that their findings "provide further evidence that legislation mandating helmet use may be an effective way of reducing injury among all wheeled-activity users."[9]

In Many Instances, Protective Gear Is Cost-Effective

In a study published in 2008 in the *Southern Medical Journal*, researchers from Cincinnati, Ohio, examined the cost-effectiveness of requiring all recreational ice hockey players to wear facial protection. The researchers surveyed 190 players, with a mean age of 34 years, at two indoor hockey rinks in Evendale, Ohio, from October 2005 to March 2006. On average, they had been playing hockey for 17 years. Forty-six percent of the hockey players reported experiencing a serious injury during the previous five years. Yet, 25 percent of those surveyed did not wear face protection, which only cost $48 per person. "Individuals with face protection reported significantly more sprains and strains that resulted in significantly more physician office visits and specialty physician visits." According to the researchers, over a five-year period, face protection would prevent seven facial lacerations and three facial bone fractures. That would be a savings of about $15,000 (in 2008 dollars). The researchers concluded that "wearing face protection is cost-effective due to the prevention of facial injuries."[10]

BARRIERS AND PROBLEMS

People Using Protective Gear May Take More Risks

In a study published in 2007 in *Accident Analysis & Prevention*, researchers from Canada examined the notion that school-age children who wore protective gear engaged in more risk-taking practices. The cohort consisted of 100 children in four groups. One group had 25 boys between the ages of seven and nine years; a second group had 25 girls of the same age. The third and fourth groups had 25 boys between the ages of 10 and 12 years and 25 girls of the same age. Each child navigated an obstacle course twice, once with protective gear and a second time without. To minimize the potential for practice effects, the second navigation was completed in the reverse direction. Children and parents independently completed questionnaires. The researchers found that when the children were wearing protective gear, they had more "reckless and risky behaviors." When they were wearing their protective gear, "children went faster through the obstacle course and behaved more recklessly, as indicated by tripping and falling and banging into things more frequently." Those children who were high in "sensation seeking" were more likely than the other children to take risks.[11]

In a more recent study published in 2015 in *Accident Analysis and Prevention*, researchers from Canada and Minnesota investigated whether wearing helmets in skiing and snowboarding increased risk-taking behaviors in intermediate and proficient skiers and snowboarders. The cohort consisted of 114 male and 115 female skiers or snowboarders between the ages of 19 and 40 years. The researchers found that helmet use "was a significant predictor of risk taking." So, the benefits obtained from wearing helmets may be reduced by the increases in risky behaviors. Nevertheless, "the costs of increased risk taking are not likely to outweigh the protective benefits of a helmet."[12]

All-Terrain Vehicle Safety Education Program Failed to Improve the Use of Protective Gear

In a study published in 2013 in the *Journal of Primary Care & Community Health*, researchers from Los Angeles and Peoria, Illinois, wanted to learn if a program to improve all-terrain vehicle safety was improving safety knowledge and practice among youth in rural central Illinois. The cohort consisted of 260 rural central Illinois middle and high school students. During the 2009 to 2010 school year, they received didactic and interactive training in all-terrain vehicle safety. Before and after this training, the students completed surveys, which included questions about all-terrain vehicle safety knowledge and actual riding practices.

Before the intervention, more than 200 surveys were collected; 12 to 24 weeks after the intervention, 165 surveys were collected. The researchers learned that after the educational program, there were significant increases in knowledge about safety issues. However, there was no significant increase in the use of protective gear. According to the researchers, even though the students knew what they should be doing, the "nonsignificant changes in riding practices and crash rates demonstrated that youth behavior is more difficult to impact than knowledge." The researchers suggested that a future program may be more successful if it also targets the parents.[13]

Football Helmets Do Not Always Protect Players from Concussions

In a study presented to the 66th Annual Meeting of the American Academy of Neurology, held from April 26 to May 3, 2014, in Philadelphia, researchers from Florida noted that the football helmets that are currently used provide little protection to the side of the head. The researchers conducted 330 tests on dummies to measure the ability of 10 popular football helmets to protect against traumatic brain injury. When compared to wearing no helmet, the researchers found that the football helmets reduced the risk of traumatic brain injury by only 20 percent. According to the lead researcher, Frank Conidi, MD, DO, MS, "Alarmingly, those that offered the least protection are among the most popular in the field."[14]

Some Football Helmets Appear to Be Better Than Others in Preventing Concussions

In a retrospective analysis published in 2014 in the *Journal of Neurosurgery*, researchers from multiple locations in the United States wanted to learn if some football helmet designs are better than others in preventing concussions. The cohort consisted of head impact data collected from 1,833 collegiate football players. Out of a total of 1,281,444 head impacts that were recorded, there were 64 diagnosed concussions. Different helmets appeared to place players at increased or decreased risk for sustaining a concussion. According to the researchers, "not all helmets are designed equally in their ability to rescue the head accelerations resulting from impact." As a result, "helmet designs should be optimized to reduce head acceleration over the continuum of impacts experienced by football players."[15]

NOTES

1. U.S. Centers for Disease Control, www.cdc.gov.

2. Stop Sports Injuries, www.stopsportsinjuries.org.

3. The Nemours Foundation, http://kidshealth.org.

4. Ibid.

5. Richard Keijzer, Geni F. Smith, Keith E. Georgeson, and Oliver J. Muensterer, "Watercraft and Watersport Injuries in Children: Trauma Mechanisms and Proposed Prevention Strategies," *Journal of Pediatric Surgery* 48 (2013): 1757–61.

6. Daichi Ishimaru, Hiroyasu Ogawa, Kazuhiko Wakahara et al., "Hip Pads Reduce the Overall Risk of Injuries in Recreational Snowboarders," *British Journal of Sports Medicine* 46, no. 15 (2012): 1055–58.

7. Y. Kaplan, G. Myklebust, M. Nyska et al., "The Prevention of Injuries in Contact Flag Football," *Knee Surgery, Sports Traumatology, and Arthroscopy* 22, no. 1 (2014): 26–52.

8. H. Försti, C. Haass, B. Hemmer et al., "Boxing—Acute Complications and Late Sequelae: From Concussion to Dementia," *Deutsches Ärzteblatt International* 107, no. 47 (2010): 835–39.

9. H. Lindsay and M. Brussoni, "Injuries and Hemet Use Related to Non-Motorized Wheeled Activities Among Pediatric Patients," *Chronic Diseases and Injuries in Canada* 34, no. 2–3 (2014): 74–81.

10. Scott E. Woods, John Diehl, Eric Zabat et al., "Is It Cost-Effective to Require Recreational Ice Hockey Players to Wear Face Protection?" *Southern Medical Journal* 101, no. 10 (2008): 991–95.

11. Barbara A. Morrongiello, Beverly Walpole, and Jennifer Lasenby, "Understanding Children's Injury-Risk Behavior: Wearing Safety Gear Can Lead to Increased Risk Taking," *Accident Analysis & Prevention* 39 (2007): 618–23.

12. Cynthia J. Thomson and Scott R. Carlson, "Increased Patterns of Risky Behaviours Among Helmet Wearers in Skiing and Snowboarding," *Accident Analysis and Prevention* 75 (2015): 179–83.

13. Joshua A. Novak, John W. Hafner, Jean C. Aldag, and Marjorie A. Getz, "Evaluation of a Standardized All-Terrain Vehicle Safety Education Intervention for Youth in Rural Central Illinois," *Journal of Primary Care & Community Health* 4, no. 1 (2013): 8–13.

14. Science Daily, www.sciencedaily.com/releases/2014/02/140217200751.htm.

15. Steven Rowson, Stefan M. Duma, Richard M. Greenwald et al., "Can Helmet Design Reduce the Risk of Concussion in Football?" *Journal of Neurosurgery* 120 (2014): 919–22.

REFERENCES AND RESOURCES

Magazines, Journals, and Newspapers

de Rome, L., R. Ivers, M. Fitzharris et al. "Effectiveness of Motorcycle Protective Clothing: Riders' Health Outcomes in the Six Months Following a Crash." *Injury* 43 (2012): 2035–45.

Försti, H., C. Haass, B. Hemmer et al. "Boxing—Acute Complications and Late Sequelae: From Concussion to Dementia." *Deutsches Ärzteblatt International* 107, no. 47 (2010): 835–39.

Ishimaru, Daichi, Hiroyasu Ogawa, Kazuhiko Wakahara et al. "Hip Pads Reduce the Overall Risk of Injuries in Recreational Snowboarders." *British Journal of Sports Medicine* 46, no. 15 (2012): 1055–58.

Kaplan, Y., G. Myklebust, M. Nyska et al. "The Prevention of Injuries in Contact Flag Football." *Knee Surgery, Sports Traumatology, Arthroscopy* 22, no. 1 (2014): 26–32.

Keijer, Richard, Geni F. Smith, Keith E. Georgeson, and Oliver J. Muensterer. "Watercraft and Watersport Injuries in Children: Trauma Mechanisms and Proposed Prevention Strategies." *Journal of Pediatric Surgery* 48 (2013): 1757–61.

Lindsay, H., and M. Brussoni. "Injuries and Helmet Use Related to Non-Motorized Wheeled Activities Among Pediatric Patients." *Chronic Diseases and Injuries in Canada* 34, no. 2–3 (2014): 74–81.

Morrongiello, Barbara A., Beverly Walpole, and Jennifer Lasenby. "Understanding Children's Injury-Risk Behavior: Wearing Safety Gear Can Lead to Increased Risk Taking." *Accident Analysis & Prevention* 39 (2007): 618–23.

Novak, Joshua A., John W. Hafner, Jean C. Aldag, and Marjorie A. Getz. "Evaluation of a Standardized All-Terrain Vehicle Safety Education Intervention for Youth in Rural Central Illinois." *Journal of Primary Care & Community Health* 4, no. 1 (2013): 8–13.

Rowson, Steven, Stefan M. Duma, Richard M. Greenwald et al. "Can Helmet Design Reduce the Risk of Concussion in Football?" *Journal of Neurosurgery* 120 (2014): 919–22.

Thomson, Cynthia J., and Scott R. Carlson. "Increased Patterns of Risky Behaviours Among Helmet Wearers in Skiing and Snowboarding." *Accident Analysis and Prevention* 75 (2015): 179–83.

Woods, Scott E., John Diehl, Eric Zabat et al. "Is It Cost-Effective to Require Recreational Ice Hockey Players to Wear Face Protection?" *Southern Medical Journal* 101, no. 10 (2008): 991–95.

Web Sites

Stop Sports Injuries. www.stopsportsinjuries.org.
The Nemours Foundation. http://kidshealth.org.
U.S. Centers for Disease Control. www.cdc.gov.

Use Seatbelts

OVERVIEW

Countless numbers of studies have demonstrated over and over again that seat-belts save lives in automobile accidents. While wearing a seatbelt does not guarantee that one will emerge from an accident without a scratch, it does prevent ejection from a vehicle and any related injuries.

While all states have laws governing the use of seat belts, they vary greatly in the way they are enforced. In many states, law enforcement personnel devote little attention to these laws. Moreover, according to the National Traffic Highway Safety Administration, a division of the U.S. Department of Transportation, teens use seatbelts far less often than any other age group. In 2009, 56 percent of teens and young adults between the ages of 16 and 20 years, involved in crashes, were unbuckled.[1]

Concerned about these statistics, the Children's Hospital of Philadelphia established a Web site to address the problem. It is known as Teen Driver Source. Interestingly, teens who consider their parents to be involved in their driving—establishing rules and monitoring their driving—are twice as likely to wear a seatbelt when they are driving or in the car as a passenger.[2] It is a good idea for drivers to delay turning on the ignition until everyone in the car has buckled their seatbelts. If these rules are not followed, then teens should lose their driving privileges. The failure to comply could be the differences between life, serious injury, or even death.

WHAT THE EXPERTS SAY

People Who Don't Use Seatbelts Appear to Practice Other Unsafe Driving Behaviors

In a retrospective study published in 2015 in the journal *Accident Analysis and Prevention*, researchers from Norway wrote that in their country 608 drivers of cars or vans were killed in road crashes from 2005 to 2010. In general, blood samples were taken in about 60 to 70 percent of these traffic crashes and were analyzed for alcohol and commonly used drugs. The researchers were able to obtain results for 369 drivers. All the samples were analyzed for alcohol, and 327 samples were analyzed for 15 drugs. The researchers found statistically significant associations between impairment by alcohol or amphetamines and driving unbelted or speeding. "Statistically smaller proportions of the sober drivers with a fatal outcome were unbelted or speeded."[3]

In another study published in 2010 in the *European Journal of Public Health*, researchers from Spain investigated the associations between marijuana and cocaine use, traffic injuries, and the use of protective devices such as seatbelts. The cohort consisted of a nationwide sample of 17,484 car or motorcycle drivers surveyed in 2005 in Spain. The researchers determined that 12.5 percent of the drivers had used marijuana and 3.4 percent had used cocaine during the previous 12 months. Cocaine use of at least one day per week and marijuana use of at least four days per week were associated with more traffic accidents. In addition, the researchers found a dose-response association between the frequency of cocaine use and the failure to use seatbelts. The researchers concluded that "interventions to avoid driving under the influence of drugs and to increase use of protective devices among drug users are needed."[4]

In still another study, published in 2014 in the *Southern Medical Journal*, re-searchers from Birmingham, Alabama, noted that Alabama ranks fourth in the United States for teen crash fatalities. As a result, they wanted to determine some of the risky driving behaviors practiced by teens 15 years and older in Alabama. Questionnaires were completed by 1,399 teens; slightly over half were males and 64 percent were white. Most of the respondents were 15 or 16 years old; so, they were new drivers. Yet, 58 percent of the teens reported not wearing a seatbelt during the previous 30 days. Forty-one percent reported texting while driving, 67 percent noted that they were a passenger in a car where the driver was texting, and 11 percent reported driving after drinking. Sixty percent noted that they routinely exceeded the speed limit. Clearly, these teens were engaging in a num-ber of different risky driving practices, and they were not "receiving safe driving educational messages from parents, doctors, or driver's education classes."[5]

Several Factors Appear to Influence a Driver's Decision to Use Seatbelts

In a study published in 2014 in the *Journal of Safety Research*, researchers based in Detroit, Michigan, wanted to learn more about characteristics related to the use of seatbelts and cell phones by drivers. Data were obtained from two waves of observational surveys conducted in different locations in Michigan during the spring and summer of 2010. Data collectors recorded data on seatbelt and cell phone use or nonuse as well as demographic characteristics of the drivers and vehicles. To improve accuracy, data were only collected during daylight hours. The seatbelt rate was determined to be 94.7 percent, much higher than rates in most other studies. The researchers noted that Michigan is a primary seatbelt law state, which means that drivers may be pulled over for not wearing a seatbelt. The researchers learned that drivers between the ages of 16 and 19 years were the least likely to wear seatbelts. Consistent with other findings, drivers in this age group are known for taking risks. Female drivers were more likely than male driv-ers to use seatbelts. Caucasian drivers were more likely than drivers of other races to use seatbelts. Drivers with young passengers or passengers over the age of 60 had an increased use of seatbelts. Drivers of pickup trucks were less likely than drivers of other vehicles to use seatbelts. The researchers noted that their study "provided important information to assist in guiding subsequent policies and programs aimed at addressing unsafe driver behaviors."[6]

Seatbelts Appear to Protect Kidneys in Motor Vehicle Collisions

In a retrospective study published in 2014 in the *Journal of Urology*, researchers from New York City, Houston, and Chicago wanted to learn more about the ability of seatbelts and airbags to protect the kidneys during motor vehicle collisions. The researchers used data from the National Trauma Data Bank (NTDB). A review of 466,028 motor vehicle collisions found 3,846 renal injuries. When compared to occupants using seatbelts, airbags, or seatbelts and airbags, motor vehicle occupants without these protective devices had higher rates of high grade renal injury, and they were more likely to require a nephrectomy, the surgical removal of all or part of a kidney. Reductions in injury were most often seen when seatbelts were used and airbags inflated. The researchers concluded that "protective devices such as seat belts and airbags are among the most important measures to further reduce motor vehicle occupant injuries and deaths."[7]

Use of Seatbelts Appears to Be Associated with Socioeconomic Status

In a study published in 2014 in the *Iranian Journal of Public Health*, researchers from Iran wanted to learn more about the association between socioeconomic status and the use of seatbelts in cars and helmets when motorcycling. The data used in this study were originally collected for a noncommunicable disease surveillance system in 2009 in Kurdistan. It included a total of 997 people, with a mean age of 39.77 years. Information was obtained from interviews and questionnaires. The researchers found a direct association between socioeconomic status and the nonuse of seatbelts and helmets. People with higher levels of socioeconomic status were more likely to wear seatbelts and helmets. As a result, efforts to address the needs of the most disadvantaged members of society may well increase the use of seatbelts and helmets. This may be accomplished by "reducing poverty, improving education, paying more attention to the poorer groups in society in health politics, increasing the access of disadvantaged groups, and designing special programs for reducing inequality."[8]

BARRIERS AND PROBLEMS

People Who Are Obese Are Less Likely to Use Seatbelts

In a retrospective study published in 2014 in the *American Journal of Emergency Medicine*, researchers from Buffalo, New York, examined the association between obesity and use of seatbelts. The cohort consisted of drivers in motor vehicle crashes listed in the Fatality Analysis Reporting System between 2003 and 2009, a database run by the National Highway Traffic Safety Administration. The researchers learned that the chances of seatbelt use for normal-weight people was 67 percent higher than the odds of seatbelt use for the morbidly obese. It appears that obesity is a significant risk factor for not wearing a seatbelt. The more obese the driver, the less likely seatbelts were used. This means that obese drivers are "at greater risk of being subjected to higher impact forces and being ejected from the vehicle, both of which lead to more severe injury and/or death."[9]

A study on the association between overweight teens and seatbelt use was published in 2011 in the *Journal of Community Health*. The investigation, which was conducted by researchers in Toledo, Ohio, and Jacksonville, Florida, initially included 1,966 students in grades 6 to 12 from 40 different schools. A total of 1,887 students completed the questionnaire. Almost 60 percent had a normal weight. About equal numbers of the remaining students were overweight or obese. When compared to the normal weight students, the researchers determined that the teens who were obese were less likely to wear seatbelts. The researchers wondered if the seatbelts were too small and uncomfortable for the teens to use. "Car manufacturers may need to take into consideration ergonomic factors of seat belt wearing for obese individuals."[10]

Seatbelts May Cause Harm, Especially If Used Incorrectly

In a study published in 2014 in the *Journal of Emergencies, Trauma, and Shock*, researchers from Israel conducted a retrospective analysis of injuries caused by seatbelts during automobile accidents. When these are more severe, they may require a laparotomy or a surgical incision into the abdominal cavity. The cohort consisted of 41 patients, who had a median age of 26 years. They were seen at a level 1 trauma unit in Israel between 2005 and 2010. Patients had solid organ and bowel injuries associated with malpositioned seatbelts. When compared to the drivers, passengers in a back seat of the car were significantly more likely to require a laparotomy. The researchers suggested that "seatbelts worn by passengers in the back seat of cars do tend to be malpositioned more commonly than the front seat (especially as children usually sit in the back seat)."[11]

NOTES

1. National Highway Traffic Safety Administration, www.nhtsa.gov.

2. Teen Driver Source, www.teendriversource.org.

3. Stig Tore Bogstrand, Magnus Larsson, Anders Holtan et al., "Associations Between Driving Under the Influence of Alcohol or Drugs, Speeding and Seatbelt Use Among Fatally Injured Car Drivers in Norway," *Accident Analysis and Prevention* 78 (2015): 14–19.

4. J. Pulido, G. Barrio, P. Lardelli et al., 2010. "Association Between Cannabis and Cocaine Use, Traffic Injuries and Use of Protective Devices," *European Journal of Public Health* 21, no. 6 (2010): 753–55.

5. Elizabeth Irons, Michele Nichols, William D. King et al., "Teen Driving Behaviors in a Rural Southern State," *Southern Medical Journal* 107, no. 12 (2014): 735–38.

6. Brendan J. Russo, Jonathan J. Kay, Peter T. Savolainen, and Timothy J. Gates, "Assessing Characteristics Related to the Use of Seatbelts and Cell Phones by Drivers: Application of a Bivariate Probit Model," *Journal of Safety Research* 49 (2014): 137–42.

7. Marc A. Bjurlin, Richard J. Fantus, Michele M. Mellett et al., "The Impact of Seat Belts and Airbags on High Grade Renal Injuries and Nephrectomy Rates in Motor Vehicle Collisions," *Journal of Urology* 192, no. 4 (2014): 1131–36.

8. Ghobad Moradi, Hossein Malekafzali Ardakani, Reza Majdzadeh et al., "Socio-economic Inequalities in Nonuse of Seatbelts in Cars and Helmets on Motorcycles Among People Living in Kurdistan Province, Iran," *Iranian Journal of Public Health* 43, no. 9 (2014): 1239–47.

9. Dietrich Jehle, Chirag Doshi, Jenna Karagianis et al., "Obesity and Seatbelt Use: A Fatal Relationship," *American Journal of Emergency Medicine* 32 (2014): 756–60.

10. James H. Price, Joseph A. Dake, Joyce E. Balls-Berry, and Margaret Wielinski, "Seat Belt Use Among Overweight and Obese Adolescents," *Journal of Community Health* 36 (2011): 612–15.

11. Seema Biswas, Mohamed Adileh, Gidon Almogy, and Mikosh Bala, "Abdominal Injury Patterns in Patients with Seatbelt Signs Requiring Laparotomy," *Journal of Emergencies, Trauma, and Shock* 7, no. 4 (2014): 295–300.

REFERENCES AND RESOURCES

Magazines, Journals, and Newspapers

Barr Jr., Gavin C., Kathleen E. Kane, Robert D. Barraco et al. "Gender Differences in Perceptions and Self-Reported Driving Behaviors Among Teenagers." *Journal of Emergency Medicine* 48, no. 3 (2015): 366–70.

Biswas, Seema, Mohamed Adileh, Gidon Almogy, and Miklosh Bala. "Abdominal Injury Patterns in Patients with Seatbelt Signs Requiring Laparotomy." *Journal of Emergencies, Trauma, and Shock* 7, no. 4 (2014): 295–300.

Bjurlin, Marc A., Richard J. Fantus, Michele M. Mellett et al. "The Impact of Seat Belts and Airbags on High Grade Renal Injuries and Nephrectomy Rates in Motor Vehicle Collisions." *Journal of Urology* 192, no. 4 (2014): 1131–36.

Bogstrand, Stig Tore, Magnus Larsson, Anders Holtan et al. "Associations Between Driving Under the Influence of Alcohol or Drugs, Speeding and Seatbelt Use Among Fatally Injured Car Drivers in Norway." *Accident Analysis and Prevention* 78 (2015): 14–19.

Irons, Elizabeth, Michele Nichols, William D. King et al. "Teen Driving Behaviors in a Rural Southern State." *Southern Medical Journal* 107, no. 12 (2014): 735–38.

Jehle, Dietrich, Chirag Doshi, Jenna Karagianis et al. "Obesity and Seatbelt Use: A Fatal Relationship." *American Journal of Emergency Medicine* 32 (2014): 756–60.

Moradi, Ghobad, Hossein Malekafzali Ardakani, Reza Majdzadeh et al. "Socioeconomic Inequalities in Nonuse of Seatbelts in Cars and Helmets in Motorcycles Among People Living in Kurdistan Province, Iran." *Iranian Journal of Public Health* 43, no. 9 (2014): 1239–47.

Price, James H., Joseph A. Dake, Joyce E. Balls-Berry, and Margaret Wielinski. "Seat Belt Use Among Overweight and Obese Adolescents." *Journal of Community Health* 36 (2011): 612–15.

Pulido, J., G. Barrio, P. Lardelli et al. "Association Between Cannabis and Cocaine Use, Traffic Injuries and Use of Protective Devices." *European Journal of Public Health* 21, no. 6 (2010): 753–55.

Russo, Brendan J., Jonathan J. Kay, Peter T. Savolainen, and Timothy J. Gates. "Assessing Characteristics Related to the Use of Seatbelts and Cell Phones by Drivers: Application of a Bivariate Probit Model." *Journal of Safety Research* 49 (2014): 137–42.

Web Sites

National Highway Traffic Safety Administration. www.nhtsa.gov.

Teen Driver Source. www.teendriversource.org.

Mental, Emotional, and Social Health

Build Social Connections and Friendships with Peers

OVERVIEW

People of all ages need to connect with other people and build friendships. While this is also observed in animals, forming connections and building friendships appear to be integral parts of being human. During the adolescent years, teens learn to form safe and healthy relationships with friends and even romantic partners. In fact, a circle of caring and supported peers and friends may ease the transition into early adulthood.

While building these connections and friendships, it is important to ensure that they are healthy relationships. You need to be able to speak freely and listen closely. Your communication should be based on honesty, respect, and trust. Healthy relationships help you feel good about yourself; unhealthy relationships foster feelings of anger, fear, sadness, or worry. Healthy relationships have about equal amounts of give and take; in an unhealthy relationship there are unfair imbalances.

WHAT THE EXPERTS SAY

Support from Peers, School, and Family Is Important as Students Transition to Secondary School

In a study published in 2014 in the *Journal of Adolescent Health*, researchers from Australia wanted to learn more about the support students received when they transitioned from Catholic primary to Catholic secondary schools. According to these researchers, it has been shown that students who do not transition well are at increased risk for emotional problems, depression, anxiety, and antisocial behaviors. So, the researchers collected data from 1,974 primary students prior to their transition from primary to secondary school. They collected data again during the first term of their first year of secondary school. Students were asked questions about their transition expectations and their support from peers, family, and the school. Slightly more than half of the students were female; they had a mean age of 12 years.

The researchers learned that support from peers, schools, and family members all predicted a positive transition. In grade 7, a high level of peer support was the most significant predictor of the expectation of an easy or somewhat easy transition. In grade 8, parental presence was the most significant protective predictor of an easy or somewhat easy transition experience. The researchers concluded that "students who expect and experience a positive transition to secondary school are generally well-supported by their peers, school, and family."[1]

Peers and Friends Appear to Play a Role in Adolescent Physical Activity

In an article published in 2012 in the *Journal of Adolescence*, researchers from Ireland wanted to learn more about the influence that peers and friends have on physical activity among American teens. The researchers searched seven electronic databases to identify articles published during the previous 10 years on children/teens between the ages of 10 and 18 years and found 23 studies to include in the investigation. The researchers found that peers and/or friends consistently played an important role in the physical activity of teens, and they identified six ways in which this is accomplished. These are peer and/or friend support, presence of peers and friends, peer norms, friendship quality and acceptance, peer crowds, and peer victimization. The researchers also learned that the influence of peer support appeared to be greater for at-risk and overweight youths. And, a teen's positive relationships with peers contributed significantly to physical activity participation. "Good quality friendships and a feeling of social connectedness with peers strengthen self-determined motivation for adolescents in sport and enjoyment of PA [physical activity] was increased through having more in common with one's peers." On the other hand, the researchers observed that peer victimization may create an environment in which teens feel less secure about physical activity and may result in avoidance of physically active situations. The researchers added that "there is merit in promoting the importance of PA amongst peers and friends in order to increase their PA levels."[2]

Another study on the same topic was conducted by Australian researchers and published in 2011 in *Social Science & Medicine*. During the 2008 school year, the researchers conducted three evaluations of self-reported participation in physical activity, cognition about physical activity, and friendship ties to fellow students in two cohorts of 378 Australian eighth grade students, with a mean age of 13.7 years.

As in the previous study, participation in physical activity by the adolescents was found to be influenced by the behavior of their friends, and friendship choices were significantly predicted by similarities in physical activity. Active teens tended to socialize with other active teens; inactive teens tended to be with other inactive teens. Similar physical activity levels tended "to be a stronger driver for friendship selection than behavioral similarities." The researchers concluded that the role of friendship in physical activity "provides some insights into possible intervention strategies that may be useful in establishing social contexts that support and encourage young people to be physically active."[3]

Female Teens Who Are Closer to Their Parents Have an Easier Time Making Friends in College

In a study published in 2010 in the *Journal of Youth and Adolescence*, researchers from Greensboro, North Carolina, wanted to learn more about the association between the attachment of female teens to their parents and the ease of forming friendships in college. In July 2006, before their first semester at college began, 172 incoming female freshmen completed a measurement of parental attachment survey. In December 2006, at the end of their first semester, an assessment was conducted of their ease in forming college friendships. The women were between the ages of 18 and 20 years, and 30 percent were minorities. The researchers found a positive association between a secure attachment to parents and an ease in forming friendships. This proved to be true for both the white and minority females. The researchers concluded that "attachment to parents plays an important role in the close relationship of female college students."[4]

Instant Messaging May Help Foster and Maintain Interpersonal Relationships

In a study published in 2009 in the journal *Adolescence*, researchers from Taiwan wanted to learn more about the association between instant messaging and the development of relationships in "real life." The cohort consisted of 369 Taiwanese junior high school students, with an average age of 14.58 years. Slightly more than half were male. After asking students questions about their use of instant messaging and their real-life interpersonal relationships, the researchers learned that the students used instant messaging an average of 3.66 hours three times a week. Apparently, the teens sent instant messages "to improve their interpersonal relationships in real life" and to help in the formation and maintenance of friendships. But, over time, instant messaging "became a standard communication device."[5]

BARRIERS AND PROBLEMS

Social Ties May Also Be Harmful

In a study published in 2015 in the journal *Sociological Perspectives*, researchers from Memphis, Tennessee, wanted to learn more about the relationship between social ties in early adulthood and suicide attempts and ideation. They used data derived from Wave I, Wave III, and Wave IV of the National Longitudinal Study of Adolescent Health, which contains nationally representative samples of adolescents in grades 7 to 12 in 132 middle and high schools in 80 different communities in the United States. The researchers found that young adults who have family members or friends who attempt suicide are more likely to report suicidal ideation or suicide attempts. The researchers commented that their findings "demonstrated that close social relationships can serve not just as sources of support, but also as conduits for the spread of suicidal behaviors." And, apparently, these effects may continue for many years.[6]

Teens May Encourage Their Friends to Start Smoking

In a study published in 2014 in the *Journal of Health and Social Behavior*, researchers from Pennsylvania and Arizona wanted to learn more about the influence peers have in the initiation of smoking. The researchers directed their attention to survey data from two high schools—one was an almost entirely white school located in a midsized town in the Midwest and the other was a racially and ethnically diverse high school located in a suburban community in the West. As in other studies, these researchers found strong evidence of the peer effects of smoking initiation. However, peers do not necessarily follow their peers when they stop smoking. The tendency for teens to follow their peers into smoking is stronger than the tendency to follow them to smoking cessation. "For many adolescents the decision to quit smoking often occurs in the absence of strong peer support of their choice."[7]

Best Friends May Have Negative Influences

In a study published online in 2015, in the *Journal of Clinical Child & Adolescent Psychology*, researchers from Florida and Sweden examined the influence best friends have over problematic behavior such as the consumption of alcohol and truancy. The cohort consisted of 306 Swedish males and 394 Swedish females who had same-sex best friends who were stable from year to year. At baseline, the students were in secondary school, ages 13 to 14 years, or high school, ages 16 to 17 years. Each member of the friendship dyads rated his or her satisfaction with the relationship. The researchers determined that the more satisfied friends had more influence than the less satisfied friends over the consumption of alcohol and truancy. The researchers noted that "some friends were a positive influence, and others were not. . . . Alcohol abuse and truancy increased when the more satisfied friend reported greater problems."[8]

NOTES

1. Stacey Waters, Leanne Lester, and Donna Cross, "How Does Support from Peers Compare with Support from Adults as Students Transition to Secondary School?" *Journal of Adolescent Health* 54 (2014): 543–49.

2. Amanda Fitzgerald, Noelle Fitzgerald, and Cian Aherne, "Do Peers Matter? A Review of Peer and/or Friends' Influence on Physical Activity Among American Adolescents," *Journal of Adolescence* 35 (2012): 941–58.

3. Kayla de la Haye, Garry Robins, Philip Mohr, and Carlene Wilson, "How Physical Activity Shapes, and Is Shaped by, Adolescent Friendships," *Social Science & Medicine* 73 (2011): 719–28.

4. S. H. Parade, E. M. Leerkes, and A. N. Blankson, "Attachment to Parents, Social Anxiety, and Close Relationships of Female Students Over the Transition to College," *Journal of Youth and Adolescence* 39, no. 2 (2010): 127–37.

5. Y. C. Lee and Y. C. Sun, "Using Instant Messaging to Enhance the Interpersonal Relationships of Taiwanese Adolescents: Evidence from Quantile Regression Analysis," *Adolescence* 44, no. 173 (2009): 199–208.

6. Anna S. Mueller, Seth Abrutyn, and Cynthia Stockton, "Can Social Ties Be Harmful? Examining the Spread of Suicide in Early Adulthood," *Sociological Perspectives* 58, no. 2 (2015): 204–22.

7. Steven A. Haas and David R. Schaefer, "With a Little Help From My Friends? Asymmetrical Social Influence on Adolescent Smoking Initiation and Cessation," *Journal of Health and Social Behavior* 55, no. 2 (2014): 126–43.

8. C. Hiatt, B. Laursen, H. Stattin, and M. Kerr, "Best Friend Influence Over Adolescent Problem Behaviors: Socialized by the Satisfied," *Journal of Clinical Child & Adolescent Psychology* (July 2015): 1–14.

REFERENCES AND RESOURCES

Magazines, Journals, and Newspapers

de la Haye, Kayla, Garry Robins, Philip Mohr, and Carlene Wilson. "How Physical Activity Shapes, and Is Shaped by, Adolescent Friendships." *Social Science & Medicine* 73 (2011): 719–28.

Fitzgerald, Amanda, Noelle Fitzgerald, and Cian Aherne. "Do Peers Matter? A Review of Peer and/or Friends' Influence on Physical Activity Among American Adolescents." *Journal of Adolescence* 35 (2012): 941–58.

Gommans, Rob, Gonneke, W. J. M. Stevens, Emily Finne et al. "Frequent Electronic Media Communications with Friends Is Associated with Higher Adolescent Substance Use." *International Journal of Public Health* 60 (2015): 167–77.

Haas, Steven A., and David R. Schaefer. "With a Little Help from My Friends? Asymmetrical Social Influence on Adolescent Smoking Initiation and Cessation." *Journal of Health and Social Behavior* 55, no. 2 (2014): 126–43.

Hiatt, C., B. Laursen, H. Stattin, and M. Kerr. "Best Friend Influence Over Adolescent Problem Behaviors: Socialized by the Satisfied." *Journal of Clinical Child & Adolescent Psychology* (July 2015): 1–14.

Huang, Grace C., Jennifer B. Unger, Daniel Soto et al. "Peer Influences: The Impact of Online and Offline Friendship Networks on Adolescent Smoking and Alcohol Use." *Journal of Adolescent Health* 54 (2014): 508–14.

Lee, Y. C., and Y. C. Sun. "Using Instant Messaging to Enhance the Interpersonal Relationships of Taiwanese Adolescents: Evidence from Quantile Regression Analysis." *Adolescence* 44, no. 173 (2009): 199–208.

Lev-Ari, Lilac, Inbar Baumgarten-Katz, and Ada H. Zohar. "Show Me Your Friends, and I Shall Show You Who You Are: The Way Attachment and Social Comparisons Influence Body Dissatisfaction." *European Eating Disorders Review* 22, no. 6 (2014): 463–69.

Logis, Handrea A., Philip C. Rodkin, Scott D. Gest, and Hai-Jeong Ahn. "Popularity as an Organizing Factor of Preadolescent Friendship Networks: Beyond Prosocial and Aggressive Behavior." *Journal of Research on Adolescence* 23, no. 3 (2013): 413–23.

Mueller, Anna S., Seth Abrutyn, and Cynthia Stockton. "Can Social Ties Be Harmful? Examining the Spread of Suicide in Early Adulthood." *Sociological Perspectives* 58, no. 2 (2015): 204–22.

Parade, S. H., E. M. Leerkes, and A. N. Blankson. "Attachment to Parents, Social Anxiety, and Close Relationship of Female Students Over Transition to College." *Journal of Youth and Adolescence* 39, no. 2 (2010): 127–37.

Waters, Stacey, Leanne Lester, and Donna Cross. "How Does Support from Peers Compare with Support from Adults as Students Transition to Secondary School?" *Journal of Adolescent Health* 54 (2014): 543–49.

Web Site

Common Sense Media. www.commonsensemedia.org.

Build Your Resilience

OVERVIEW

Many children are raised in less than ideal environments. They may be presented with a host of different problems, such as insufficient family resources, inadequate housing, violence-plagued neighborhoods, family dysfunction, poor educational opportunities, and physical and emotional health problems. But, not all of these children are destined to fail. In fact, large numbers of children succeed, some beyond anyone's expectation. These children demonstrate a healthy development in spite of adversity. They have a quality known as resilience. Despite the myriad of roadblocks that they face, these children manage to bounce back and move forward. Resilience appears to be dependent upon an individual's own personal resources as well as resources available from connectedness to family and community.

Resilient children and teens appear to demonstrate a number of key characteristics. They are optimistic, even when everyone around them is far less certain a situation or set of circumstances will improve. They focus on what they do well and are not discouraged when they have a disappointing experience. Resilient children and teens tend to be flexible and accepting of various outcomes. They are open to change.

WHAT THE EXPERTS SAY

Physical Activity Appears to Improve Mental Health and Resilience

In a cross-sectional study published in 2015 in the journal BMC *Pediatrics*, researchers based in Hong Kong evaluated the association between physical activity and the mental-health well-being of Chinese teens and the role that resilience and other factors may play in this relationship. Why is this so important? The researchers explained that at least 16 percent of adolescents in Hong Kong in grades 7 to 9 have psychiatric disorders and an additional 22 percent have related symptoms. Among these disorders, oppositional defiant disorder and anxiety disorder were the most common. Learning ways to prevent some of this illness is of prime importance. The cohort consisted of 775 Chinese students in grades 7 and 8. All the students completed questionnaires. The researchers learned that physical activity was significantly correlated with the adolescent's mental well-being and resilience. Apparently, resilience mediated most of this association. The researchers concluded that "promoting physical activities that build up resilience could be a promising way to improve adolescent mental health."[1]

A Positive Youth Development Approach May Play a Role in Building Resilience

In a study published in 2015 in *Child Abuse & Neglect*, researchers from New Zealand and Canada wanted to evaluate the ability of Positive Youth Development practices to improve the resilience of at-risk youth. The key elements of Positive Youth Development programs are the encouragement of personal agency, the respectful approach to youth and families, the focus on the strengths and competencies of children and teens, and the recognition of the risks and challenges that these children and teens may face. The cohort consisted of 605 New Zealand teens between the ages of 12 and 17 years who were clients of two or more services systems (child welfare, juvenile justice, educational support, and/or mental health) during the previous six months. The teens completed self-reported questionnaires that were administered individually. The researchers found that the service systems that used a positive youth development approach had significantly higher levels of teen resilience. Moreover, increased resilience in the teens was related to increased indicators of well-being. The researchers concluded that professional practices that provide spaces for youth engagement and decision making and that work in respectful ways taking account of youth circumstances, bring benefits in terms of enhanced resilience.[2]

A Teacher-Delivered Intervention May Reduce the Post-Traumatic Reaction from Exposure to Violence and Increase Resilience

In an article published in 2013 in the *Israel Journal of Psychiatry and Related Sciences*, researchers from Israel and New Haven, Connecticut, commented that Jewish and Arab Israeli students were traumatized by the rocket attacks during the 2006 Lebanon War. Could a teacher intervention help them? The cohort consisted of 1,372 children from both ethnic groups who were in fourth and fifth grade. All of the students were exposed to the rocket attacks. During the 14-session intervention program, the topics included processing positive and negative experiences, managing stress, dealing with emotions, correcting negative cognitions, and implementing adaptive coping mechanisms such as humor. Both before and after the program, the children were assessed for stressful life events, symptoms, and parental concerns. Before the program, the Arab children showed more severe symptoms. By the end of the program, all of the children had significant decreases in symptoms. The researchers concluded that "school-based programs with teachers as clinical mediators could be a valuable, cost-effective cross-cultural model of intervention after mass trauma."[3]

Resilient People Have a Number of Common Characteristics

In a study published in 2014 in the *European Journal of Psychotraumatology*, researchers based in New York City noted that the response of people to trauma may range from resilience to severe psychopathology, including post-traumatic stress disorder, depressive disorders, and substance use disorders. That is why it is important to identify those core psychosocial elements that appear to support resilience. One of the key elements of resilience is optimism; while the situation may initially appear bleak, a resilient person believes that the outcome will ultimately be favorable. Another important element is cognitive flexibility or the ability to reappraise and reframe one's situation. Resilient people have active coping skills and maintain a social support network. They keep as physically active as they can, and they hold a set of core beliefs that are positive about themselves. The researchers noted that "these factors can be cultivated even before exposure to traumatic events, or they can be conceptualized and targeted in interventions for individuals recovering from trauma exposure."[4]

BARRIERS AND PROBLEMS

People with Bipolar Disorder Tend to Have Low Levels of Resilience

In a study published in 2015 in the *Journal of Affective Disorders*, researchers from Korea wanted to learn more about the association between resilience and bipolar disorder. The researchers noted that stress plays an important role in the onset and recurrence of bipolar disorder, and resilience helps people cope with stress or adversity. But, there is little research on resilience in bipolar disorder. The cohort consisted of 62 people with bipolar disorder who were stabilized as a result of treatment and 62 matched healthy people. Everyone completed questionnaires and were interviewed by a psychiatrist. When compared to the people in the control group, the researchers determined that the people with bipolar disorder had significantly higher levels of impulsivity and lower levels of resilience. Their low levels of resilience were associated to an increased number of depressive episodes, which increased their risk for illness recurrence. The researchers commented that there is a need to develop resilience enhancing programs for people with bipolar disorder.[5]

People with Depression and/or Anxiety Tend to Have Lower Resilience

In a 12-month study published in 2013 in the journal *Quality of Life Research*, researchers from Korea wanted to learn more about the association between depression and/or anxiety and levels of resilience. The cohort consisted of 121 outpatients diagnosed with depression and/or anxiety disorders. Eighty of the patients had depressive disorders and 41 had anxiety disorders. The researchers learned that a low level of spirituality was the key independent predictor of low resilience in people with depressive and/or anxiety disorders. In addition, low purpose in life and less frequent exercise were associated with low and medium resilience, respectively. The researchers commented that their findings added to "the understanding of resilience and provided potential targets of resilience-focused intervention in these patients."[6]

Rural Lesbian Youth Face Additional Resilience Challenges

In a study published in 2010 in the *Journal of Lesbian Studies* researchers from Virginia reviewed some of the resilience challenges faced by lesbian rural youth. The researchers noted that, on average, lesbian girls identify at age 14 to 16 years, two or three years later than their gay counterparts. But, they are living in an environment that tends to adhere to traditional gender roles. In rural settings, female teens are often expected to conform to the heterosexual-normative model of female development—birth, marriage, children, and death. So, isolation is not an uncommon situation for rural lesbian teens, who lack a visible lesbian social network. And, these teens are at increased risk for problem behaviors, such as drinking and driving, and they have many additional barriers to resilience. However, lesbian teens may gain additional resilience through a strong relationship with at least one parent. Yet, parent/lesbian teen relationships are frequently far more strained than those between a parent and heterosexual teen. Peer relationships and school environments are often the source of still more problems.

For many lesbians living in rural communities, there are clearly numerous barriers to resilience.[7]

NOTES

1. Frederick Ka Wing Ho, Lobo Hung Tak Louie, Chun Bong Chow et al., "Physical Activity Improves Mental Health Through Resilience in Hong Kong Chinese Adolescents," *BMC Pediatrics* 15 (2015): 48+.

2. Jackie Sanders, R. Munford, T. Thimasarn-Anwar et al., "The Role of Positive Youth Development in Building Resilience and Enhancing Wellbeing for At-Risk Youth," *Child Abuse & Neglect* 42 (2015): 40–53.

3. Leo Wolmer, Daniel Hamiel, Michelle Slone et al., "Post-Traumatic Reaction of Israeli Jewish and Arab Children Exposed to Rocket Attacks Before and After Teacher-Delivered Intervention," *Israel Journal of Psychiatry and Related Sciences* 50, no. 3 (2013): 165–72.

4. Brian M. Iacoviello and Dennis S. Charney, "Psychosocial Facets of Resilience: Implications for Preventing Posttrauma Psychopathology, Treating Trauma Survivors, and Enhancing Community Resilience," *European Journal of Psychotraumatology* 5 (2014): 23970.

5. Jae-Won Choi, Boseok Cha, Jihoon Jang et al., "Resilience and Impulsivity in Euthymic Patients with Bipolar Disorder," *Journal of Affective Disorders* 170 (2015): 172–77.

6. Jung-Ah Min, Young-Eun Jung, Dai-Jin Kim et al., "Characteristics Associated with Low Resilience in Patients with Depression and/or Anxiety Disorders," *Quality of Life Research* 22, no. 2 (2013): 231–41.

7. Tracy J. Cohn and Sarah L. Hastings, "Resilience Among Rural Lesbian Youth," *Journal of Lesbian Studies* 14, no. 1 (2010): 71–79.

REFERENCES AND RESOURCES

Magazines, Journals, and Newspapers

Carr, Walter, Devvon Bradley, Alan D. Ogle et al. "Resilience Training in a Population of Deployed Personnel." *Military Psychology* 25, no. 2 (2013): 148–55.

Choi, Jae-Won, Boseok Cha, Jihoon Jang et al. "Resilience and Impulsivity in Euthymic Patients with Bipolar Disorder." *Journal of Affective Disorders* 170 (2015): 172–77.

Cohn, Tracy J., and Sarah L. Hastings. "Resilience Among Rural Lesbian Youth." *Journal of Lesbian Studies* 14, no. 1 (2010): 71–79.

Diab, Marwan, Kirsi Peltonen, Samir R. Qouta et al. "Effectiveness of Psychosocial Intervention Enhancing Resilience Among War-Affected Children and the Moderating Role of Family Factors." *Child Abuse & Neglect* 40 (2015): 24–35.

Ho, Frederick Ka Wing, Lobo Hung Tak Louie, Chun Bong Chow et al. "Physical Activity Improves Mental Health Through Resilience in Hong Kong Chinese Adolescents." *BMC Pediatrics* 15 (2015): 48+.

Iacoviello, Brian M., and Dennis S. Charney. "Psychosocial Facets of Resilience: Implications for Preventing Posttrauma Psychopathology, Treating Trauma Survivors, and Enhancing Community Resilience." *European Journal of Psychotraumatology* 5 (2014): 23970.

Min, Jung-Ah, Young-Eun Jung, Dai-Jin Kim et al. "Characteristics Associated with Low Resilience in Patients with Depression and/or Anxiety Disorders." *Quality of Life Research* 22, no. 2 (2013): 231–41.

Okvat, Heather A., and Alex J. Zautra. "Community Gardening: A Parsimonious Path to Individual, Community, and Environmental Resilience." *American Journal of Community Psychology* 47 (2011): 374–87.

Sanders, J. R. Munford, T. Thimasarn-Anwar et al. "The Role of Positive Youth Development in Building Resilience and Enhancing Wellbeing for At-Risk Youth." *Child Abuse & Neglect* 42 (2015): 40–53.

Wolmer, Leo, Daniel Hamiel, Michelle Slone et al. "Post-Traumatic Reaction of Israeli Jewish and Arab Children Exposed to Rocket Attacks Before and After Teacher-Delivered Intervention." *Israel Journal of Psychiatry and Related Sciences* 50, no. 3 (2013): 165–72.

Zhao, J., P. Chi, X. Li et al. "Extracurricular Interest as a Resilience Building Block for Children Affected by Parental HIV/AIDS." *AIDS Care* 26, no. 6 (2014): 758–62.

Web Site

American Psychological Association. www.apa.org.

Don't Become a Bully

OVERVIEW

Bullies demonstrate a number of different bad behaviors. They call their peers names with negative connotations, they threaten to cause bodily harm, they spread rumors about other people, and they exclude certain people from their associates. Bullies may also physically attack others.

In an article published in 2015 in the *Archives of Public Health*, researchers from Sweden wanted to learn more about how teens defined bullying. Web-based questionnaires were completed by a diverse group of 128 teens, and the researchers conducted four single-gender focus group interviews with 21 students (8 females and 13 males) between the ages of 13 and 15 years. The students considered bullying to be something as small as a single hurtful or harmful incident, even one on the Internet. They also addressed the health consequences of bullying. When compared to the younger students, older students reported more types of behaviors as bullying. Males reported fewer bullying behaviors than females. The researchers noted that their findings indicated that "the traditional criteria included in most definitions of bullying may not fully reflect adolescents' understanding and definition of bullying." Since teens appeared to have a broader definition of bullying, researchers may actually be failing to identify all bullying that is taking place.[1]

It is important to remember that bullying may occur in many different places, including inside schools, outside on playgrounds, at the mall, at a job, and during sporting events. People may be bullied electronically. That is known as electronic bullying or cyberbullying. According to the Web site stopbullying.gov, between

1 in 4 and 1 in 3 students report that they have been bullied in school. Most bullying appears to happen in middle school. Young people who are thought to be different from their peers appear to be at highest risk for bullying. Bullying is normally not a simple interaction between a single bully and a single victim. More often, it is groups of students bullying others. In addition, it is not uncommon for victims of bullies to turn around and become bullies, a truly vicious circle.[2]

WHAT THE EXPERTS SAY

School-Based Programs and Teachers May Help Students Avoid Becoming Bullies

In a study published in 2012 in the journal *Archives of Pediatrics & Adolescent Medicine*, researchers from Baltimore, Maryland, wanted to determine the impact of a bullying prevention program, known as School-Wide Positive Behavioral Intervention and Supports (SWPBIS), on students during their transition into early adolescence. The intervention attempted to accomplish a number of goals, including promoting a positive school environment based on respect, consistent discipline, the positive reinforcement of desired behaviors, and consequences for inappropriate behaviors. Four years of data were obtained from 37 Maryland public elementary schools involving 12,344 children. Slightly over half the children were male; 45.1 percent were African American, and 46.1 percent were white. When the study began, the children were in kindergarten, first grade, and second grade. As the children grew older, their risk for bullying and peer rejection increased. Yet, the researchers learned that the children in the 21 schools that implemented SWPBIS had lower rates of teacher reported bullying, both as victim and perpetrator, and peer rejection than in the 16 schools without SWPBIS. The researchers commented that "as a result of exposure to SWPBIS in elementary school, we anticipate that these children will make the transition to adolescence with a reduced risk for involvement in bullying." Moreover, "a universal SWPBIS model is a promising approach for preventing bullying."[3]

In a study published in 2014 in the *Journal of Educational Psychology*, researchers from the Netherlands, Finland, and Australia wanted to learn more about the role that teachers may play in reducing the development of bullying in their students. The cohort consisted of data on 2,776 Finnish students in fourth to sixth grades in 31 different schools. There were almost equal numbers of males and females. Students completed Internet-based questionnaires in which they were asked about the ability of their teachers to reduce bullying. When students perceived that their teachers effectively reduced bullying with a relatively low level of effort, there were reductions in bullying. "If teachers are seen to be efficacious, they are likely to prevent bullying." The researchers noted that their findings "show that teachers can play an important role in antibullying programs and should be seen as targets of intervention."[4]

Parenting Style Has an Impact on the Development of Bullying

In a study published in 2012 in the *Journal of School Violence*, a researcher from Greece examined the association between parenting styles and the development of bullying in early adolescence. The researcher noted that previous studies have found that an insecure parenting attachment style and inappropriate parenting tend to predispose children to become bullies. The cohort consisted of 601 Greek preadolescents, almost the same number of boys and girls, between the ages of 10 and 12 years. The researchers found that parenting appeared to play an important role in determining whether a preadolescent became a bully. While the students who reported themselves as being securely attached had less involvement in bullying, the students who saw their parents as cold and indifferent or actually hostile and rejecting were at increased risk for bullying. The researchers concluded that parents need to become educated about family cohesion and conflict resolution. Their increased knowledge may "have a potential impact on children's behavior and may serve as an indirect intervention in bullying incidents at school." And, school efforts to prevent bullying should include parents. "Children who perceive low emotional parental warmth, over protection, and high rejection are more likely to exhibit bullying behaviors."[5]

BARRIERS AND PROBLEMS

The Children and Teens of Parents Who Display Negative Parenting Behavior Are at Increased Risk for Becoming Victims or Victims Who Bully Others

In a meta-analysis published in 2013 in the journal *Child Abuse & Neglect*, researchers from the United Kingdom wanted to learn more about the association between negative parenting behavior and the risk of becoming a victim or a victim who bullies others. The researchers conducted a systematic review of the relevant literature. Seventy studies were included in the final analysis. These studies represented a total of 208,778 children, teens, and young adults between the ages of 4 and 25 years. The researchers learned that victims and bullies who become victims were more likely to have been exposed to negative parenting, such as abuse, neglect, and maladaptive parenting. The researchers suggested that intervention programs that target children exposed to harsh or abusive parenting may help reduce the risk of a negative outcome.[6]

Teens Who Have a Negative Body Image Are More Likely to Become Bullies

In a study published in 2015 in the *European Journal of Pediatrics*, researchers from Slovakia, the Czech Republic, and the Netherlands assessed the association between body image dissatisfaction and involvement in bullying. Data were obtained from the Health Behaviour in School-Aged Children study conducted in 2010 in Slovakia. The cohort consisted of 8,050 adolescents between the ages of 11 and 15 years, with a mean age of 13.57 years. Less than half of the cohort was male. More than 20 percent of the sample reported being involved in bullying. Males were more likely than females to bully. While more than half of the sample thought that their bodies were the "right size," the remaining reported dissatisfaction with their bodies. Their bodies were either too thin or too fat. The researchers found a significant association between body dissatisfaction and involvement in bullying. That is why, the researchers commented, it is necessary for schools to incorporate programs that support positive self-perceptions into the curriculum. "The target group should include all adolescents, not only those who are dissatisfied with their body image."[7]

Bullies Appear to Have Some Advantages

In a study published online in 2015 in the *Journal of Interpersonal Violence*, researchers from Canada examined evolutionary aspects of adolescent bullying behaviors. Over a two-week period of time in February 2014, the researchers administered questionnaires to 133 teens, between the ages of 13 and 16 years, from one secondary school in metro Vancouver, British Columbia. The vast majority of the students were white. The students were then placed in one of four groups—bullies, victims, bully/victims, or bystanders. The researchers classified 15 students as bullies or 11 percent of the total sample. Almost three-quarters of the bullies were males. The students were evaluated for depression, self-esteem, social status, and social anxiety. The researchers determined that the bullies had the most positive scores on mental health measures and held the highest social rank in the school environment. According to the researchers, maybe that is why programs that attempt to alter bullying behavior are not always effective and why this "pervasive problem" continues to exist. Intervention programs tend to take away the rewards of bullying without offering any way that bullies may reach their goals. The researchers commented that bullying may well be "a natural phenomenon that works to establish rank and maximize survival of the species." The researchers advocated "shifting the scope to implement strategies that allow 'bullying' to occur with a lower level of harm."[8]

Children from Socioeconomically Disadvantaged Families Have an Increased Risk of Involvement in Bullying

In a study published in 2012 in BMC *Public Health*, researchers based in the Netherlands examined the prevalence and socioeconomic disparities of bullying behavior among young elementary school children. The cohort was derived from a large population-based survey in the Netherlands. Teacher reports of bullying behavior and socioeconomic status of families and schools were available for

6,379 children between the ages of five and six years. The researchers found that one-third of the children were involved in bullying. Of these, 17 percent were bullies. The researchers found that the children from disadvantaged families had a particularly high risk for involvement in bullying. The researchers noted that their findings "suggest the need of timely bullying preventions and interventions that should have a special focus on children of families with a low socioeconomic background."[9]

NOTES

1. L. Hellström, L. Persson, and C. Hagquist, "Understanding and Defining Bullying—Adolescents' Own Views," *Archives of Public Health* 73, no. 1 (2015): 4+.

2. stopbullying.gov.

3. Tracy E. Waasdorp, Catherine P. Bradshaw, and Philip J. Leaf, "The Impact of Schoolwide Positive Behavioral Interventions and Supports on Bullying and Peer Rejection," *Archives of Pediatrics & Adolescent Medicine* 166, no. 2 (2012): 149–56.

4. R. Veenstra, S. Lindenberg, G. Huitsing et al., "The Role of Teachers in Bullying: The Relation Between Antibullying Attitudes, Efficacy, and Efforts to Reduce Bullying," *Journal of Educational Psychology* 106, no. 4 (2014): 1135–43.

5. Constantinos M. Kokkinos, "Bullying and Victimization in Early Adolescence: Associations with Attachment Style and Perceived Parenting," *Journal of School Violence* 12 (2013): 174–92.

6. Suzet Tanya Lereya, Muthanna Samara, and Dieter Wolke, "Parenting Behavior and the Risk of Becoming a Victim and a Bully/Victim: A Meta-Analysis Study," *Child Abuse & Neglect* 37 (2013): 1091–108.

7. Jana Holubcikova, Peter Kolarcik, Andrea Madarasova Geckova et al., "Is Subjective Perception of Negative Body Image Among Adolescents Associated with Bullying?" *European Journal of Pediatrics* 174, no. 8 (2015): 1035–41.

8. Jun-Bin Koh and Jennifer S. Wong, "Survival of the Fittest and the Sexiest: Evolutionary Origins of Adolescent Bullying," *Journal of Interpersonal Violence* (July 2015).

9. Pauline W. Jansen, Marina Verlinden, Anke Dommisse-van Berkel et al., "Prevalence of Bullying and Victimization Among Children in Early Elementary School: Do Family and School Neighborhood Socioeconomic Status Matter?" BMC *Public Health* 12 (2012): 494+.

REFERENCES AND RESOURCES

Magazines, Journals, and Newspapers

Bowllan, Nancy M. "Implementation and Evaluation of a Comprehensive, School-Wide, Bullying Prevention Program in an Urban/Suburban Middle School." *Journal of School Health* 81, no. 4 (2011): 167–73.

Hellström, L., L. Persson, and C. Hagquist. "Understanding and Defining Bullying—Adolescents' Own Views." *Archives of Public Health* 73, no. 1 (2015): 4+.

Holubcikova, Jana, Peter Kolarcik, Andrea Madarasova Geckova et al. "Is Subjective Perception of Negative Body Image Among Adolescents Associated with Bullying?" *European Journal of Pediatrics* 174, no. 8 (2015): 1035–41.

Jansen, Pauline W., Marina Verlinden, Anke Dommisse-van Berkel et al. "Prevalence of Bullying and Victimization Among Children in Early Elementary School: Do Family and School Neighborhood Socioeconomic Status Matter?" BMC Public Health 12 (2012): 494+.

Koh, Jun-Bin, and Jennifer S. Wong. "Survival of the Fittest and the Sexiest: Evolutionary Origins of Adolescent Bullying." Journal of Interpersonal Violence (July 2015).

Kokkinos, Constantinos M. "Bullying and Victimization in Early Adolescence: Associations with Attachment Style and Perceived Parenting." Journal of School Violence 12 (2013): 174–92.

Lereya, Suzet Tanya, Muthanna Samara, and Dieter Wolke. "Parenting Behavior and the Risk of Becoming a Victim and a Bully/Victim: A Meta-Analysis Study." Child Abuse & Neglect 37 (2013): 1091–108.

Veenstra, R., S. Lindenberg, G. Huitsing et al. "The Role of Teachers in Bullying: The Relation Between Antibullying Attitudes, Efficacy, and Efforts to Reduce Bullying." Journal of Educational Psychology 106, no. 4 (2014): 1135–43.

Verinden, M., P. W. Jansen, R. Veenstra et al. "Preschool Attention-Deficit/Hyperactivity and Oppositional Defiant Problems as Antecedents of School Bullying." Journal of the American Academy of Child & Adolescent Psychiatry 54, no. 7 (2015): 571–79.

Waasdorp, Tracy E., Catherine P. Bradshaw, and Philip J. Leaf. "The Impact of Schoolwide Positive Behavioral Interventions and Supports on Bullying and Peer Rejection." Archives of Pediatrics & Adolescent Medicine 166, no. 2 (2012): 149–56.

Young, Kevin C., Todd B. Kashdan, Patrick E. McKnight et al. "Happy and Unhappy Adolescent Bullies: Evidence for Theoretically Meaningful Subgroups." Personality and Individual Differences 75 (2015): 224–28.

Web Site

Stopbullying.gov.

Improve Self-Esteem

OVERVIEW

Self-esteem consists of the thoughts and feelings we have about ourselves. For most people, it is an ever-evolving process. Some days, such as the one when we finally pass the driving test and earn a driver's license, we feel very good about what we have accomplished. Other days, such as the one when we forgot to complete a homework assignment, our self-esteem may be lower. Occasional bouts with low self-esteem are to be expected. But, people who have low self-esteem most of the time have less ability to function effectively.

It is not uncommon for people with low self-esteem to be unaware that they are thinking negatively about themselves. Without such knowledge, one is unable to transform negative thoughts about oneself into positive thoughts. More positive thinking about oneself is useful for increasing self-esteem. For example, it is important to stop being your own worst critic. People who focus only on their shortcomings, reinforce low self-esteem. It is crucial to accept that mistakes happen to everyone. Instead of concentrating on what was done incorrectly, consider mistakes as an opportunity to learn an improved way of accomplishing a goal.

WHAT THE EXPERTS SAY

Cyberprogram 2.0 Appears to Be Useful for Solving Conflict and Improving Self-Esteem

In a study published in 2015 in the *Journal of Adolescent Health*, researchers from Spain wanted to determine if an antibullying program, known as Cyberprogram 2.0, was also useful for improving self-esteem. The cohort consisted of a randomly selected sample of 176 Spanish teens between the ages of 13 and 15 years. The intervention group had 93 teens; the control group had 83. The sample was recruited from three schools with varying socioeconomic levels—low, medium, and high. Assessment instruments were administered before and after the program, which consisted of 19 one-hour sessions carried out during the school term. The researcher learned that the program increased the use of conflict resolution strategies, decreased aggressive and avoidant strategies, and increased self-esteem. The change was similar in the males and females. The researchers concluded that the improvements in self-esteem were the result of "behavioral improvements caused by the intervention."[1]

The Girls on the Go! Program Appears to Raise Self-Esteem in Girls and Teens

In a study published in 2015 online in the *American Journal of Health Promotion*, researchers based in Australia wanted to learn if an out of school intervention known as "Girls on the Go!" actually raised self-esteem and addressed other problems such as poor body image and low levels of self-confidence. The cohort consisted of 122 primary and secondary female students between the ages of 10 and 16 years. The 10-week program was held at a community health center located in a culturally diverse area of Melbourne, Australia. It employed an empowerment model that included interactive and experiential approaches.

Weekly themes included body image, self-esteem, safety, assertiveness, trust, and confidence. The researchers found that the program led to significant increases in self-esteem and self-efficacy. After six months, a follow-up determined that the students retained these improvements. The researchers concluded that the intervention was "a successful means of improving self-esteem among girls from diverse cultural backgrounds."[2]

Multiple Social Identifications Appears to Raise Teens' Self-Esteem

In a longitudinal, cross-sectional, and cross-cultural study published in 2015 in the *Journal of Adolescence*, researchers from Israel and Germany investigated the relationship between multiple social identifications in teens and self-esteem. Their cohort consisted of 2,337 early adolescents (mean age of 11.4) and mid-adolescents (mean age of 15.9) from Israel and Germany. Completing question-naires, the teens described their social identification as students, family members, and as members of the majority national group, and reported on their degrees of self-esteem. The researchers found that the students with multiple social identifications had more self-esteem, and the multiple social identifications appeared to have an accumulative effect. The researchers noted that the fact that the studies in the two distinct countries had identical results shows the "robustness of the findings." The researchers concluded that "both parents and educators should work to increase adolescents' group engagement, in the hope that involvement with these groups will have a positive effect on adolescents' self-esteem."[3]

Positive Self-Images Appear to Improve Self-Esteem in People with Social Anxiety

In a study published in 2012 in the journal *Cognitive Behaviour Therapy*, re-searchers from the United Kingdom and Australia wanted to learn more about the ability of positive self-images to improve self-esteem in people with social anxiety. They asked 44 participants with high levels of social anxiety and 44 participants with low levels of social anxiety to generate either positive or negative self-images and complete measurements of explicit (conscious) and implicit (automatic) self-esteem. The participants who had negative self-images reported lower levels of positive implicit self-esteem. They also noted that they had lower positive explicit and higher negative explicit self-esteem. And, all participants having positive self-images reported higher levels of explicit self-esteem than those holding negative self-images.[4]

A Group Mindfulness Program May Improve Adolescent Self-Esteem

In a study published in 2015 in the journal *Child and Adolescent Mental Health*, researchers from Australia wanted to learn more about the association between teen participation in a mindfulness program and improvements in certain condi-tions including levels of self-esteem. (Mindfulness involves the process of being aware of one's thoughts.) The researchers recruited 80 teens between the ages of 13 and 18 years from three community mental health clinics. The teens were randomly placed in an intervention group or a control group. Although all the teens received their usual treatments, the teens in the intervention group participated in a five-week mindfulness-training program. Assessments were conducted at baseline, after the program ended, and at a three-month follow-up. At the three-month follow-up, the teens in the intervention group showed significant improvements in self-esteem and other aspects of mental health. The researchers noted that the changes were consistent with mindfulness theory.[5]

There Appears to Be a Strong Association between Body Dissatisfaction and Self-Esteem in Teens

In a school-based study published in 2010 in the *Journal of Adolescent Health*, researchers from Texas, Minnesota, and Australia learned more about the association between body dissatisfaction and self-esteem in teens. The cohort consisted of a diverse samples of 4,746 adolescents between the ages of 11 and 18 years who lived in the Minneapolis–St. Paul area of Minnesota. Five years later, the teens were resurveyed through the mail; the response to the second survey was 2,516 teens and young adults. The researchers found a strong and significant relationship between body dissatisfaction and self-esteem in both the males and females, and there was no significant difference between the genders. As a result of their findings, the researchers noted that "adolescents who express overly negative evaluations of their bodies or appearance should be considered at risk for lowered self-esteem."[6]

BARRIERS AND PROBLEMS

Childhood Exposure to Violence Appears to Result in a Lowering of Adult Self-Esteem

In a study published in 2015 in the journal *Violence and Victims*, a researcher from Israel wanted to learn more about the effects of violence between parents and/or parent-to-child violence and adult self-esteem. Data were obtained from a sample of 352 university students between the ages of 18 and 30 years. Most of the participants were born in Israel or moved to Israel, primarily from the former Soviet Union, when they were young children. The researcher learned that the students not exposed to family violence in childhood had the highest levels of self-esteem. The students who experienced one type of childhood violence, generally parent-to-child violence, had lower self-esteem. The lowest self-esteem was seen in students who experienced both types of family violence. Self-esteem was also associated with the frequency of family violence. The researcher noted that the findings "demonstrated that the presence and frequency of family violence experiences have a negative accumulative effect on adult self-esteem."[7]

A Child's Chronic Physical Illness May Result in Lower Self-Esteem

In a study published in 2015 in the *Journal of Abnormal Child Psychology*, researchers from Canada examined the association between chronic physical illness in children and a number of other factors including self-esteem. Why is this important? Chronic physical illness among children is actually fairly common. According to the researchers, almost 20 percent of children have some type of chronic physical illness such as asthma or diabetes. As a result, millions of children and their families deal with these problems every day. To learn more, the researchers examined data from the National Longitudinal Survey of Children, a study of Canadian children from birth to early adulthood (n=10,646). The researchers found that childhood chronic physical illness was directly associated with maternal depression and family dysfunction "leading to declines in child self-esteem." So, children dealing with chronic illness may have lower levels of self-esteem.[8]

People with Generalized Social Anxiety Disorder Have an Increased Risk of Self-Esteem Instability

In a study published in 2014 in the journal *Clinical Psychological Science*, researchers from George Mason University in Virginia wanted to learn more about the association between social anxiety disorder and self-esteem. (Social anxiety disorder is a condition in which a person fears being evaluated by others and avoids social situations.) The cohort consisted of 40 people (25 women) who had been diagnosed with social anxiety disorder and 39 matched healthy controls. The participants were asked to provide two weeks of end-of-day reports on their affect and self-esteem. The researchers found that compared to the healthy adults, the participants with social anxiety disorder had unstable low self-esteem. In addition, people with social anxiety disorder were three times more likely to have acute shifts in self-esteem. The researchers theorized that self-esteem instability "may be an important marker for social anxiety symptoms."[9]

NOTES

1. Maite Garaigordobil and Vanesa Martínez-Valderrey, "The Effectiveness of Cyberprogram 2.0 on Conflict Resolution Strategies and Self-Esteem," *Journal of Adolescent Health* 57 (2015): 229–34.

2. L. Tirlea, H. Truby, and T. P. Haines, "Pragmatic, Randomized Controlled Trials of the Girls on the Go! Program to Improve Self-Esteem in Girls," *American Journal of Health Promotion* (May 2015).

3. Maya Benish-Weisman, Ella Daniel, David Schiefer et al., "Multiple Social Identifications and Adolescents' Self-Esteem," *Journal of Adolescence* 44 (2015): 21–31.

4. Natalie Hulme, Colette Hirsch, and Lusia Stopa, "Images of the Self and Self-Esteem: Do Positive Self-Images Improve Self-Esteem in Social Anxiety?" *Cognitive Behaviour Therapy* 41, no. 2 (2012): 163–73.

5. Lucy Tan and Graham Martin, "Taming the Adolescent Mind: A Randomised Controlled Trial Examining Clinical Efficacy of an Adolescent Mindfulness-Based Group Programme." *Child and Adolescent Mental Health* 20, no. 1 (2015): 49–55.

6. Patricia A. van den Berg, Jonathan Mond, Marla Eisenberg et al., "The Link Between Body Dissatisfaction and Self-Esteem in Adolescents: Similarities Across Gender, Age, Weight Status, Race/Ethnicity, and Socioeconomic Status," *Journal of Adolescent Health* 47 (2010): 290–96.

7. Zeev Winstok, "Effects of Childhood Experience of Violence Between Parents and/ or Parent-to-Child Violence on Young Israeli Adults' Global Self-Esteem," *Violence and Victims* 30, no. 4 (2015): 699–713.

8. Mark A. Ferro and Michael H. Boyle, "The Impact of Chronic Physical Illness, Maternal Depressive Symptoms, Family Functioning, and Self-Esteem on Symptoms of Anxiety and Depression in Children," *Journal of Abnormal Child Psychology* 43 (2015): 177–87.

9. Antonia S. Farmer and Todd B. Kashdan, "Affective and Self-Esteem Instability in the Daily Lives of People with Generalized Social Anxiety Disorder," *Clinical Psychological Science* 2, no. 2 (2014): 187–201.

REFERENCES AND RESOURCES

Magazines, Journals, and Newspapers

Abbott, Rebecca A., Anne J. Smith, Erin K. Howie et al. "Effects of Home Access to Active Videogames on Child Self-Esteem, Enjoyment of Physical Activity, and Anxiety Related to Electronic Games: Results From a Randomized Controlled Trial." *Games for Health Journal* 3, no. 4 (2014): 260–66.

Benish-Weisman, Maya, Ella Daniel, David Schiefer et al. "Multiple Social Identifications and Adolescents' Self-Esteem." *Journal of Adolescence* 44 (2015): 21–31.

Ciccolo, Joseph T., Nicholas J. SantaBarbara, Shira I. Dunsiger et al. "Muscular Strength Is Associated with Self-Esteem in College Men But Not Women." *Journal of Health Psychology* (July 2015).

Farmer, Antonina S., and Todd B. Kashdan. "Affective and Self-Esteem Instability in the Daily Lives of People with Generalized Social Anxiety Disorder." *Clinical Psychological Science* 2, no. 2 (2014): 187–201.

Ferro, Mark A., and Michael H. Boyle. "The Impact of Chronic Physical Illness, Maternal Depressive Symptoms, Family Functioning, and Self-Esteem on Symptoms of Anxiety and Depression in Children." *Journal of Abnormal Child Psychology* 43 (2015): 177–87.

Garaigordobil, Maite, and Vanesa Martínez-Valderrey. "The Effectiveness of Cyberprogram 2.0 on Conflict Resolution Strategies and Self-Esteem." *Journal of Adolescent Health* 57 (2015): 229–34.

Hulme, Natalie, Colette Hirsch, and Lusia Stopa. "Images of the Self and Self-Esteem: Do Positive Self-Images Improve Self-Esteem in Social Anxiety?" *Cognitive Behaviour Therapy* 41, no. 2 (2012): 163–73.

Tan, Lucy, and Graham Martin. "Taming the Adolescent Mind: A Randomised Controlled Trial Examining Clinical Efficacy of an Adolescent Mindfulness-Based Group Programme." *Child and Adolescent Mental Health* 20, no. 1 (2015): 49–55.

Tirlea, L., H. Truby, and T. P. Haines. "Pragmatic, Randomized Controlled Trials of the Girls on the Go! Program to Improve Self-Esteem in Girls." *American Journal of Health Promotion* (May 2015).

van den Berg, Patricia A., Jonathan Mond, Marla Eisenberg et al. "The Link Between Body Dissatisfaction and Self-Esteem in Adolescents: Similarities Across Gender, Age, Weight Status, Race/Ethnicity, and Socioeconomic Status." *Journal of Adolescent Health* 47 (2010): 290–96.

Winstok, Zeev. "Effects of Childhood Experience of Violence Between Parents and/or Parent-to-Child Violence on Young Israeli Adults' Global Self-Esteem." *Violence and Victims* 30, no. 4 (2015): 699–713.

Web Site

The Nemours Foundation. www.kidshealth.org.

Maintain a Healthy Body Image

OVERVIEW

During the teen and young adult years, when both young men and young women are bombarded with a host of different physiological and psychological changes and challenges, it is especially important to try to maintain a healthy body image. Body image actually includes a number of different factors. It is how we see our bodies and how we feel about our appearance. Body image is also how we think other people view our bodies and the degree to which we are connected to our bodies. And, thinking about body image is not a rare occurrence. In fact, both male and female teens and young adults think about their body image often. According to the Brown University Web site, one study of college students found that 74.4 percent of normal weight women indicated that they thought about their weight or appearance either all the time or frequently; the same study found that 46 percent of the normal weight men responded in the same way. Yet, paradoxically, the more focus is placed on body image, the worse people tend to feel about themselves.[1] And, poor body image is associated with a number of medical problems, including extreme dieting and/or exercising, self-induced vomiting, abuse of laxatives, and ingestion of anabolic steroids.

And the preoccupation with body image is not only a problem in the United States. In a study published in 2013 in *Nutrición Hospitalaria*, researchers from Brazil examined a cohort of 852 females and 642 males between the ages of 11 and 17 years. All of the members of the cohort, who were public school students in Salvador, Brazil, completed questionnaires. The researchers found that body image dissatisfaction was present in almost one-fifth of the students. Prevalence was 26.6 percent among the girls and 10 percent among the boys. The researchers noted that these findings indicated "a high occurrence of body image dissatisfaction" among the students they studied.[2]

WHAT THE EXPERTS SAY

An Unhealthy Body Image May Increase the Risk of Major Depression

In a study published in 2013 in the *Journal of Psychiatric Research*, researchers from Houston, Texas, and Hanoi, Vietnam, examined the association between major depression, obesity, and body image among adolescents. The cohort consisted of 4,175 teens between the ages of 11 and 17 years. The teens completed questionnaires and had their weight and height measured. There were two measurements of body image—perceived weight and body satisfaction. The researchers found that the actual weight of the teens was less important than their perceived body weight. And, both the males and females who thought they were overweight had an increased risk for major depression. The researchers concluded that "perceived weight is more important than weight in terms of risk for major depression." They recommended that greater attention be paid to how teens "feel about their weight and body."[3]

Physical Activity Appears to Reduce Dissatisfaction with Body Image

In a study published in 2011 in the journal *Psychology of Sport and Exercise*, researchers from Portugal evaluated the association between physical activity and dissatisfaction with body image. The cohort consisted of 234 students between the ages of 10 and 17 years. Trained interviewers took measurements, such as height and weight, and they assessed students' level of physical activity and body image perceptions. The researchers found that more females than males (68.1 percent versus 52.9 percent) were dissatisfied with their body image. Close to 72 percent of both male and female students demonstrated body image distortion. As their body mass index levels rose, so did body image distortion. Still, there was a hopeful finding. Higher levels of physical activity were associated with lower levels of body image dissatisfaction in males and females. According to the researchers, it has long been known that regular physical activity has a number of benefits. Now these include improvements in body image dissatisfaction.[4]

Caucasian Women Are More Likely Than African American Women to Have a Negative Body Image

In a study published in 2015 in *Eating Behaviors*, researchers from American University in Washington, D.C., investigated the hypothesis that African American women have less body dissatisfaction than Caucasian women. The cohort consisted of 202 women between the ages of 18 and 45 who identified themselves as African American or Caucasian. The participants viewed 10 advertisements showing ethnically similar thin models, ethnically different thin models, ethnically similar plus-sized models, and ethnically diverse plus-sized models. After exposure, body image was measured. The researchers found that the African American women had less body dissatisfaction than the Caucasian women. African American women had similar responses when exposed to thin and plus models. On the other hand, Caucasian women had greater body dissatisfaction when exposed to the plus-sized models than the thin models. The researchers concluded that "African American women experience less body dissatisfaction than Caucasian women even following exposure to an ethnically similar thin model."[5]

A School-Based Intervention May Improve Body Image in Females

In a study published in 2010 in the *International Journal of Eating Disorders*, researchers from Australia evaluated the efficacy of Happy Being Me, a school-based body image intervention program for young female teens. The cohort consisted of 194 female seventh-grade students from two Catholic secondary schools in Melbourne, Australia. The students in one school became the intervention group, and the students in the other school became the control group. The students in the intervention group participated in three 50-minute interactive body image sessions; the goal was to teach the students about the negative consequences of poor body images and to develop strategies to combat forces promoting negative images. The students in the control group attended their normal classes. Questionnaires were administered at baseline, postintervention, and at a three-month follow-up. The researchers learned that the students in the intervention group had significantly more positive outcomes on a number of different measures than the students in the control group. The researchers concluded that their work provided proof that this school-based program was effective and had proven results.[6]

BARRIERS AND PROBLEMS

Female Models Often Do Not Look Like Most Women

In a study published in 2013 in the journal *Body Image*, researchers from the University of Massachusetts in Amherst had 44 female college students, with a mean age of 20.2 years, view a slideshow of very thin models. After two weeks, they watched a second slideshow of healthy weight models. After each slideshow, the researchers measured the participants' body image, anxiety, happiness, and depression. The researchers found that when the students viewed the healthy weight models, their notion of ideal body types was larger than when they viewed the thinner models. This effect was significantly stronger in those with high levels of baseline anxiety. These students "also had significantly more positive affect after viewing healthy weight models than after viewing thin models." The researchers concluded that "a movement toward healthy weight models in popular media may provide a substantial benefit to mental health."[7]

The Media's Portrayal of the Post-Baby Bodies of Celebrities Negatively Impacts the Body Image of Women

In a study published in 2014 in the journal *Sex Roles*, a researcher from Urbana, Illinois, used a Korean research firm to learn how the post-baby bodies of celebrities influenced Korean women who had given birth. The research firm sent email questionnaires to women in their twenties and thirties who had experienced childbirth within three years of the study. The researchers later decided to include only the women who gave birth within a year. That left 345 women in the cohort; their average age was just under 30 years. The researchers found a positive association between women who were interested in the postpregnancy bodies of celebrities and women who compared their bodies to others. That association was positively linked to body dissatisfaction and the drive for thinness among postpartum Korean women. The researchers noted that their findings "confirm the effect of media representations of postpartum celebrities as a beauty standard for non-celebrities."[8]

Teasing by Parents, Siblings, and Peers May Negatively Impact Body Image

In a cross-sectional study published in 2014 in *Eating Behaviors*, researchers from the North Dakota State University examined the association between "appearance-related teasing" and body image during the teen years. The cohort consisted of 80 girls and 78 boys in seventh, eighth, and ninth grades in a Midwestern middle school. Over 90 percent were white. The researchers used specific scales to measure teasing and body image. In general, the group experienced relatively low levels of teasing. The highest levels of teasing came from peers. Siblings teased more often than parents. However, parents who engaged in appearance-related teasing had siblings who teased more often. In fact, when parents teased, siblings were almost 10 times more likely to tease. And, this teasing was significantly associated with the body dissatisfaction of the girls' and the boys' drive for muscularity. Because of the potential negative impact of teasing, the researchers recommended that "teasing needs to be addressed with family members and peers through therapy, research, and prevention and intervention programs."[9]

Excessive Use of Facebook May Foster Negative Body Image

In a study published in 2015 in *Body Image*, researchers from Australia examined the association between use of Facebook and body image concerns among 227 first-year female university psychology students at a large public university in eastern Australia. The researchers found that the students most often compared their appearance to distant peers. Next, they compared themselves about as often to close friends and celebrities. They compared themselves significantly less frequently to female family members. Interestingly, when the students compared themselves to female celebrities, they rated themselves with the most negativity. That was followed by close friends and distant peers. They rated themselves with the least negativity when comparing themselves to female family members. Except when they compared themselves to family members, in all the other comparisons, the students rated their bodies as worse. The researchers advised future research to "identify ways to minimize any possible negative consequences of Facebook usage for young women's body image concerns."[10]

NOTES

1. Brown University, www.brown.edu.

2. Mônica L. P. Santana, Rita de Cássia Silva, Ana M.O. Assis et al., "Factors Associated with Body Image Dissatisfaction Among Adolescents in Public Schools Students in Salvador, Brazil," *Nutrición Hospitalaria* 23, no. 3 (2013): 747–55.

3. Robert E. Roberts and Hao T. Duong, "Perceived Weight, Not Obesity, Increases Risk for Major Depression Among Adolescents," *Journal of Psychiatric Research* 47 (2013): 1110–17.

4. Marisa J. Monteiro Gaspar, Teresa F. Amaral, Bruno M.P.M. Oliveira, and Nuno Borges, "Protective Effect of Physical Activity on Dissatisfaction with Body Image in Children—A Cross-Sectional Study," *Psychology of Sport and Exercise* 12 (2011): 563–69.

5. Gina L. Bruns and Michele M. Carter, "Ethnic Differences in the Effects of Media on Body Image: The Effects of Priming with Ethnically Different of Similar Models," *Eating Behaviors* 17 (2015): 33–36.

6. Shanel M. Richardson and Susan J. Paxton, "An Evaluation of a Body Image Intervention Based on Risk Factors for Body Dissatisfaction: A Controlled Study with Adolescent Girls," *International Journal of Eating Disorders* 43, no. 2 (2010): 112–22.

7. Rebecca Owen and Rebecca M. C. Spencer, "Body Ideals in Women After Viewing Images of Typical and Healthy Weight Models," *Body Image* 10, no. 4 (2013): 489–94.

8. Jiyoung Chae, "Interest in Celebrities' Post-Baby Bodies and Korean Women's Body Image Disturbance After Childbirth," *Sex Roles* 71 (2014): 419–35.

9. Mallary K. Schaefer and Elizabeth H. Blodgett Salafia, "The Connection of Teasing By Parents, Siblings, and Peers with Girls' Body Dissatisfaction and Boys' Drive for Muscularity: The Role of Social Comparison as a Mediator," *Eating Behaviors* 15 (2014): 599–608.

10. Jasmine Fardouly and Lenny R. Vartanian, "Negative Comparisons About One's Appearance Mediate the Relationship Between Facebook Usage and Body Image Concerns," *Body Image* 12 (2015): 82–88.

REFERENCES AND RESOURCES

Magazines, Journals, and Newspapers

Bruns, Gina L., and Michele M. Carter. "Ethnic Differences in the Effects of Media on Body Image: The Effects of Priming with Ethnically Different or Similar Models." *Eating Behaviors* 17 (2015): 33–36.

Chae, Jiyoung. "Interest in Celebrities' Post-Baby Bodies and Korean Women's Body Image Disturbance After Childbirth." *Sex Roles* 71 (2014): 419–35.

Fardouly, Jasmine, and Lenny R. Vartanian. "Negative Comparisons About One's Appearance Mediate the Relationship Between Facebook Usage and Body Image Concerns." *Body Image* 12 (2015): 82–88.

Gaspar, Marisa J. Monteiro, Teresa F. Amaral, Bruno M.P.M. Oliveira, and Nuno Borges. "Protective Effect of Physical Activity on Dissatisfaction with Body Image in Children—A Cross-Sectional Study." *Psychology of Sport and Exercise* 12 (2011): 563–69.

Hayes, Jacqueline F., Kristen E. D'Anci, and Robin B. Kanarek. "Foods That Are Perceived as Healthy or Unhealthy Differentially Alter Young Women's State Body Image." *Appetite* 57 (2011): 384–87.

Nicoli, Marina G., and Raphael D. R. Liberatore Junior. "Binge Eating Disorder and Body Image Perception Among University Students." *Eating Behaviors* 12, no. 4 (2011): 284–88.

Okeke, Nnenna L., Margaret R. Spitz, Michele R. Forman, and Anna V. Wilkinson. "The Associations of Body Image, Anxiety, and Smoking Among Mexican-Origin Youth." *Journal of Adolescent Health* 53 (2013): 209–14.

Owen, Rebecca, and Rebecca M. C. Spencer. "Body Ideals in Women After Viewing Images of Typical and Healthy Weight Models." *Body Image* 10, no. 4 (2013): 489–94.

Richardson, Shanel M., and Susan J. Paxton. "An Evaluation of a Body Image Intervention Based on Risk Factors for Body Dissatisfaction: A Controlled Study with Adolescent Girls." *International Journal of Eating Disorders* 43, no. 2 (2010): 112–22.

Roberts, Robert E., and Hao T. Duong. "Perceived Weight, Not Obesity, Increases Risk for Major Depression among Adolescents." *Journal of Psychiatric Research* 47 (2013): 1110–17.

Santana, Mônica L. P., Rita de Cássia R. Silva, Ana M. O. Assis et al. "Factors Associated with Body Image Dissatisfaction Among Adolescents in Public Schools Students in Salvador, Brazil." *Nutrición Hospitalaria* 28, no. 3 (2013): 747–55.

Schaefer, Mallary K., and Elizabeth H. Blodgett Salafia. "The Connection of Teasing By Parents, Siblings, and Peers with Girls' Body Dissatisfaction and Boys' Drive for Muscularity: The Role of Social Comparison as a Mediator." *Eating Behaviors* 15 (2014): 599–608.

Web Site

Brown University. www.brown.edu.

Practice Mindfulness

OVERVIEW

Mindfulness is the moment-by-moment awareness of thoughts, feelings, body sensations, and the surrounding environment. It involves paying close attention to thoughts and feelings without judging them; it does not allow thinking about events that took place in the past or that may occur in the future.

Although mindfulness has roots in Buddhist meditation, Jon Kabat-Zinn, who founded the Mindfulness-Based Stress Reduction program at the University of Massachusetts Medical School in 1979, introduced the intervention to modern culture. Kabat-Zinn emphasized the need to pay attention to one's breathing, especially during times of intense emotion. He also stressed the importance of noticing sights, sounds, and smells that may change in a moment. Kabat-Zinn is probably best known for the raisin exercise. He encouraged members of his groups to use all of their senses to observe and then taste a single raisin.

Mindfulness advocates believe that it is associated with a number of different physical and psychological benefits. These include stress relief, cardiovascular support, reductions in blood pressure and pain, and improved sleep and gastrointestinal health. In addition, mindfulness has sometimes been included in treatments for depression, substance abuse, eating disorders, anxiety disorders, and obsessive-compulsive disorder.[1]

WHAT THE EXPERTS SAY

Practicing Mindfulness Appears to Improve Emotional Well-Being

In a pilot study published in 2015 in the journal *Explore*, researchers from Chapel Hill, North Carolina, and Knoxville, Tennessee, wanted to learn more about the effect mindfulness would have on the emotional well-being of a community sample of teens. Twenty-eight teens, between the ages of 10 and 18 years, participated. All of them took part in a mindfulness curriculum designed for teens; it was taught in six 90-minute sessions, each dealing with a specific theme—body, thoughts, emotions, attention, loving kindness, and healthy habits. More than half of the teens were females and 79 percent were white. Surveys were conducted before the program began and after it concluded. The researchers found that after participating in the mindfulness classes the teens demonstrated small to moderate positive changes in emotional well-being. They noted that their findings suggested "that mindfulness may be an effective intervention for improving indicators of emotional well-being among an adolescent population."[2]

Mindfulness Appears to Be Useful for At Least Some Psychiatric Disorders

In an open trial published in 2015 in the *Journal of Alternative and Complementary Medicine*, researchers from Durham, North Carolina; Philadelphia, Pennsylvania; Canada; and the United Kingdom wanted to learn more about the association between mindfulness and depression. The initial cohort consisted of 322 adults who were enrolled in an eight-week community-based mindfulness program held at a large academic integrative medical center. Most of the participants were educated white women, and they completed Internet questionnaires before the course began and after they completed it. From the first questionnaire, it was evident that half of the participants had some degree of clinical depression. The researchers found that after completing the mindfulness program the severity of the depressive symptoms "decreased significantly." The researchers commented that "the magnitude of change in depressive symptoms fell in the medium range across nearly all participant subgroups, indicating significance for real-world practice."[3]

In a study published in 2015 online in the journal *Early Intervention in Psychiatry*, researchers from Cincinnati, Ohio, noted that children and teens who have a parent with bipolar disease are at increased risk for anxiety disorders. Yet, medications used to treat anxiety may increase the risk of mania in these children. As a result, the researchers wanted to learn if mindfulness would be useful with these youth. The cohort consisted of eight females and two males with a mean age of 13.2 years. They all had generalized, social, and/or separation anxiety disorders and at least one parent with bipolar disorder. The subjects participated in 12 weekly sessions of mindfulness therapy for children. The researchers learned that increases in the practicing of mindfulness were associated with decreases in anxiety. According to the researchers, "the fact that this correlation is statistically significant in such a small sample is quite compelling."[4]

Mindfulness May Reduce Binge Eating and Emotional Eating

In an analysis published in 2014 in the journal *Eating Behaviors*, researchers from Chicago and Louisville, Kentucky, wanted to determine if mindfulness programs would be useful for binge eating, emotional eating, and weight loss. So, they reviewed the literature and located 14 relevant studies published in peer-reviewed journals. Most of the studies were conducted in the United States; the participants ranged in age from 18 to 75 years. The researchers found that mindfulness interventions significantly reduced binge eating across a range of populations. "Given that binge eating decreased despite such variability in the target population and intervention, mindfulness may be a powerful tool in treating this behavior." And, mindfulness appeared to be useful for people who reported elevated levels of emotional eating. "In addition to reducing binge eating, it appears that mindfulness meditation reduces emotional eating for those who are engaging in this behavior." The evidence on the association between mindfulness and weight loss was mixed and inconclusive. For example, several of the studies failed to find an association between mindfulness and weight loss in the short term, but the researchers commented that "it remains unknown whether mindfulness meditation impacts long-term weight change."[5]

Koru, a Mindfulness Training Program for College Students and Emerging Adults, Is Effective

In a study published in 2014 in the *Journal of American College Health*, researchers from Durham, North Carolina, and Swarthmore, Pennsylvania, wanted to determine the effectiveness of Koru, a mindfulness training program for college students and other emerging adults. Between the fall of 2012 and the spring of 2013, 90 students were assigned to participate in Koru mindfulness training classes, or they were placed on a wait-list control group. (The students in the wait-list control group were offered an opportunity to participate in a Koru class later in the semester.) Almost three-quarters of the students attended a graduate or professional school, and 66 percent of the participants were female. The researchers hypothesized that Koru would reduce perceived stress and sleep problems and increase mindfulness, self-compassion, and gratitude. Before beginning the four-week program, the participants completed an online questionnaire. In addition, the Koru program required that participants meditate for at least 10 minutes a day, complete and return a daily meditation log, and read the required chapters in the course book. The researchers found that after completing the Koru program students had improvements in perceived stress, sleep quality, mindfulness, and self-compassion. The researchers concluded that their findings "supported Koru as a viable intervention for student counseling centers and other agencies that seek to provide cost-effective, low-stigma interventions for students suffering from unmanageable levels of stress."[6]

BARRIERS AND PROBLEMS

Mindfulness Programs May Need to Be Specially Designed to Meet the Needs of Ethnically Diverse At-Risk Teens

In a study published in 2016 in the journal *Mindfulness*, researchers from Chapel Hill, North Carolina; Austin, Texas; and University Park, Pennsylvania, wanted to learn more about the use of mindfulness in ethnically diverse at-risk teens. As a result, the researchers conducted a randomized pilot study of a school-based mindfulness program used with teens who attended an alternative high school in North Carolina for students in grades 9 to 12. Before attending this alternative program, all of the students had struggled academically in traditional high schools. Twenty-seven students were assigned to either a mindfulness program or substance abuse control class. These classes were held for 50 minutes, once a week, for a semester. A number of different modifications were made to accommodate students who had "experienced frequent and often profound disappointments by adults over the course of their lives." For example, the classes were generally held in the gym. Regular classrooms had negative associations for these students. Gym space was linked with positive experiences. More time was devoted to mindfulness body activities and less to sitting activities. The mindfulness instructor often stayed after class to eat lunch with the students. She also visited the school on a second day each week and participated in an elective class, generally involving either sports or board games. As the students developed a relationship with this teacher, "qualitative data revealed that the mindfulness class helped them feel less stressed." At first, the students considered the mindfulness class to be less credible than the substance abuse class. During the course of the semester, the credibility of the mindfulness class increased while the credibility of the substance abuse class decreased. This indicated that the students "grew stronger in their belief that their [mindfulness] class was effective." By the end of the trial, the researchers found small to moderate difference between the two groups for changes in mindfulness, anxiety, and perceived stress and a large difference between the two groups for changes in depression. The researchers commented that the teens who participated in the mindfulness classes appeared to have acquired more protection from their ongoing challenges and appeared to have more resilience to adversity.[7]

A Mindfulness Intervention May Not Reduce Portion Size, So It May Not Support Weight Loss

In a study published in 2014 in the journal *Appetite*, researchers from the Netherlands examined the ability of a brief mindfulness-based intervention to foster healthy eating and reduce portion sizes. The cohort consisted of 110 undergraduate students, with a mean age of 20.9 years. After listening to the 14-minute introduction to an audio-book (not related to health, food, or weight) or performing an audio mindfulness exercise for 14 minutes, the students answered questions about their moods and their audio-recordings. Then, the students were served a small or large portion of chocolate chip cookies, and they were able to eat as many cookies as they wanted. After 10 minutes, the cookies were removed. Whether or not they participated in the mindfulness intervention, the students given the larger portion of cookies ate more than the students with the small portions. The mindfulness intervention did not appear to influence portion size "even when the mindfulness intervention had increased awareness of body sensations."[8]

NOTES

1. Helpguide.org.

2. Karen Bluth, Patricia N. E. Roberson, and Susan A. Gaylord, "A Pilot Study of a Mindfulness Intervention for Adolescents and the Potential Role of Self-Compassion in Reducing Stress," *Explore* 11, no. 4 (2015): 292–95.

3. Jeffrey M. Greeson, Moria J. Smoski, Edward C. Suarez et al., "Decreased Symptoms of Depression After Mindfulness-Based Stress Reduction: Potential Moderating Effects of Religiosity, Spirituality, Trait Mindfulness, Sex, and Age," *Journal of Alternative and Complementary Medicine* 21, no. 3 (2015): 166–74.

4. S. Cotton, C. M. Luberto, R. W. Sears et al., "Mindfulness-Based Cognitive Therapy for Youth with Anxiety Disorders at Risk for Bipolar Disease: A Pilot Trial," *Early Intervention in Psychiatry* (January 2015).

5. Shawn N. Katterman, Brighid M. Kleinman, Megan M. Hood et al., "Mindfulness Meditation as an Intervention for Binge Eating, Emotional Eating, and Weight Loss: A Systematic Review," *Eating Behaviors* 15 (2014): 197–204.

6. J. M. Greeson, M. K. Juberg, M. Maytan et al., "A Randomized Controlled Trial of Koru: A Mindfulness Program for College Students and Other Emerging Adults," *Journal of American College Health* 62, no. 4 (2014): 222–33.

7. Karen Bluth, Rebecca A. Campo, Sarah Pruteanu-Malinici et al., "A School-Based Mindfulness Pilot Study for Ethnically Diverse At-Risk Adolescents," *Mindfulness* 7, no. 1 (2016): 90–94.

8. David Marchiori and Esther K. Papies, "A Brief Mindfulness Intervention Reduces Unhealthy Eating When Hungry, but Not the Portion Size Effect," *Appetite* 75 (2014): 40–45.

REFERENCES AND RESOURCES

Magazines, Journals, and Newspapers

Bluth, Karen, Patricia N. E. Roberson, and Susan A. Gaylord. "A Pilot Study of a Mindfulness Intervention for Adolescents and the Potential Role of Self-Compassion in Reducing Stress." *Explore* 11, no. 4 (2015): 292–95.

Bluth, Karen, Rebecca A. Campo, Sarah Pruteanu-Malinici et al. "A School-Based Mindfulness Pilot Study for Ethnically Diverse At-Risk Adolescents." *Mindfulness* 7, no. 1 (2016): 90–94.

Cotton, S., C. M. Luberto, R. W. Sears et al. "Mindfulness-Based Cognitive Therapy for Youth with Anxiety Disorders At Risk for Bipolar Disorder: A Pilot Trial." *Early Intervention In Psychiatry* (January 2015).

Greeson, J. M., M. K. Juberg, M. Maytan et al. "A Randomized Controlled Trial of Koru: A Mindfulness Program for College Students and Other Emerging Adults." *Journal of American College Health* 62, no. 4 (2014): 222–33.

Greeson, Jeffrey M., Moria J. Smoski, Edward C. Suarez et al. "Decreased Symptoms of Depression After Mindfulness-Based Stress Reduction: Potential Moderating Effects of Religiosity. Spirituality, Trait Mindfulness, Sex, and Age." *Journal of Alternative and Complementary Medicine* 21, no. 3 (2015): 166–74.

Katterman, Shawn N., Brighid M. Kleinman, Megan M. Hood et al. "Mindfulness Meditation as an Intervention for Binge Eating, Emotional Eating, and Weight Loss: A Systematic Review." *Eating Behaviors* 15 (2014): 197–204.

Marchiori, David, and Esther K. Papies. "A Brief Mindfulness Intervention Reduces Unhealthy Eating When Hungry, but Not the Portion Size Effect." *Appetite* 75 (2014): 40–45.

Olson, KayLoni L., and Charles F. Emery. "Mindfulness and Weight Loss: A Systematic Review." *Psychosomatic Medicine* 77 (2015): 59–67.

Ussher, Michael, Amy Spatz, Claire Copland et al. "Immediate Effects of a Brief Mindfulness-Based Body Scan on Patients with Chronic Pain." *Journal of Behavioral Medicine* 37 (2014): 127–34.

Web Site

Helpguide.org.

Sex and Dating

Get Screened for STIs

OVERVIEW

All teens and young adults who are sexually active need to use protection, such as a condom, and should be tested for sexually transmitted infections. Not all sexually transmitted infections have recognizable signs and symptoms that will trigger a visit to a medical provider. While they may have no signs or symptoms, untreated sexually transmitted infections may exact a toll on the body. STIs that can be tested for include herpes, human papillomavirus (HPV), human immunodeficiency virus (HIV), chlamydia, gonorrhea, and syphilis. Depending on the STI, screening may be done via a blood or urine test or a swab and cell culture.

WHAT THE EXPERTS SAY

Chlamydia Test Results Were Associated with Behavior Changes

In a study published in 2015 in *Sexually Transmitted Diseases*, researchers from the Netherlands wanted to learn how the results of a chlamydia test influenced subsequent sexual risk behavior. The cohort consisted of men and women, between the ages of 16 and 19 years, who participated in at least two of the four rounds (n= 6,802) of the Chlamydia Screening Implementation. The researchers found that those who tested positive for chlamydia were more likely to practice more protective behaviors. And, those who had negative results were more likely to practice riskier behaviors. Large differences between the two groups were seen on condom use with a casual partner. Specifically, people who had tested positive for chlamydia were far less likely to report that they never used a condom with a causal partner, and people who had tested negative for chlamydia were less likely to indicate that they always used a condom with a casual partner. The researchers concluded that the chlamydia test results "were associated with subsequent sexual risk behavior." They advised more research into the responses to the negative test.[1]

Concurrent Sexual Relationships Increase the Risk of HIV for Young Adults Who Are Heterosexual

In a study published in 2015 in *Sexually Transmitted Diseases*, researchers from several locations in the United States wanted to learn more about the association between HIV and the frequency and types of sexual concurrency in young adults. They also examined other factors, such as condom use. The researchers recruited 261 men and 275 women between the ages of 18 and 30 years from community locations in Los Angeles. During a 12-month period, the participants completed four in-person interviews. Data were collected on four types of dating concurrency. Transitional concurrency occurred when a second relationship began before the first one ended. Single-day concurrency took place when a single-day relationship happened while a person was already in a relationship. Contained concurrency is the beginning and ending of a relationship while still in another relationship. And, multiple concurrency is when someone is in three or more relationships at the same time. At baseline, 47 percent of the men and 32 percent of the women reported some form of concurrency during the previous four months. A striking 26 percent of the men and 10 percent of the women reported multiple concurrencies. Condom use ranged from 56 percent to 64 percent, with the highest in the transitional concurrency. All types of concurrency appeared to increase the risk of acquiring and spreading sexually transmitted infections. Given such high numbers, the researchers suggested that there is a need for more preventive interventions. "It is critical that health care providers discuss the risk of concurrency with their young adult patients." In addition, "broader media campaigns . . . could be used to raise awareness of the potential consequences of involvement in extended sexual networks and the part concurrency plays in persistent epidemics of STIs [sexually transmitted infections] in the United States."[2]

Self-Collected Samples May Help Screen Women at Increased Risk

In a study published in 2015 online in the journal *Sexually Transmitted Infections*, researchers from several locations in the United States noted that women who are behaviorally bisexual (women who have sex with men and women) are more likely than women who have sex exclusively with women or exclusively with men to report a history of sexually transmitted infections. As a result, the researchers wanted to determine if these women would be willing to collect their own oral, vaginal, and anal samples for testing. The initial cohort consisted of 80 women from two Midwestern locations. After these women completed an online questionnaire, 54 women were interviewed and asked to self-collect the samples. They ranged in age between 18 and 46 years. Only a small percentage of the samples was positive. Still, the researchers found that the women were compliant in submitting the samples. The researchers commented that self-collection may be especially useful for these women who may not have disclosed to their healthcare providers that they had sex with men and women. This has the potential to "increase testing and treatment among an underserved and often invisible population of women."[3]

Pharmacists May Also Play a Role in Screening for Sexually Transmitted Infections

In a study published in 2013 in *Sexually Transmitted Diseases*, researchers from Kansas City, Missouri, investigated the role that pharmacists may serve in screening and treatment for sexually transmitted infections. Participants were recruited from a Kansas City free health clinic between May 3, 2010, and October 14, 2010. A confidential survey was completed by 164 participants. Of these, 86.3 percent indicated an "overwhelming acceptance" of a pharmacist as their treatment provider. The participants were most comfortable with the pharmacist running a urine screen, treating sexually transmitted infections, and discussing the results of the tests. They were a little less comfortable with the pharmacists performing physical examinations. But, almost everyone approved of pharmacists working in collaboration with a physician. The researchers commented that "a pharmacist prepared with the clinical skills to screen a patient for STIs, discuss test results, and then recommend, select, administer, and manage STI medication therapy could prove an invaluable resource and asset to the public health care team."[4]

BARRIERS AND PROBLEMS

Opportunities to Screen for HIV May Be Missed

In a study published in 2009 in *AIDS Patient Care and STDs*, researchers based in Oakland, California, noted that in 2005 the Department of Emergency Medicine at Alameda County Medical Center implemented an HIV testing program. Was the program working? They did not know. So, the researchers conducted a review of medical records and attempted to identify screening opportunities that were missed. The researchers learned that from April 1, 2005, to November 31, 2006, there were 112,544 age-eligible Emergency Department visits, and 9,130 HIV tests were performed. Ninety-five previously undiagnosed patients tested positive. Of these, 66 were diagnosed during their first emergency visit, but 29 people made a total of 59 visits before testing positive. The researchers noted that "missed opportunities for earlier HIV diagnosis occurred frequently despite an HIV screening program."[5]

Medical Providers May Not Be Ordering All the Tests That They Should

In a study published in 2014 in *Sexually Transmitted Diseases*, researchers from Atlanta, Georgia, noted that men who have sex with other men are at increased risk for sexually transmitted infections. To protect their health and the health of other men, these men need more screening for these infections. Yet, it has become apparent that these men are receiving suboptimal levels of screening. The researchers wanted to better understand the barriers to these needed medical services. So, they conducted 40 semistructured interviews with medical providers of HIV-infected men who have sex with men (at eight large HIV clinics in six U.S. cities). Providers were asked about their screening procedures for sexually transmitted infections and the barriers they had to conducting sexual risk assessments of their patients. While the medical providers screened frequently for syphilis, the screenings for chlamydia and gonorrhea did not happen as often. The researchers found that the obstacles that prevented these tests included time constraints, problems with obtaining a sexual history, language and cultural barriers, and patient confidentially concerns. The researchers concluded that "providers reported many obstacles to routine chlamydia and gonorrhea screening." Therefore, "interventions are needed to help mitigate barriers to STD screening, such as structural and patient-directed health series models that might facilitate increased testing coverage of these important preventive services."[6]

Out-of-Pocket Costs to Patients May Play a Role in Limiting Tests

In a study published in 2013 in the *International Journal of STD & AIDS*, researchers from New Orleans; Wilmington, Delaware; and Columbia, South Carolina, wanted to determine if the out-of-pocket costs associated with chlamydia and gonorrhea screening tests were barriers to follow-up and annual screening. The researchers used data from a major health insurance claims database (2006–2010). When they compared the chlamydia patients without out-of-pocket expenses, the researchers found that those with out-of-pocket expenses of $30 or more "had significantly reduced likelihood of receiving re-screening and annual screening." The researchers found similar results for gonorrhea patients. They concluded that out-of-pocket costs "served as a significant barrier to re-screening and annual screening."[7]

NOTES

1. Loes C. Soetens, Birgit H. B. van Benthem, and Eline L. M. Op de Coul, "Chlamydia Test Results Were Associated with Sexual Risk Behavior Change Among Participants of the Chlamydia Screening Implementation in the Netherlands," *Sexually Transmitted Diseases* 42, no. 3 (2015): 109–14.

2. Jocelyn T. Warren, S. Marie Harvey, Isaac Joel Washburn et al., "Concurrent Sexual Partnerships Among Young Heterosexual Adults at Increased HIV Risk: Types and Characteristics," *Sexually Transmitted Diseases* 42, no. 4 (2015): 180–84.

3. Vanessa Schick, Barbara Van Der Pol, Brian Dodge et al., 2015. "A Mixed Methods Approach to Assess the Likelihood of Testing for STI Using Self-Collection Samples

Among Behaviourally Bisexual Women," *Sexually Transmitted Infections* 91, no. 5 (2015): 329–33.

4. Sara J. Deppe, Chessa R. Nyberg, Brooke Y. Patterson et al., "Expanding the Role of a Pharmacist as a Sexually Transmitted Infection Provider in the Setting of an Urban Free Health Clinic," *Sexually Transmitted Diseases* 40, no. 9 (2013): 685–88.

5. Douglas A. E. White, Otis U. Warren, Alicia N. Scribner, and Bradley W. Frazee, "Missed Opportunities for Earlier HIV Diagnosis in an Emergency Department Despite an HIV Screening Program," *AIDS Patient Care and STDs* 23, no. 4 (2009): 245–50.

6. Jarvis W. Carter, Geoffrey D. Hart-Cooper, Mary O. Butler et al., "Provider Barriers Prevent Recommended Sexually Transmitted Disease Screening of HIV-Infected Men Who Have Sex With Men," *Sexually Transmitted Diseases* 41, no. 2 (2014): 137–42.

7. L. Shi, Y. Xie, J. Liu et al., "Is Out-of-Pocket Cost a Barrier to Receiving Repeat Tests for Chlamydia and Gonorrhoea?" *International Journal of STD & AIDS* 24 (2013): 301–6.

REFERENCES AND RESOURCES

Magazines, Journals, and Newspapers

Bechtel, Mark A., and Wayne Trout. "Sexually Transmitted Diseases." *Clinical Obstetrics and Gynecology* 58, no. 1 (2015): 172–84.

Carter, Jarvis W., Geoffrey D. Hart-Cooper, Mary O. Butler, et al. "Provider Barriers Prevent Recommended Sexually Transmitted Disease Screening of HIV-Infected Men Who Have Sex With Men." *Sexually Transmitted Diseases* 41, no. 2 (2014): 137–42.

Chan, Philip A., Justine Maher, Daniele Poole et al. "Addressing the Increasing Burden of Sexually Transmitted Infections in Rhode Island." *Rhode Island Medical Journal* 98, no. 1 (2015): 31–34.

Deppe, Sara J., Chessa R. Nyberg, Brooke Y. Patterson et al. "Expanding the Role of a Pharmacist as a Sexually Transmitted Infection Provider in the Setting of an Urban Free Health Clinic." *Sexually Transmitted Diseases* 40, no. 9 (2013): 685–88.

Falasinnu, T., M. Gilbert, P. Gustafson, and J. Shoveller. "Deriving and Validating a Risk Estimation Tool for Screening Asymptomatic Chlamydia and Gonorrhea." *Sexually Transmitted Diseases* 41, no. 12 (2014): 706–12.

Li, De-Kun, Marsha A. Raebel, T. Craig Cheetham et al. "Genital Herpes and Its Treatment in Relation to Preterm Delivery." *American Journal of Epidemiology* 180, no. 11 (2014): 1109–17.

Schick, Vanessa, Barbara Van Der Pol, Brian Dodge et al. "A Mixed Methods Approach to Assess the Likelihood of Testing for STI Using Self-Collected Samples Among Behaviourally Bisexual Women." *Sexually Transmitted Infections* 91, no. 5 (2015): 329–33.

Shi, L., Y. Xie, J. Liu et al. "Is Out-of-Pocket Cost a Barrier to Receiving Repeat Tests for Chlamydia and Gonorrhoea?" *International Journal of STD & AIDS* 24 (2013): 301–6.

Soetens, Loes C., Birgit H. B. van Benthem, and Eline L. M. Op de Coul. "Chlamydia Test Results Were Associated with Sexual Risk Behavior Change Among Participants of the Chlamydia Screening Implementation in the Netherlands." *Sexually Transmitted Diseases* 42, no. 3 (2015): 109–14.

Warren, Jocelyn T., S. Marie Harvey, Isaac Joel Washburn et al. "Concurrent Sexual Partnerships Among Young Heterosexual Adults at Increased HIV Risk: Types and Characteristics." *Sexually Transmitted Diseases* 42, no. 4 (2015): 180–84.

White, Douglas A. E., Otis U. Warren, Alicia N. Scribner, and Bradley W. Frazee. "Missed Opportunities for Earlier HIV Diagnosis in an Emergency Department Despite an HIV Screening Program." *AIDS Patient Care and STDs* 23, no. 4 (2009): 245–50.
Yehia, Baligh R., Wanjun Cui, William W. Thompson et al. "HIV Testing Among Adults with Mental Illness." *AIDS Patient Care and STDs* 28, no. 12 (2014): 628–34.

Web Sites

Centers for Disease Control and Prevention. www.cdc.gov.
Planned Parenthood. www.plannedparenthood.org.

Get Vaccinated for HPV (Human Papillomavirus)

OVERVIEW

The human papillomavirus or HPV is the most common sexually transmitted infection. In fact, it is so common that just about all sexually active males and females will contract it at some point in their lives. About 79 million Americans are now infected with HPV. The association between HPV and genital warts and cervical cancer is well established. So, it should surprise no one that every year, about 360,000 people in the United States are diagnosed with genital warts and about 11,000 women are diagnosed with cervical cancer.

HPV may be transmitted via vaginal, anal, or oral sex. There are many different varieties of this virus. Some types are not associated with health problems. However, others have been found to be related to the previously noted genital warts and cervical cancer as well cancers of the vulva, vagina, penis, anus, tongue, and/or back of the throat (oropharyngeal cancer). And, symptoms may appear shortly after exposure or take years to emerge. At present, it is unclear why certain people with HPV develop symptoms and others do not. It is thought that people with weakened immune symptoms are at increased risk. Most people with HPV do not realize they are infected until symptoms appear.

The U.S. Advisory Committee on Immunization Practices (ACIP) recommends that male and female preteens, aged 11 or 12 years, be vaccinated with a licensed HPV vaccine. Vaccination is also recommended for females aged 13 through 26 years and males 13 through 21 years.[1] Currently, there are three vaccines—Cervarix, Gardasil, and Gardasil 9. Because all the vaccines provide protection from cervical cancer, females may be vaccinated with any of these three vaccines. Gardasil and Gardasil 9 provide additional safeguards. In females, they also protect against genital warts, and vulvar, vaginal, and anal cancers. In males, they protect against genital warts and anal cancer. Males should be vaccinated with Gardasil or Gardasil 9. For those males who have sex with males or who are immunocompromised or have HIV, the ACIP recommends vaccination through age 26 years.[2]

The vaccines are given in three separate shots over a six-month period of time. To obtain the maximum effectiveness, you must have all three shots. There are also "catch-up" vaccines, which are recommended for males up to 21 years and females through 26 years. These are for males and females who were not vaccinated when they were younger.[3] According to an article published in 2015 in *Primary Care: Clinics in Office Practice*, the vaccines "have been shown [to] be highly efficacious." But, they are expensive. At present, each dose costs between $130 and $170, which does not include administration charges. While most health insurance plans cover these costs, there are some that do not. Eligible uninsured and underinsured children under the age of 19 may be covered by the U.S. Government's Vaccines for Children Program.[4]

WHAT THE EXPERTS SAY

HPV Vaccination Does Not Appear to Be Associated with Riskier Sexual Behaviors

In a study published in 2014 in *Pediatrics*, researchers from New York City, Ohio, and Indiana commented that some people have raised concerns that the use of the HPV vaccine will trigger higher rates of risky sexual behaviors. The cohort consisted of 339 females between the ages of 13 and 21 years who were patients at a hospital-based adolescent primary care center. They completed questionnaires immediately after HPV vaccination and two and six months later. However, not everyone returned for the follow-ups. There were 280 (82.6 percent) for the two-month follow-up and 258 (76.1 percent) for the six-month follow-up. The researchers found no association between risk perceptions immediately after vaccination and sexual risk behaviors over the subsequent six months in sexually experienced and inexperienced young women. The researchers commented that their study offered "reassuring evidence that changes in risk perceptions after vaccination are not associated with riskier sexual behaviors, providing additional support for the increasing evidence that HPV vaccination does not lead to changes in sexual behaviors among adolescents."[5]

Implementation of HPV Vaccine Reduced Incidence of Genital Warts

In a study published in 2013 in *Sexually Transmitted Diseases*, researchers from Denmark noted that about 90 percent of genital warts are caused by HPV. Since Denmark has been providing HPV vaccines for several years, it is a good place to check the vaccine's effectiveness against genital warts. Using data from the Danish

National Patient Register, the researchers found that since the introduction of the vaccine program in 2008 and 2009 the incidence of genital warts has been declining. The decrease was greatest for younger women, especially those who were 17 years old and younger. The researchers concluded that their findings "provide strong, plausible indications for a protective effect of the . . . HPV vaccine at general population level."[6]

The HPV Vaccine Appears to Be Very Safe

In a study published in 2013 in *Human Vaccine & Immunotherapeutics*, researchers from Italy wanted to learn more about the safety of the HPV vaccine. So, they recruited 271 women who were all 25 years old to have the HPV vaccines. Only 213 of these women received all three doses of the vaccine. Still, there were no serious adverse events related to the vaccine. The most common side effect was localized pain at the vaccination site. That was followed by localized swelling and the elevation of body temperature (fever). The researchers noted that their results were similar to previous studies conducted on preadolescent Italian girls. "Fever and local pain were however more frequently registered in our sample of adult women."[7]

School-Based Educational Programs Increase Knowledge About HPV and HPV Vaccine

In an article published in 2011 in *Cancer Epidemiology, Biomarkers & Prevention*, researchers from Ohio and North Carolina conducted one-time HPV education sessions with groups of people who have close contact with adolescent females. These included sessions with 376 parents, 118 healthcare staff, and 456 school staff. And, the participants completed self-administered surveys. Before the sessions, the participants knew little about HPV and HPV vaccines. Following the sessions, all the participants knew a great deal more. In fact, more than 90 percent of the school staff members "believed HPV and HPV vaccine education is worthwhile for school personnel and that middle schools are an appropriate venue for this education." And, 97 percent of parents and 85 percent of school staff members noted that they would support school-based vaccination clinics. "Education interventions represent a simple yet potentially effective strategy for increasing HPV vaccination and garnering support for school-based vaccination clinics."[8]

BARRIERS AND PROBLEMS

In the United States Rates of HPV Vaccination Remain Low, Especially in Certain Groups

In a study published in 2013 in *Human Vaccines & Imunotherapeutics*, researchers from Boston noted that there are relatively low rates of HPV vaccination among all adolescents in the United States, and the rates are even worse among minority and low-income adolescents. Thus, according to these researchers, when compared to white women, the incidence and mortality of cervical cancer in black women are, respectively, 25 percent and 95 percent higher. In Latino women, the incidence and mortality are, respectively, 53 percent and 41 percent higher. Moreover, the incidence of cervical cancer is twice as high in counties with poverty levels above 20 percent than it is in counties with poverty levels below 10 percent. And, since chronic HPV infection causes 99.7 percent of invasive cervical cancers, higher vaccination rates are needed. Only about 53 percent of female adolescents start the HPV vaccine process and only about 35 percent complete it. When compared to their white counterparts, black females are half as likely to complete their HPV vaccinations. These poor rates of HPV vaccination contrast sharply with other countries such as England and Canada where the rates have as many as 80 percent of the female teens obtaining all three doses. The researchers concluded that there is a need for more patient-targeted interventions that focus on completing all three HPV vaccinations. "With an integrated initiative focused on HPV awareness, widespread vaccination should be achievable across all races and demographics."[9]

Healthcare Providers May Not Be Sufficiently Persuasive in Encouraging a Timely Administration of HPV

In a study published in 2014 in *Pediatrics*, researchers from several locations in Massachusetts investigated the reasons parents or guardians give for delaying the administration of the HPV vaccine in their daughters aged 11 to 17 years. The researchers conducted interviews with 124 parents/guardians in one public clinic and three private practice settings. The research also included 37 providers. The most often cited reason for not vaccinating their daughters was the lack of a physician recommendation. Apparently, providers were delaying the recommendation in girls whom they perceived to be at a low risk for sexual activity. On the other hand, providers who vaccinate more people described the HPV vaccine as a routine vaccine with a proven safety record used to prevent cancer. When presented in that framework, parents responded positively. According to the researchers, by connecting HPV vaccination to the onset of sexual activity, providers miss opportunities to vaccinate. "Routine recommending HPV vaccination as cancer prevention to be coadministered with other vaccines at age 11 years can improve vaccination rates."[10]

Insurance and Financial Barriers to HPV Vaccination

In a study published 2012 in the *American Journal of Managed Care*, researchers based in Los Angeles examined the role that insurance and income play in the rates of HPV vaccination. The researchers used data from the 2007 California Health Interview Survey, a representative random-dial telephone survey of more than 53,600 households, including about 51,000 adults. Since the interviews were conducted in a number of different languages, including English, Spanish, Mandarin, Cantonese, Korean, and Vietnamese, the data was obtained from people with diverse backgrounds. The cohort consisted of 1,840 females between the ages of 18 and 26 years and 5,765 females between the ages of 8 and 17 years. The questions were answered by the parents. The researchers learned that most of the parents had heard about the HPV vaccine. However, only 16 percent of the older females and 21 percent of the younger females had received at least one dose. When compared to those who had private HMO (health maintenance organization) coverage, the uninsured were less likely to have had this dose. "Disparities in receipt of the HPV vaccine are likely to continue without targeted outreach to more vulnerable populations."[11]

NOTES

1. Advisory Committee on Immunization Practices, www.cdc.gov/vaccines/acip.

2. Ibid.

3. Centers for Disease Control and Prevention, www.cdc.gov.

4. Lisa S. Gilmer, "Human Papillomavirus Vaccine Update," *Primary Care: Clinics in Office Practice* 42 (2015): 17–32.

5. Allison Mayhew, Tanya L. Kowalczyk Mullins, Lili Ding et al., "Risk Perceptions and Subsequent Sexual Behaviors After HPV Vaccination in Adolescents," *Pediatrics* 133 (2014): 404–11.

6. Louise Baandrup, Maria Blomberg, Christian Dehlendorff et al., "Significant Decrease in the Incidence of Genital Warts in Young Danish Women After Implementation of a National Human Papillomavirus Vaccination Program," *Sexually Transmitted Diseases* 40, no. 2 (2013): 130–35.

7. Miriam Levi, Paolo Bonanni, Elena Burroni et al., "Evaluation of Bivalent Human Papillomavirus (HPV) Vaccine Safety and Tolerability in a Sample of 25 Year Old Tuscan Women," *Human Vaccines & Immunotherapeutics* 9, no. 7 (2013): 1407–12.

8. Paul L. Reiter, Brenda Stubbs, Catherine A. Panozzo et al., "HPV and HPV Vaccine Education Intervention: Effects on Parents, Healthcare Staff, and School Staff," *Cancer Epidemiology, Biomarkers & Prevention* 20, no. 11 (2011): 2354–61.

9. Patricia Jeudin, Elizabeth Liveright, Marcela G. del Carmen, and Rebecca B. Perkins, "Race, Ethnicity and Income as Factors for HPV Vaccine Acceptance and Use," *Human Vaccines & Immunotherapeutics* 9, no. 7 (2013): 1413–20.

10. Rebecca B. Perkins, Jack A. Clark, Gauri Apte et al., "Missed Opportunities for HPV Vaccination in Adolescent Girls: A Qualitative Study," *Pediatrics* 134, no. 3 (2014): e666–e674.

11. Nadereh Pourat and Jenna M. Jones, "Role of Insurance, Income, and Affordability in Human Papillomavirus Vaccination," *American Journal of Managed Care* 18, no. 6 (2012): 320–30.

REFERENCES AND RESOURCES

Magazines, Journals, and Newspapers

Baandrup, Louise, Maria Blomberg, Christian Dehlendorff et al. "Significant Decrease in the Incidence of Genital Warts in Young Danish Women After Implementation of a National Human Papillomavirus Vaccination Program." *Sexually Transmitted Diseases* 40, no. 2 (2013): 130–35.

Gerend, Mary A., and Janet E. Shepherd. "Correlates of HPV Knowledge in the Era of HPV Vaccination: A Study of Unvaccinated Young Adult Women." *Women & Health* 51, no. 1 (2011): 25–40.

Gilmer, Lisa S. "Human Papillomavirus Vaccine Update." *Primary Care: Clinics in Office Practice* 42 (2015): 17–32.

Jeudin, Patricia, Elizabeth Liveright, Marcela G. del Carmen, and Rebecca B. Perkins. "Race, Ethnicity and Income As Factors for HPV Vaccine Acceptance and Use." *Human Vaccines & Immunotherapeutics* 9, no. 7 (2013): 1413–20.

Kharbanda, Elyse Olshen, Emily Parker, James D. Nordin et al. "Receipt of Human Papillomavirus Vaccine Among Privately Insured Adult Women in a U. S. Midwestern Health Maintenance Organization." *Preventive Medicine* 57 (2013): 712–14.

Langer-Gould, A., L. Qian, S. Y. Tartof, S. M. Bara et al. "Vaccines and the Risk of Multiple Sclerosis and Other Central Nervous System Demyelinating Diseases." *JAMA Neurology* 71, no. 12 (2014): 1506–13.

Levi, Miriam, Paolo Bonanni, Elena Burroni et al. "Evaluation of Bivalent Human Papillomavirus (HPV) Vaccine Safety and Tolerability in a Sample of 25 Year Old Tuscan Women." *Human Vaccines & Immunotherapeutics* 9, no. 7 (2013): 1407–12.

Mayhew, Allison, Tanya L. Kowalczyk Mullins, Lili Ding et al. "Risk Perceptions and Subsequent Sexual Behaviors After HPV Vaccination in Adolescents." *Pediatrics* 133 (2014): 404–11.

Perkins, Rebecca B., Jack A. Cark, Gauri Apte et al. "Missed Opportunities for HPV Vaccination in Adolescent Girls: A Qualitative Study." *Pediatrics* 134, no. 3 (2014): e666–e674.

Pourat, Nadereh, and Jenna M. Jones. "Role of Insurance, Income, and Affordability in Human Papillomavirus." *American Journal of Managed Care* 18, no. 6 (2012): 320–30.

Reiter, Paul, Noel T. Brewer, Annie-Laurie McRee et al. "Acceptability of HPV Vaccine Among a National Sample of Gay and Bisexual Men." *Sexually Transmitted Diseases* 37, no. 3 (2011): 197–203.

Reiter, Paul L., Brenda Stubbs, Catherine A. Panozzo et al. "HPV and HPV Vaccine Education Intervention: Effects on Parents, Healthcare Staff, and School Staff." *Cancer Epidemiology Biomarkers & Prevention* 20, no. 11 (2011): 2354–61.

Topan, Aysel, Ozlem Ozturk, Hulya Eroglu et al. "Knowledge Level of Working and Student Nurses on Cervical Cancer and Human Papilloma Virus Vaccines." *Asian Pacific Journal of Cancer Prevention* 16, no. 6 (2014): 2515–19.

Web Sites

Advisory Committee on Immunization Practices. www.cdc.gov/vaccines/acip.
Centers for Disease Control and Prevention. www.cdc.gov.

Cultivate Healthy Dating Relationships

OVERVIEW

During the adolescent years, it is perfectly normal to have a number of different dating relationships. That is how teens learn what they like and dislike in a boyfriend or girlfriend and in a dating relationship. When dating, it is important to create healthy relationships. Healthy relationships may take a variety of forms, but they tend to include a few key components, such as mutual respect and trust. Other elements are honesty, support in good and bad times, good communication, and fairness. It is also important to maintain a sense of independence. A healthy relationship does not require being together every free moment. In fact, in a healthy relationship each person pursues his or her own individual responsibilities, friends, and interests. These characteristics are in contrast to an unhealthy relationship, which may include mean, disrespectful, controlling, and/or abusive behavior.

Although there are many long-married adults who met as teens and have been together for decades, most teen dating relationships do not continue for extended periods of times. Teens are still growing and changing. It is not uncommon for teens to evolve out of a relationship. That is part of the teen dating process.

Whenever possible, it is a good idea for teens to discuss healthy relationships with their parents. And, it is an equally good idea for parents to try to model healthy relationships for their teens.

WHAT THE EXPERTS SAY

Teens Cite Specific Characteristics They Want in a Healthy Dating Relationship

In a study published in 2014 in the *Journal of Primary Prevention*, researchers from Baltimore and College Park, Maryland, wanted to learn more about how teens characterize healthy dating relationships. So, they conducted one-on-one, semistructured, in-depth interviews with 33 African American girls between the ages of 15 and 18 years, from public and private schools. The three most commonly mentioned characteristics were trust, good communication, and honesty. They were followed by respect, self-confidence, individuality, understanding, and compromise. The researchers commented that the "girls possessed a general understanding of qualities that they should look for in healthy romantic relationships." Why is that so important? "Given the potential for unhealthy relationships to negatively affect adolescent functioning, it is critically important to help girls identify healthy relationships and encourage their participation in dating relationships that are free of harm."[1]

A Community-Based Interactive Theater Program May Help Middle School Students Learn to Form Healthier Relationships

In an article published in 2010 in the *Journal of Community Health Nursing*, a researcher from Austin, Texas, described a community-based interactive theater program designed to help middle school students learn to form healthier relationships. The cohort consisted of 114 primarily Hispanic seventh-grade health class students who lived in an underserved rural school district in Central Texas.

The program included three consecutive theater performances and one follow-up performance; each was about 50 minutes in length. A total of 24 performances took place during a three-week period of time. The topics of respect, bullying, and sexual harassment were interwoven into the play. Qualitative responses from the students indicated that the majority considered the program to be "a positive experience." Based on what they had learned, the students anticipated that their future behavior would change. The researcher noted that "creative, appealing programs using community-based participatory research (CBPR) methods can be an effective means of teaching youth how to recognize and form healthy peer and beginning romantic relationships."[2]

A College-Based Course on Relationship Education May Improve Relationships

In a study published in 2010 in the *Journal of Family Psychology*, researchers from Utah and Florida investigated the effectiveness of college-based relationship education on improving the fidelity of college students in committed romantic relationships. The cohort consisted of 380 college students. The intervention group had about five times as many students as the control group. For the intervention group, the relationship education program was integrated into existing college courses. It included information on partner selection, healthy relationship transitions, communication skills, and the potentially negative consequences of cheating and how to prevent cheating from occurring. The students in the control group did not receive relationship education. At baseline, 11 percent of the students admitted to having sexual intercourse with someone other than their romantic partner, 13 percent said they had sexual behavior but not sex, 44 percent indicated they caressed and hugged, and 22 percent noted that they kissed. When compared to the students in the control group, the students who received the intervention were less likely to commit unfaithful acts. As a result, the researchers concluded that this educational intervention reduced the overall frequency of acts of infidelity over the course of a semester. This was especially true for females.[3]

People in Healthier Same-Sex Relationships Have Fewer Depressive Symptoms

In a study published in 2014 in the *Journal of Family Psychology*, researchers from the University of Cincinnati examined the association between the healthfulness of a same-sex romantic relationship and depressive symptoms. The cohort consisted of a geographically diverse sample of 571 adults (62 percent women) in the United States who are in same-sex relationships. They completed online surveys that asked several questions about their relationships and individual characteristics. The researchers found a moderately negative association between relationship quality and depressive symptoms, which is similar to results obtained from heterosexual couples. There were no gender differences. The researchers commented that "the robust association between relationship quality and depressive symptoms observed in this sample highlights the potential importance of intimate relationships to the well-being of LGBT adults."[4]

Sisters Teach Each Other About Healthy Dating Relationships

In an observational study published in 2014 in the journal *Family Relations*, researchers from the University of Missouri investigated sibling communication about dating and sexuality. The cohort consisted of 28 dyads who were recruited through community organizations and videotaped during their conversations. All of the younger sisters were in high school. On average, the younger sisters were 15.76 years, and the older sisters were 19.03 years. The average age gap between the sisters was 3.28 years.

The researchers determined that the sisters functioned in three different roles—confidants, sources of support, and mentors. While older and younger sisters served as confidants and sources of support for each other, the older sisters were more likely to be mentors for their younger sisters. The researchers emphasized that their findings indicated "the potential importance of sisters in the formation of adolescent girls' ideas about romantic relationships and sexuality." In addition, because of older sisters' mentoring role, they may be useful "in prevention intervention programs focused on reducing adolescent sexual risk behaviors and promoting healthy romantic relationships and sexual development."[5]

BARRIERS AND PROBLEMS

Frequent Users of Facebook Have an Increased Risk of Problematic Relationships

In a study published in 2013 in *Cyberpsychology, Behavior, and Social Networking*, researchers from Missouri, Hawaii, and Texas wanted to learn more about the association between using the social networking site Facebook and the inability to maintain healthy relationships. The researchers surveyed 205 Facebook users, between the ages of 18 and 82 years, about their use of Facebook and negative relationship outcomes. The researchers found an association between high levels of Facebook use and negative relationship outcomes for people who have been together three years or less. The high level of Facebook use appears to play a role in damaging interpersonal relationships. Moreover, these relationships were mediated by Facebook-related conflict. The researchers suggested that Facebook use may contribute to emotional and physical cheating and/or break-ups. The researchers concluded that "high levels of Facebook use, when mediated by Facebook-related conflict, significantly predict negative relationship outcomes."[6]

There Is a Prevailing Fear of Dating Violence and Relationship Abuse

In a study published in 2014 in the journal *Research in Nursing & Health*, researchers from Florida wanted to learn more about the perceptions Cuban American teens and their parents have about dating relationships. The researchers held a total of eight focus groups that included 29 ninth-grade teens, 29 parents or primary caretakers, and 16 school personnel. The teens, the parents/caretakers, and the school personnel each had separate groups that only included their peers. All the teens, who were between the ages of 13 and 16 years, attended an urban public high school in Miami-Dade County where 97 percent the population was of Hispanic origin. Most frequently, the students reported that they were of Cuban descent. During the focus groups, parents, students, and school personnel all expressed concern about teen dating violence in their community. And, they maintained that adolescents of Hispanic origin had an increased risk for dating violence because of factors such as early sexual initiation. Furthermore, the participants noted generational differences in dating norms, and the influences of school, community, and society presented challenges to maintaining healthy relationships. For example, while parents viewed relationships that included sex to be serious, the teens considered sex to be a normal part of the relationship. The teens felt that abuse was a frequent part of relationships, and they reported that boyfriends and girlfriends often embarrassed each other in public and used "foul" language in their communication.[7]

In Some High-Risk Urban Areas Middle School Students Are Faced with High Rates of Teen Dating Violence

In a study published in 2015 in the *Journal of Adolescent Health*, researchers from Georgia and Illinois wanted to learn more about the prevalence of teen dating violence in a sample of middle school students from high-risk urban communities. The cohort consisted of 1,653 middle school students from Alameda County, California; Baltimore, Maryland; Broward County, Florida; and Chicago. All of the students had dated, and there were slightly more females than males.

The results were truly stunning. Seventy-seven percent of the students reported perpetrating verbal/emotional abuse; 32 percent reported perpetrating physical abuse; 20 percent reported threatening a partner; 15 percent reported perpetrating sexual abuse. Smaller percentages were involved in relational abuse and stalking. The researchers noted that their findings found that teen dating violence "is a serious problem in the high-risk middle schools included in our sample," and there is a need for programming to address this problem.[8]

NOTES

1. Debnam Katrina J., Donna E. Howard, and Mary A. Garza, "'If You Don't Have Honesty in a Relationship, Then There Is No Relationship': African American Girls' Characterization of Healthy Dating Relationships, A Qualitative Study," *Journal of Primary Prevention* 35, no. 6 (2014): 397–407.

2. Nina M. Fredland, "Nurturing Healthy Relationships Through a Community-Based Interactive Theater Program," *Journal of Community Healthy Nursing* 27, no. 2 (2010): 107–18.

3. Scott R. Braithwaite, Nathaniel M. Lambert, Frank D. Fincham, and Kay Pasley, "Does College-Based Relationship Education Decrease Extradyadic Involvement in Relationships?" *Journal of Family Psychology* 24, no. 6 (2010): 740–45.

4. Sarah W. Whitton and Amanda D. Kuryluk, "Associations Between Relationship Quality and Depressive Symptoms in Same-Sex Couples," *Journal of Family Psychology* 28, no. 4 (2014): 571–76.

5. Sarah L. Killoren and Andrea L. Roach, "Sibling Conversations About Dating and Sexuality: Sisters as Confidants, Sources of Support, and Mentors," *Family Relations* 63, no. 2 (2014): 232–43.

6. Russell B. Clayton, Alexander Nagurney, and Jessica R. Smith, "Cheating, Breakup, and Divorce: Is Facebook Use to Blame?" *Cyberpsychology, Behavior, and Social Networking* 16, no. 10 (2013): 717–20.

7. R. M. Gonzalez-Guarda, A. M. Cummings, K. Pino et al., "Perceptions of Adolescents, Parents, and School Personnel from a Predominantly Cuban American Community Regarding Dating and Teen Dating Violence Prevention," *Research in Nursing & Health* 37, no. 2 (2014): 117–27.

8. Phyllis Holditch Niolon, Alana M. Vivolo-Kantor, Natasha E. Latzman et al., "Prevalence of Teen Dating Violence and Co-Occurring Risk Factors Among Middle School Youth in High-Risk Urban Communities," *Journal of Adolescent Health* 56 (2015): S5–S13.

REFERENCES AND RESOURCES

Magazines, Journals, and Newspapers

Braithwaite, Scott R., Nathaniel M. Lambert, Frank D. Fincham, and Kay Pasley. "Does College-Based Relationship Education Decrease Extradyadic Involvement in Relationships?" *Journal of Family Psychology* 24, no. 6 (2010): 740–45.

Clayton, Russell B., Alexander Nagurney, and Jessica R. Smith. "Cheating, Breakup, and Divorce: Is Facebook Use to Blame?" *Cyberpsychology, Behavior, and Social Networking* 16, no. 10 (2013): 717–20.

Debnam, Katrina J., Donna E. Howard, and Mary A. Garza. "'If You Don't Have Honesty in a Relationship, Then There Is No Relationship': African American Girls' Characterization of Healthy Dating Relationships, A Qualitative Study." *Journal of Primary Prevention* 35, no. 6 (2014): 397–407.

Fredland, Nina M. "Nurturing Healthy Relationships Through a Community-Based Interactive Theater Program." *Journal of Community Health Nursing* 27, no. 2 (2010): 107–18.

Gonzalez-Guarda, R. M., A. M. Cummings, K. Pino et al. "Perceptions of Adolescents, Parents, and School Personnel from a Predominantly Cuban American Community Regarding Dating and Teen Dating Violence Prevention." *Research in Nursing & Health* 37, no. 2 (2014): 117–27.

Haglund, Kristin, Ruth Ann Belknap, and Juanita Terrie Garcia. "Mexican American Female Adolescents' Perceptions of Relationships and Dating Violence." *Journal of Nursing Scholarship* 44, no. 3 (2012): 215–22.

Killoren, Sarah L., and Andrea L. Roach. "Sibling Conversations about Dating and Sexuality: Sisters as Confidants, Sources of Support, and Mentors." *Family Relations* 63, no. 2 (2014): 232–43.

Macauda, Mark M., Pamela I. Erickson, Merrill C. Singer, and Claudia C. Santelices. "A Cultural Model of Infidelity Among African American and Puerto Rican Young Adults." *Anthropology & Medicine* 18, no. 3 (2011): 351–64.

Niolon, Phyllis Holditch, Alana M. Vivolo-Kantor, Natasha E. Latzman et al. "Prevalence of Teen Dating Violence and Co-Occurring Risk Factors Among Middle School Youth in High-Risk Urban Communities." *Journal of Adolescent Health* 56 (2015): S5–S13.

Ward, Karen M., Julie P. Atkinson, Curtis A. Smith, and Richard Windsor. "A Friendships and Dating Program for Adults with Intellectual and Developmental Disabilities: A Formative Evaluation." *Intellectual and Developmental Disabilities* 51, no. 1 (2013): 22–32.

Whitton, Sarah W., and Amanda D. Kuryluk. "Associations Between Relationship Quality and Depressive Symptoms in Same-Sex Couples." *Journal of Family Psychology* 28, no. 4 (2014): 571–76.

Web Site

The Nemours Foundation. www.kidshealth.org.

Practice Safer Sex

OVERVIEW

Many people believe that almost all teens have sex. While it may come as a surprise, that is not true. Less than half of all high school students have sex. Large numbers of teens want to delay having sex until they are older or meet "the right one." It is okay not to have sex. Teens who began having sex before they were ready often wish they had waited. Complete and total protection from pregnancy and sexually transmitted infections (also known as sexually transmitted diseases) is only possible with abstinence. Nevertheless, since most people will eventually have sex, it is important to address the issue of safer sex.

There are two main risks associated with sex. When sex is between a male and a female, there is a risk for pregnancy and a risk for sexually transmitted infections. Obviously, there is no risk for pregnancy in sex between two men or two women, but there is still a risk of sexually transmitted infections. Perhaps the easiest and most convenient way to provide greater protection from pregnancy and sexually transmitted infections is to use a condom. There are condoms for both males and females. Male condoms, which are usually made from latex or polyurethane, should be used for vaginal, anal, or oral sex. (Avoid condoms that say they are "natural" or made from lambskin. They may allow the transmission of sexual infections.) Female condoms, which have a ring on each end, are used only for vaginal sex. The condom is held in place by the inside ring. The outside ring stays outside the vagina.

Birth control pills and intrauterine devices (IUD) provide protection from pregnancy, but they offer no protection from sexually transmitted infections. While condoms are sold at pharmacies and other retail locations, your medical provider must write a prescription for birth control pills or insert an IUD into the uterus. Remaining in a monogamous relationship reduces the risk of sexually transmitted infections, but there is always the risk of pregnancy.

WHAT THE EXPERTS SAY

There Are Interventions That Support the Use of Condoms

In a study published in 2014 in *Worldviews on Evidence-Based Nursing*, researchers from Columbus, Ohio, noted that condoms are a primary means to reduce the incidence of sexually transmitted infections, a major public health concern. The researchers decided to conduct a review of behavioral intervention studies on increasing the use of condoms, ultimately including a total of 13 meta-analyses or systematic reviews that represented 248 studies. The researchers found that behavioral interventions were very successful in promoting condom use and reducing sexually transmitted infections. However, they were not useful in promoting abstinence. The programs worked best when they were designed for specific populations and included skill-building exercises. "The evidence suggests that tailoring content based on ethnicity, culture, and gender—incorporating personal and interpersonal skill building exercises—and exposure to content are important in obtaining effective health outcomes."[1]

Adding an Emotional Component to Safer Sex Education Increases Efficacy

In a study published in 2011 in *Health Psychology*, researchers from Maryland and Connecticut wanted to learn if the addition of an emotional component to traditional safer sex education increased intervention efficacy. The researchers recruited 198 college students. Only students who had ever had sex were invited to participate. That left 189 students. The trial consisted of a baseline assessment, a 120-minute intervention, an online follow-up at three months, and a second online follow-up at six months. Sixty-eight students had an intervention that included an emotional component; 67 students had the regular intervention, and 64 students had no intervention beyond the standard material offered by the university. At the six-month follow-up, there were still 160 participants. When compared to the other two groups, the students who were part of the emotional intervention group reported increased condom use. The researchers commented that their findings offer "preliminary evidence to suggest that incorporating an emotional education component into a social-cognitive intervention may help to facilitate sexual risk reduction."[2]

Culturally Sensitive Media Messages May Play a Role in Safer Sex

In a study published in 2011 in the *Journal of Adolescent Health*, researchers from multiple locations in the United States wanted to learn the long-term effects of a mass media intervention that employed "culturally and developmentally appropriate messages" to enhance safer sex, particularly in regard to the prevention of the transmission of the human immunodeficiency virus (HIV) in high risk African American teens. For three years, the researchers coordinated the delivery of television and radio messages in Syracuse, New York, and Macon, Georgia. They focused on channels that were popular with African American teens. The cities of Providence, Rhode Island, and Columbia, South Carolina, served as controls. Over a 16-month period, the researchers recruited 1,710 African-American adolescents between the ages of 14 and 17 years from these four cities. After the teens completed computer-assisted self-interviews lasting about 45 minutes, there were follow-up assessments at 3, 6, 12, and 18 months. The researchers found that the media interventions improved condom-use negotiation among the teens. In addition, the adolescents ages 16 and 17 years who were exposed to the media programs "showed less risky age trajectory of unprotected sex than those in the nonmedia cities." The researchers concluded that "culturally tailored mass media messages that are delivered consistently over time have the potential to reach a large audience of high-risk adolescents, to support changes in HIV-prevention beliefs, and to reduce HIV-associated risk behaviors among older youth."[3]

Online Focus Groups May Reinforce Safer Sex

In a study published in 2014 in *AIDS Education and Prevention*, researchers from several cities in the United States but based in San Clemente, California, examined the ability of online focus groups to alter the sexual behavior of gay, queer, and bisexual male teens between the ages of 14 and 18 years. The researchers conducted two rounds of online focus groups. The first round, in November 2012, had 37 teens, and the second round, in January 2013, had 38 teens. The results were notable. Most of the sexually experienced teens indicated that "participation positively changed their views and behavioral intentions." Some of the participants noted that the focus group increased their ability to talk about sex in comfort and helped them make better choices, such as negotiating condoms. Sexually inexperienced participants said that the group decreased their sense of isolation. A number of participants indicated that they intended to become more vocal advocates for abstinence and/or safer sex. The researcher noted that their findings indicated "that online focus groups or moderated-led social support groups could be further explored as a low cost intervention for this vulnerable population of young people."[4]

BARRIERS AND PROBLEMS

It May Be Difficult for Women to Negotiate Safer Sex, Even If They Have a Sexually Transmitted Infection

In a study published in 2012 in the *Journal of Clinical Nursing*, a researcher from New Zealand investigated the challenges women may encounter in negotiating the use of a condom, even when they have a sexually transmitted disease. The researcher conducted interviews with 12 clinicians with experience in the sexual health field and 26 women with a diagnosis of either herpes simplex or human papilloma virus. Only a small number of the women with sexually transmitted infections had received any safer sex instruction from their clinicians, and they wanted their clinicians to initiate these talks. The women noted that talking about safer sex had become more difficult since their diagnosis. "Women's dilemmas were whether to disclose the diagnosis as part of insisting on condom use, whether condom use mitigated the obligation to disclose or whether any talk or condom use was avoided as too 'risky' to feminine identity." The women indicated that they wanted their clinicians to offer advice, and they noted that if the women themselves did not raise the topic of safer sex, it was not addressed. Only a small number of women felt that they could initiate the topic. The researcher concluded that "nurses need training in sexual history taking and communication skills to address the gendered complexities of safer sex."[5]

There May Be Financial Pressure for Disadvantaged Teens to Avoid Using Condoms

In a study published in 2012 in the *Journal of Adolescent Health*, researchers from Maryland and Georgia wanted to determine if female teens who received economic benefits from their boyfriends were more likely to avoid using condoms. Data were obtained from a longitudinal HIV prevention intervention study that included 715 African American teen females, between the ages of 15 and 21 years, in urban Atlanta. The teens, who all had low socioeconomic status, were interviewed at baseline, six months, and 12 months. At baseline, 83.6 percent of the teens reported having a boyfriend, and four of the teens had a child or children. Twenty-four percent of the women said that their boyfriend was their primary source of spending money. These women were 50 percent more likely never to use condoms. Interestingly, women whose boyfriend had been their primary source of spending money but who found another source of spending money were more likely to start using condoms. And, women who had boyfriends who owned cars were more likely never to use condoms. The researchers noted that safer sex may be undermined when teen females receive spending money from their boyfriends. Clinicians working with this at-risk population "should consider that adolescents who receive spending money from their boyfriends may be at risk for coercive relationships or unsafe sex."[6]

Depressed Young Women Are at Increased Risk for Less Safe Sex

In a study published in 2011 in the *Journal of Pediatric & Adolescent Gynecology*, researchers from Boston noted that depressed young women are at increased risk for sexually transmitted infections. As a result, the researchers wanted to learn more about this association. Their cohort consisted of 45 depressed young women between the ages of 15 and 22 years. Over a two-week period, 31 of these women reported at least one sex event in which a condom was used. A total of 143 condom use events were reported. During 51 percent of these condom events, the condoms were used incorrectly. The most common error was the failure to hold the condom during withdrawal. The researchers commented that "even if they use condoms, depressed adolescents and young adult women are at increased risk of STIs [sexually transmitted infections] because they frequently use condoms incorrectly."[7]

Women Who Have Sex with Other Women May Not Use Protection

In a study published in 2013 in the *International Journal of Gynecology and Obstetrics*, researchers from San Francisco and Davis, California, wanted to determine the frequency and associations of barrier protection used during sexual activity in women who have sex with other women. The cohort consisted of 1,557 women from throughout the world who were 17 years old or older and had sex with other women. The majority of responses (67.4 percent) were from women living in the United States. While the vast majority of women (82.4 percent) were in monogamous relationships, 19.5 percent of the women reported that they had sexual relationships with women they "did not know well." As might be expected, the women in the monogamous relationships were less likely to use barrier protection. Still, the researchers noted that it is not uncommon for women to underestimate their risk for sexually transmitted infections. The researchers advised healthcare providers and public health researchers to devote more attention to fostering safer sex practices among women who have sex with other women.[8]

NOTES

1. Victoria von Sadovszky, Breana Draudt, and Samantha Boch, "A Systematic Review of Reviews of Behavioral Interventions to Promote Condom Use," *Worldviews on Evidence-Based Nursing* 11, no. 2 (2014): 107–17.

2. Rebecca A. Ferrer, Jeffrey D. Fisher, Ross Buck, and K. Rivet Amico, "Pilot Test of an Emotional Education Intervention Component for Sexual Risk Reduction," *Health Psychology* 30, no 5 (2011): 656–60.

3. Sharon Sznitman, Peter A. Vanable, Michael P. Carey et al., "Using Culturally Sensitive Media Messages to Reduce HIV-Associated Sexual Behavior in High-Risk African American Adolescents: Results from a Randomized Trial," *Journal of Adolescent Health* 49 (2011): 244–51.

4. Michele L. Ybarra, Zachary DuBois, Jeffrey T. Parsons et al., "Online Focus Groups as an HIV Prevention Program for Gay, Bisexual, and Queer Adolescent Males," *AIDS Education and Prevention* 26, no. 6 (2014): 554–64.

5. Catherine Cook, "'Nice Girls Don't': Women and the Condom Conundrum," *Journal of Clinical Nursing* 21, no. 3–4 (2012): 535–43.

6. Janet Rosenbaum, Jonathan Zenilman, Eve Rose et al., "Cash, Cars, and Condoms: Economic Factors in Disadvantaged Adolescent Women's Condom Use," *Journal of Adolescent Health* 51 (2012): 233–41.

7. Lydia A. Shrier, Courtney Walls, Christopher Lops, and Henry A. Feldman, "Correlates of Incorrect Condom Use Among Depressed Young Women: An Event-Level Analysis," *Journal of Pediatric & Adolescent Gynecology* 24, no. 1 (2011): 10–14.

8. Tami S. Rowen, Benjamin N. Breyer, Tzu-Chin Lin et al., "Use of Barrier Protection for Sexual Activity Among Women Who Have Sex with Women," *International Journal of Gynecology and Obstetrics* 120 (2013): 42–45.

REFERENCES AND RESOURCES

Magazines, Journals, and Newspapers

Cook, Catherine. "'Nice Girls Don't': Women and the Condom Conundrum." *Journal of Clinical Nursing* 21, no. 3–4 (2012): 535–43.
Ferrer, Rebecca A., Jeffrey D. Fisher, Ross Buck, and K. Rivet Amico. "Pilot Test of an Emotional Education Intervention Component for Sexual Risk Reduction." *Health Psychology* 30, no. 5 (2011): 656–60.

Fowler, Patrick J., Darnell Motley, Jinjin Zhang et al. "Adolescent Maltreatment in the Child Welfare System and Developmental Patterns of Sexual Risk Behaviors." *Child Maltreatment* 20, no. 1 (2015): 50–60.

Kuo, Kelly, Tao Y. Zhu, Shandhini Raidoo et al. "Partnering with Public Schools: A Resident-Driven Reproductive Health Education Initiative." *Journal of Pediatric & Adolescent Gynecology* 27 (2014): 20–24.

Lawrence, Ryan E., Kenneth A. Rasinski, John D. Yoon, and Farr A. Curlin. "Obstetrician-Gynecologists' Beliefs About Safe-Sex and Abstinence Counseling." *International Journal of Gynecology and Obstetrics* 114 (2011): 281–85.

Rosenbaum, Janet, Jonathan Zenilman, Eve Rose et al. "Cash, Cars, and Condoms: Economic Factors in Disadvantaged Adolescent Women's Condom Use." *Journal of Adolescent Health* 51 (2012): 233–41.

Rowen, Tami S., Benjamin N. Breyer, Tzu-Chin Lin et al. "Use of Barrier Protection for Sexual Activity Among Women Who Have Sex with Women." *International Journal of Gynecology and Obstetrics* 120 (2013): 42–45.

Shrier, Lydia A., Courtney Walls, Christopher Lops, and Henry A. Feldman. "Correlates of Incorrect Condom Use Among Depressed Young Women: An Event-Level Analysis." *Journal of Pediatric & Adolescent Gynecology* 24, no. 1 (2011): 10–14.

Sznitman, Sharon, Peter A. Vanable, Michael P. Carey et al. "Using Culturally Sensitive Media Messages to Reduce HIV-Associated Sexual Behavior in High-Risk African American Adolescents: Results from a Randomized Trial." *Journal of Adolescent Health* 49 (2011): 244–51.

von Sadovszky, Victoria, Breana Draudt, and Samantha Boch. "Systematic Review of Reviews of Behavioral Interventions to Promote Condom Use." *Worldviews on Evidence-Based Nursing* 11, no. 2 (2014): 107–17.

Ybarra, Michele, L. Zachary DuBois, Jeffrey T. Parsons et al. "Online Focus Groups as an HIV Prevention Program for Gay, Bisexual, and Queer Adolescent Males." *AIDS Education and Prevention* 26, no. 6 (2014): 554–64.

Web Site

Planned Parenthood. www.plannedparenthood.org.

Use Emergency Contraception When Necessary

OVERVIEW

The statistics are truly stunning. In the United States, about half of all pregnancies are unintended. Four out of 10 unintended pregnancies are terminated by abortion. Of the women who have these abortions, 54 percent used a method of contraception during the month that they became pregnant.[1]

Emergency contraception is useful for a number of different situations. These include the incorrect use or failure of birth control, the failure to use birth control while sexually active, the breakage of a condom, and as a victim of sexual assault or rape. All of these situations increase the risk of becoming pregnant. The use of emergency contraception pills appears to work by delaying the release of an egg from the woman's ovaries and prevents the sperm from fertilizing an already released egg.

There are two types of emergency contraception that may be purchased without a prescription. They contain a synthetic form of the hormone progesterone called levonorgestrel. Plan B One-Step is a single tablet of 1.5 mg levonorgestrel; Next Choice, also known as Plan B, is taken as two doses. Each dose is .75 mg of levonorgestrel. These doses may be taken together or 12 hours apart, up to five days after sex. These pills prevent a pregnancy from occurring, but they do not terminate a pregnancy that has already implanted. They are most effective when used within 24 hours of sex. Emergency contraception should not be used if a teen may be pregnant for several days or when there is vaginal bleeding. There is a prescription medication, ulipristal acetate (Ella), which is taken as a single tablet. It works by delaying ovulation. It requires a prescription from a medical provider. It may be taken up to five days after unprotected sex.

A copper intrauterine device (IUD) is the most effective method of emergency contraception, and it may also be used for regular contraception. It may be inserted into the uterus by a medical provider up to five days after unprotected sex. It may work by inhibiting sperm movement or by other mechanisms that inhibit fertilization and implantation.

WHAT THE EXPERTS SAY

Emergency Contraception Saves Lives

In a study published in 2014 in the *Indian Journal of Medical Research*, a researcher from India commented that "many unwanted pregnancies end in unsafe abortions." To help control the number of abortions, greater effort needs to be made to make people more aware of emergency contraception. According to this researcher, each year there are about 210 million pregnancies worldwide. About 22 million (22 percent) of these pregnancies end in induced abortions and 20 million in unsafe abortions. The vast majority of these (95 percent) occur in developing countries. Moreover, 13 percent of pregnancy-related deaths are the result of unsafe abortions. While the researcher acknowledged that emergency contraception is not a substitute for the correct use of contraception, it "is an important method for women whose contraception has failed or who have unprotected sex." And, because emergency contraception is most effective when used as early as possible after sex, it is a good idea to have a supply on hand. Still, women should be aware that emergency contraception may have side effects including nausea, vomiting, abdominal pain, breast tenderness, headache, dizziness, and fatigue. (If vomiting occurs within two hours of the ingestion of a dose, a re-peat dose is recommended.) Most side effects usually resolve within a day. It is common to have a temporary disruption of the menstrual cycle. According to the researcher, it is important to remember that "emergency contraception is a wom-an's last chance to prevent unintended pregnancy." Increased access to emergency contraception does not lead to riskier sexual practice, but it does lower rates of abortion. "All women may need a last-minute chance to prevent unwanted preg-nancy by making emergency contraception accessible as a back-up method."[2]

Exposure to Emergency Contraception Does Not Harm Physical and Mental Development of Children

In a study published in 2014 in the journal *Biology of Reproduction*, researchers from China examined the effect on the physical and mental development of chil-dren born after the failure of emergency contraception. The researchers com-pared a group of 195 children exposed to emergency contraception to a matched group of 214 children who were never exposed to emergency contraception. Over a two-year period, the physical and mental health of the two groups were evalu-ated. The researchers found no statistically significant differences between the two groups of children in weight, height, head circumference, and intelligence scores. "The values of all parameters of both groups were similar to those of the national standards." The researchers concluded that emergency contraception had "no effect on the physical growth, mental development, or occurrence of birth defects in children born from pregnancies in which EC [emergency contra-ception] failed."[3]

BARRIERS AND PROBLEMS

College Students May Have Little Information About Emergency Contraception

In a study published in 2011 in *Contraception*, a researcher from Edinboro University in Pennsylvania wanted to determine what male and female under-graduates knew about emergency contraception. A survey was conducted during the Spring 2008 semester; it included 358 females and 338 males. The researcher learned that 83 percent of the students had experienced sexual intercourse; of these students or their partners, 52 percent had feared pregnancy at least once. Only 17 percent of the students or their partners had used emergency con-traception. While 74 percent of the students had heard about emergency contra-ception, less than one-third knew any specifics, such as potential side effects. And, only 16 percent were aware that emergency contraception was available at their college health center. According to the researcher, if emergency contra-ception is to be better utilized as a tool against unintended pregnancy and abor-tion, college students and others need to be more informed. The researcher concluded that college students have a "poor" level of knowledge about emergency contraception.[4]

There Are Some Serious Barriers to Emergency Contraception

In a study published in 2015 in the *Indian Journal of Community Medicine*, researchers from New Delhi interviewed a number of experts in the field of emergency contraception to determine some of the reasons that it is so infrequently used. In addition, the researchers conducted a review of the literature on the topic. A number of key barriers emerged. The vast majority of the sales of emergency contraception are in the cities. In fact, 71 percent of the total sales are in urban areas, but urban areas comprise only 29.8 percent of the population of India. And, emergency contraception does not appear to be readily available in many rural areas. Moreover, many physicians have incorrect information about emergency contraception. For example, though it has proven to be untrue, some physicians believe that these products may trigger an ectopic pregnancy or an abortion. Some gynecologists have negative views of women who use emergency contraception. For example, they thought that these women have multiple sexual partners and/or risky sexual behaviors. There is also the issue of cost. Some of the most popular brands are expensive, and all women may not find them to be affordable. The researchers recommended an educational campaign involving the media and improvements in access to emergency contraception, with the ultimate goal of "mainstreaming" these treatments.[5]

The Efficacy Rates of Emergency Contraception May Vary

In a study published in 2011 in *Contraception*, researchers from Scotland; Bethesda, Maryland; and Paris noted that emergency contraception does not always work. To learn why this occurs, they examined data from a meta-analysis of two randomized controlled trials. When compared to women with normal body mass index (BMI), the risk of pregnancy after using emergency contraception was three times higher in women who were obese. This is a very important finding for overweight and obese women who want to avoid pregnancy. The second finding was more anticipated. Even after taking emergency contraception, the risk of pregnancy was highest when sex took place near ovulation. When compared to women who had sex outside the fertile times of the month, the women who had sex the day before the estimated day of ovulation had a fourfold increase risk of pregnancy. According to the researchers, women who are overweight or obese and women who have unprotected sex near ovulation should have a medical provider insert a copper intrauterine device.[6] While this may appear to be a readily available solution, an emergency appointment with a medical provider is not necessarily available, especially to a teen who may have little experience navigating medical systems.

Males May Encounter Problems Purchasing Emergency Contraception

In a study published in 2014 in *Contraception*, New York City researchers wanted to learn more about the ability of males to purchase emergency contraception in the three New York City neighborhoods of Washington Heights, East Harlem, and the Upper East Side. In July 2012 three male research assistants, aged 19, 25, and 28 years, were sent to ask about purchasing these products. (Because of a lack of resources, they did not actually purchase the items.) In each of the 158 pharmacies that they visited, the research assistants explained to the pharmacist or pharmacy technician that the condom had broken during sex with their partner, and the partner now required emergency contraception. Of the 128 pharmacies, 81 percent indicated that emergency contraception was available for sale. Although this represented a very solid majority, the researchers noted that young men had a one in five chance of not having emergency contraception available. Also disturbing was the fact that the research assistants were, on occasion, given incorrect information. One pharmacist noted that emergency contraception caused miscarriages and abortions. Another pharmacist said that it was associated with birth defects. The researchers added that the costs associated with emergency contraception may be high for those living in lower socioeconomic areas, and the pharmacies may not have extended hours on the weekend, when unprotected sex is more likely to occur. An even more serious concern is the possibility that some pharmacists may be finding ways to refuse to dispense emergency contraception because of their own personal beliefs. "Cost and timely access are still important issues that remain today."[7]

NOTES

1. Pelin Batur, "Emergency Contraception: Separating Fact from Fiction," *Cleveland Clinic Journal of Medicine* 79, no. 11 (2012): 771–76.

2. Suneeta Mittal, "Emergency Contraception: Potential for Women's Health," *Indian Journal of Medical Research* 140, Supplement (2014): 45–52.

3. Lin Zhang, Weiping Ye, Wen Yu et al., "Physical and Mental Development of Children After Levonorgestrel Emergency Contraception Exposure: A Follow-Up Prospective Cohort Study," *Biology of Reproduction* 91, no. 1 (2014): 27.

4. Laura M. Miller, "College Student Knowledge and Attitudes Toward Emergency Contraception," *Contraception* 83 (2011): 68–73.

5. Anvita Dixit, M. E. Khan, and Isha Bhatnagar, "Mainstreaming of Emergency Contraception Pill in India: Challenges and Opportunities," *Indian Journal of Community Medicine* 40, no. 1 (2015): 49–55.

6. Anna Glasier, Sharon T. Cameron, Diana Blithe et al., "Can We Identify Women at Risk of Pregnancy Despite Using Emergency Contraception? Data From Randomized Trials of Ulipristal Acetate and Levonorgestrel," *Contraception* 84 (2011): 363–67.

7. David Bell, Elvis J. Camacho, and Andrew B. Velasquez, "Male Access to Emergency Contraception in Pharmacies: A Mystery Shopper Survey," *Contraception* 90 (2014): 413–15.

REFERENCES AND RESOURCES

Magazines, Journals, and Newspapers

Batur, Pelin. "Emergency Contraception: Separating Fact from Fiction." *Cleveland Clinic Journal of Medicine* 79, no. 11 (2012): 771–76.

Bell, David L., Elvis J. Camacho, and Andrew B. Velasquez. "Male Access to Emergency Contraception in Pharmacies: A Mystery Shopper Survey." *Contraception* 90 (2014): 413–15.

Dixit, Anvita, M. E. Khan, and Isha Bhatnagar. "Mainstreaming of Emergency Contraception Pill in India: Challenges and Opportunities." *Indian Journal of Community Medicine* 40, no. 1 (2015): 49–55.

Glasier, Anna, Sharon T. Cameron, Diana Blithe et al. "Can We Identify Women at Risk of Pregnancy Despite Using Emergency Contraception? Data From Randomized Trials of Ulipristal Acetate and Levonorgestrel." *Contraception* 84 (2011): 363–67.

Gudka, Sajni, Aline Bourdin, Kim Watkins et al. "Self-Reported Risk Factors for Chlamydia: A Survey of Pharmacy-Based Emergency Contraception Consumers." *International Journal of Pharmacy Practice* 22 (2014): 13–19.

Hickey, Mary T., and Jane White. "Female College Students' Experiences with and Perceptions of Over-the-Counter Emergency Contraception in the United States." *Sexual & Reproductive Healthcare* 6 (2015): 28–32.

Miller, Laura M. "College Student Knowledge and Attitudes Toward Emergency Contraception." *Contraception* 83 (2011): 68–73.

Mittal, Suneeta. "Emergency Contraception—Potential for Women's Health." *Indian Journal of Medical Research* 140, Supplement (2014): 45–52.

Palermo, J. Bleck, and E. Westley. "Knowledge and Use of Emergency Contraception: A Multicountry Analysis." *International Perspectives on Sexual and Reproductive Health* 40, no. 2 (2014): 79–86.

Zhang, Lin, Weiping Ye, Wen Yu et al. "Physical and Mental Development of Children After Levonorgestrel Emergency Contraception Exposure: A Follow-Up Prospective Cohort Study." *Biology of Reproduction* 91, no. 1 (2014): 27.

Web Site

Planned Parenthood. www.plannedparenthood.org.

Other Lifestyle Choices

Avoid Electronic Cigarettes

OVERVIEW

Also known as e-cigarettes or electronic nicotine delivery systems, electronic cigarettes are generally battery-operated devices that are designed to deliver nicotine, flavorings, and chemicals in the form of a vapor. Most often, puffing activates the heating device, which vaporizes the liquid in the cartridge. The resulting aerosol or vapor is inhaled; this is called "vaping."

Electronic cigarettes are intended to simulate the act of smoking by producing an aromatic aerosol that looks and feels like tobacco smoke without the toxic chemicals associated with the burning of tobacco. Electronic cigarettes tend to be marketed as a healthier alternative to tobacco cigarettes. But like tobacco, they contain nicotine, which is addictive, and other chemicals, which may be harmful. Surely, using these products does not support health. Yet, among teens, electronic cigarettes appear to be gaining popularity. And, they are readily available; they may easily be purchased online. Another possible reason for concern about electronic cigarettes is that they need to be refilled. When refilling these cigarettes, users may be exposing themselves to toxic levels of nicotine.[1]

WHAT THE EXPERTS SAY

Large Numbers of Young Adults Are Using Electronic Cigarettes

In a study published in 2015 in *Addictive Behaviors*, researchers from San Francisco, Oakland, and Palo Alto, California, examined the prevalence of electronic cigarette use in three different samples, collected between 2009 and 2013, of young adult smokers between the ages of 18 and 25 years. The researchers found the percentage of people using electronic cigarettes was higher in each subsequent sample. So, the most recent sample had the largest numbers of people using electronic cigarettes. Many of the young adults reported using electronic cigarettes to reduce or quit conventional smoking. In fact, in the third sample, 38 percent reported using electronic cigarettes for those goals. And, the people who smoked more frequently were more likely to have used electronic cigarettes during the previous month. The researchers speculated that "heavier smokers may have been exploring new ways to consume tobacco regardless of intention to quit smoking." And, they concluded that "e-cigarette use is increasingly common among young adults."[2]

Use of Electronic Cigarettes in Teens Does Not Discourage, and May Encourage, Use of Tobacco Cigarettes

In a study published in 2014 in JAMA *Pediatrics*, researchers based in San Francisco wanted to learn more about the use of electronic and tobacco cigarettes in adolescents. As a result, they used the 2011 and 2012 National Youth Tobacco Surveys to conduct cross-sectional analyses of a representative sample of U.S. middle and high school students, from grade 6 to grade 12. Their 2011 sample had 17,353 students, and their 2012 sample had 22,529 students; the students lived in all 50 states and the District of Columbia. The researchers learned that smoking electronic cigarettes was associated with higher odds of smoking tobacco cigarettes. Use of electronic cigarettes was also associated with lower odds of abstinence from tobacco cigarettes. According to these researchers, "e-cigarette use is aggravating rather than ameliorating the tobacco epidemic among youths." And, they noted that their findings "called into question claims that e-cigarettes are effective as smoking cessation aids."[3]

Nicotine in Electronic Cigarettes May Be Dangerous for a Growing Fetus

In a study published in the journal *Birth Defects Research. Part A, Clinical and Molecular Teratology*, researchers from Texas noted that electronic cigarettes and other nicotine-containing products are often used by women of reproductive age. That is why it is important to determine the effect nicotine has on a growing fetus. It is known that nicotine easily crosses the placenta and enters fetal circulation. From animal studies, the researchers learned that nicotine is associated with adverse effects for the lungs, cardiovascular systems, and brains. Lung problems included reduce surface area, weight, and volume. Fetuses exposed to nicotine may develop into adults with high blood pressure, pulmonary disorders such as asthma, and, possibly, a predisposition to diabetes. The researchers concluded that "no amount of nicotine is known to be safe during pregnancy."[4]

In an article published in 2015 in the *American Journal of Preventive Medicine*, researchers from Atlanta underscored the potential adverse effects nicotine has on a growing fetus. Yet, these researchers noted that the adverse effects of nicotine have largely been absent from the public discussion on electronic cigarettes. Electronic cigarettes are widely available and are sold legally to minors in many states. Electronic cigarettes with very high amounts of nicotine may be purchased on the Internet. Unlike tobacco cigarettes, there is generally no warning label. The researchers suggested the implementation of several regulatory and policy measures for electronic cigarettes and other nicotine-containing products. There must be prohibitions that forbid the marketing of these products to children and teens, similar to those that are already in place for tobacco products. The products should have health warnings and special packaging to prevent accidental poisonings. And, there is a need for protection from exposure to secondhand electronic cigarette aerosol. Moreover, higher pricing may help minimize youth initiation and use. The researchers noted that "in the absence of appropriate restrictions, millions of youth could become addicted to nicotine and many more pregnant women, children, and adolescents unnecessarily exposed."[5]

Smoking Electronic Cigarettes Leaves Nicotine in the Environment

In a study published in 2015 in the journal *Nicotine & Tobacco Research* researchers from Buffalo, New York, noted that when people smoke electronic cigarettes, nicotine remains on nearby surfaces. Nicotine reacts with oxidizing chemicals in the air and forms secondary pollutants, such as cancer-causing nitrosamines. The researchers filled three brands of electronic cigarettes with varying concentrations of nicotine. They released 100 puffs of each product directly into an exposure chamber. Surface wipe samples were taken pre- and postrelease of the vapors. The researchers found that three of their four experiments showed significant increases in the amount of nicotine on all the surfaces. The largest increases in nicotine were seen on the floors and glass windows. The researchers noted that their findings "indicated that there is a risk for thirdhand exposure to nicotine from e-cigarettes."[6]

BARRIERS AND PROBLEMS

Electronic Cigarettes Are Associated with Other Problematic Behaviors in Teens

In a cross-sectional survey published in 2015 in the journal *BMC Public Health*, researchers from the United Kingdom wanted to learn more about the characteristics of teens who are accessing electronic cigarettes. The cohort consisted of 16,193 students in northwest England between the ages of 14 and 17 years. The researchers examined associations between electronic cigarette access and demographics, conventional smoking behaviors, alcohol consumption, and methods of accessing cigarettes and alcohol. One out of every five teens reported having access to electronic cigarettes. The prevalence was highest among smokers, though 15.8 percent of the teen who had access to electronic cigarettes had never smoked tobacco cigarettes. Access to electronic cigarettes was associated with being male, having parents/guardians who smoke, and the use of alcohol. When compared to nondrinkers, the teens who drank alcohol at least once per week and binge drank were more likely to have accessed electronic cigarettes. Among teen drinkers, access to electronic cigarettes was related to drinking to be drunk, alcohol-related violence, consumption of alcohol, the self-purchase of alcohol, and the recruitment of adults to purchase alcohol. The researcher concluded that "there is an urgent need for controls on the promotion and sale of e-cigarettes to children." According to these researchers, teens are using electronic cigarettes more for experimentation than smoking cessation. In addition, "those most likely to access e-cigarettes may already be familiar with illicit methods of accessing age-restricted substances."[7]

Despite Concerns, Electronic Cigarette Use Is Increasing and Linked to Heavy Alcohol Consumption in College Students

In a study published in 2015 in the *Journal of American College Health*, researchers from Lubbock, Texas, examined the use of electronic cigarettes in college students in relation to gender, race/ethnicity, traditional tobacco use, and heavy drinking. The cohort, which consisted of 599 college students enrolled in General Psychology at a state university in Texas, completed questionnaires in January 2014. Sixty-five percent of the cohort was female; the cohort had a mean age of 19.19 years. Twenty-nine percent of the students reported prior use of electronic cigarettes, with 14 percent using in the previous 30 days. Males were more likely than females to use electronic cigarettes, but the use was not associated with race or ethnicity. Use of both tobacco and electronic cigarettes was associated with heavier use of both types of cigarettes and heavy drinking. The researchers concluded that "e-cigarette use among college students is exponentially on the rise and its co-use with alcohol may contribute to negative outcomes in this population."[8]

NOTES

1. National Institute on Drug Abuse, www.drugabuse.gov.
2. Danielle Ramo, Kelly C. Young-Wolff, and Judith J. Prochaska, "Prevalence and Correlates of Electronic-Cigarette Use in Young Adults: Findings from Three Studies Over Five Years," *Addictive Behaviors* 41 (2015): 142–47.
3. Lauren M. Dutra and Stanton A. Glantz, "Electronic Cigarettes and Conventional Cigarette Use Among US Adolescents: A Cross-Sectional Study," *JAMA Pediatrics* 168, no. 7 (2014): 610–17.
4. Melissa A. Suter, Joan Mastrobattista, Maike Sachs, and Kjersti Aagaard, "Is There Evidence for Potential Harm of Electronic Cigarette Use in Pregnancy?" *Birth Defects Research. Part A, Clinical and Molecular Teratology* 103, no. 3 (2015): 186–95.
5. Lucinda J. England, Rebecca E. Bunnell, Terry F. Pechacek et al., "Nicotine and the Developing Human: A Neglected Element in the Electronic Cigarette Debate," *American Journal of Preventive Medicine* 49 (2015): 286–93.
6. Maciej L. Goniewicz and Lily Lee, "Electronic Cigarettes Are a Source of Thirdhand Exposure to Nicotine," *Nicotine & Tobacco Research* 17, no. 2 (2015): 256–58.

7. Karen Hughes, Mark A. Bellis, Katherine A. Hardcastle et al., "Associations Between E-Cigarette Access and Smoking and Drinking Behaviours in Teenagers," BMC Public Health 15 (2015): 244+.

8. Andrew K. Littlefield, Joshua C. Gottlieb, Lee M. Cohen, and David R. M. Trotter, "Electronic Cigarette Use Among College Students: Links to Gender, Race/Ethnicity, Smoking, and Heavy Drinking," Journal of American College Health 63 (2015): 523.

REFERENCES AND RESOURCES

Magazines, Journals, and Newspapers

Brose, Leonie, Sara C. Hitchman, Jamie Brown et al. "Is the Use of Electronic Cigarettes While Smoking Associated with Smoking Cessation Attempts, Cessation and Reduced Cigarette Consumption? A Survey with a 1-Year Follow-Up." Addiction 110 (2015): 1160–68.

Bullen, Christopher, Colin Howe, Murray Laugesen et al. "Electronic Cigarettes for Smoking Cessation: A Randomised Controlled Trial." Lancet 382 (2013): 1629–37.

Dutra, Lauren M., and Stanton A. Glantz. "Electronic Cigarettes and Conventional Cigarette Use Among US Adolescents: A Cross-Sectional Study." JAMA Pediatrics 168, no. 7 (2014): 610–17.

England, Lucinda J., Rebecca E. Bunnell, Terry F. Pechacek et al. "Nicotine and the Developing Human: A Neglected Element in the Electronic Cigarette Debate." American Journal of Preventive Medicine 49 (2015): 286–93.

Goniewicz, Maciej L., and Lily Lee. "Electronic Cigarettes Are a Source of Thirdhand Exposure to Nicotine." Nicotine & Tobacco Research 17, no. 2 (2015): 256–58.

Hughes, Karen, Mark A. Bellis, Katherine A. Hardcastle et al. "Associations Between E-Cigarette Access and Smoking and Drinking Behaviours in Teenagers." BMC Public Health 15 (2015): 244+.

Lee, Yong Hee, Michal Gawron, and Maciej Lukasz Goniewicz. "Changes in Puffing Behavior Among Smokers Who Switched from Tobacco to Electronic Cigarettes." Addictive Behaviors 48 (2015): 1–4.

Littlefield, Andrew K., Joshua C. Gottlieb, Lee M. Cohen, and David R. M. Trotter. "Electronic Cigarette Use Among College Students: Links to Gender, Race/Ethnicity, Smoking, and Heavy Drinking." Journal of American College Health 63 (2015): 523.

Popova, Lucy, and Pamela M. Ling. "Alternative Tobacco Product Use and Smoking Cessation: A National Study." American Journal of Public Health 103, no. 5 (2013): 923–30.

Ramo, Danielle E., Kelly C. Young-Wolff, and Judith J. Prochaska. "Prevalence and Correlates of Electronic-Cigarette Use in Young Adults Findings From Three Studies over Five Years." Addictive Behaviors 41 (2015): 142–47.

Suter, Melissa A., Joan Mastrobattista, Maike Sachs, and Kjersti Aagaard. "Is There Evidence for Potential Harm of Electronic Cigarette Use in Pregnancy?" Birth Defects Research. Part A, Clinical and Molecular Teratology 103, no. 3 (2015): 186–95.

Web Site

National Institute on Drug Abuse. www.drugabuse.gov.

Avoid Indoor Tanning Beds

OVERVIEW

For decades, it has been well known that there is a strong correlation between the use of tanning beds, which emit ultraviolet rays, and skin cancer. Yet, tanning beds are widely used and readily available in communities throughout the United States and in other countries. In fact, according to an article published in 2015 in the *American Journal of Preventive Medicine*, almost 30 percent of white female high school students and 13 percent of all high school students reported tanning indoors during the previous year, and about 25 percent of the high school tanners had used a tanning bed more than 20 times during that same time period. The tanning rates rise dramatically during the teen years. Seven percent of teens who are 14 years old use indoor tanners; by the time they are 17 years old, the rate has risen to 35 percent. The article noted that "the popularity of indoor tanning beds has risen amid mounting evidence of adverse health consequences."[1] Clearly, the use of tanning beds among younger people has become a serious public health concern.

WHAT THE EXPERTS SAY

There Appears to Be an Association between Indoor Tanning and Psychiatric and Addictive Symptoms in Young Adult Females

In a study published in 2014 in the *American Journal of Health Promotion*, researchers from Pennsylvania, Oregon, and New Jersey wanted to learn more about the association between indoor tanning in young adult females and psychiatric and addictive symptoms. The cohort consisted of 306 female university students between the ages of 18 and 25 years, with an average age of 19.9 years. All of the women completed questionnaires and telephone interviews. The researchers found that 46 percent of the women reported a history of indoor tanning; of these, 25 percent were classified as "tanning dependent." There was also a significant association between indoor tanning and the symptoms of alcohol use disorders and generalized anxiety and a marginal association with the symptoms of seasonal affective disorder. The researchers underscored the importance of their findings. "Not only is the association between tanning and skin cancer a significant public health concern, but the association between tanning and psychiatric and substance use disorders may represent an important mental health concern."[2]

There Seems to Be a Strong Association between the Use of Tanning Beds and the Incidence of Skin Cancer

In a study published in 2012 in the *Journal of Clinical Oncology*, researchers from Boston and China wanted to evaluate the association between the use of sun tanning beds and skin cancer in teens and young adults. The cohort consisted of 73,494 female nurses who were followed for 20 years from 1989 to 2009 in the United States. During follow-up, 5,506 nurses were diagnosed with basal cell carcinoma, 403 with squamous cell carcinoma, and 349 with melanoma. The researchers found a dose-response relationship between frequency of tanning bed use and risk of skin cancers. So, more frequent tanning bed users had higher rates of the three most common types of skin cancer; this was most evident with the incidence of basal cell carcinoma. And, the association was strongest for people who used tanning beds at younger ages. The researchers advised policy makers to "promote restrictions on the indoor tanning industry."[3]

In a study published in 2012 in the *Journal of the American Academy of Dermatology*, researchers from New Haven, Connecticut, examined the association between early exposure to indoor tanning and the early onset of basal cell cancer. The researchers identified 376 people with basal cell cancer and another 390 with minor benign skin conditions; all of the participants were under the age of 40 years and almost 70 percent were female. The participants provided detailed information on their use of indoor tanning. The researchers learned that the people who had ever used an indoor tanner had a 69 percent increased risk of early-onset basal cell cancer. The risk increased in those with years of regular indoor tanning, number of overall burns, and burns to biopsy site. According to the researchers, about 27 percent of all early onset basal cell cancers could be prevented if people never used indoor tanners. Moreover, women who tanned indoors were two times more likely to have basal cell cancer than women who never tanned indoors. In addition, indoor tanning was strongly associated with basal cell cancers that were located on the trunk and extremities, body sites that are particularly exposed during indoor tanning. The researchers concluded that "both policy-based and behavioral interventions to restrict or reduce indoor tanning in young people are needed to alter the increasing incidence of this most common human malignancy."[4]

BARRIERS AND PROBLEMS

Tanning Beds Are Easy to Find on or near Many College Campuses

In a study published in 2015 in *JAMA Dermatology*, researchers from Massachusetts and Tennessee wanted to evaluate the availability of indoor tanning facilities on and near college and university campuses in the United States. The cohort consisted of the top 125 U.S. colleges and universities listed in the *US News and World Report*. The researchers noted that they selected those schools because they "represented the most highly regarded colleges in the United States, ones that may be viewed as trendsetters for US undergraduate education." The researchers searched Web sites of the colleges and universities and nearby housing and contacted them by telephone to ask about tanning services. The researchers found that 48 percent of the 125 colleges and universities had indoor tanning facilities either on campus or in off-campus housing. In addition, 14.4 percent of the colleges and universities allowed campus cash cards to be used to pay for tanning. Indoor tanning was available on campus in 12 percent of the colleges and universities and in off-campus housing in 42.4 percent of the college and universities. Almost all of the off-campus housing facilities with indoor tanning provided it free to tenants. The highest prevalence of indoor tanning on campus was found in the Midwest, and the highest prevalence of indoor tanning in off-campus housing was found in the South. The West had no colleges that offered on-campus tanning. The researchers concluded that "the presence of indoor tanning facilities on and near college campuses may passively reinforce indoor tanning in college students, thereby facilitating behavior that will increase their risk for skin cancer both in the short term and later in life."[5]

Not All Tanning Salons Obey the Underage Rules and Some Salons Provide Incorrect Information

In a study published in 2013 in the *Journal of the American Academy of Dermatology*, researchers from Pennsylvania and California noted that in 2011 California became the first state to pass a ban on indoor tanning for those under the age of 18 years. Since then, several other states have followed. But has the ban actually prevented younger people from tanning? A researcher posing as a 17-year-old teen contacted 338 tanning operations throughout California and asked to make an appointment. When she noted her age, 77 percent of the tanning salons refused to schedule a time. That means that in almost one-quarter of the salons the researcher could schedule tanning. Of these, 12 percent said that she could come and 11 percent said that she could come with parental consent. One facility indicated that she could tan with a doctor's note and another said to come and discuss the situation in person. Even more alarming is the fact that almost 80 percent of the tanning facilities told the researcher that when she turned 18, she could tan daily, as often as she wanted. When asked about any risks associated with tanning, 61 percent of the facilities denied there was any danger. Almost half of the facilities noted that tanning increased the body's production of vitamin D. Some indicated that tanning was useful for medical conditions such as acne, eczema, psoriasis, depression, and arthritis. The researchers commented that "California has substantial work ahead to achieve more uniform compliance."[6]

Some Researchers Contend That Indoor Tanning Has the Potential to Be Addictive

In an article published in 2015, a researcher from the University of Kansas noted that despite the negative impact indoor tanning has on the body, the rates are increasing at record levels, and the industry is making extraordinary profits. According to this researcher, it has become obvious that frequent indoor tanning users have trouble quitting the practice. They report that tanning makes them feel healthier and that people perceive them as being healthier. And, indoor tanners are far more focused on the present benefits of tanning than the long-term negative consequences. Moreover, they experience withdrawal symptoms similar to those seen in substance-related disorders, such as nausea and jitteriness. In fact, indoor tanners are more likely to practice other risky behaviors, such as smoking, binge drinking, illicit drug use, unhealthy weight control practices, steroid use, and sex with multiple partners. Left unchecked, the many people demonstrating addictive indoor tanning behaviors "could become a major burden on the health care industry."[7]

In a study published in 2010 in the journal *Clinical and Experimental Dermatology*, researchers from Dallas, Texas, assessed the presence of addictive-like behaviors in people who frequently use indoor tanning facilities. The cohort consisted of 64 women and 36 men who completed two questionnaires; their mean age was 29.3 years. In total, 41 of the subjects met the criteria of tanning addictive behavior and an additional 33 met the criteria for problematic tanning behavior. That means that 74 of the 100 participants reported some level of aberrant tanning behaviors. The researchers concluded that "a high percentage of subjects who tan frequently in indoor salons experience behaviours and consequences to their tanning consistent with other identified addictive disorders."[8]

NOTES

1. Andrew B. Seidenberg, Aditya Mahalingam-Dhingra, Martin A. Weinstock et al., "Youth Indoor Tanning and Skin Cancer Prevention," *American Journal of Preventive Medicine* 48, no. 2 (2015): 188–94.

2. Carolyn J. Heckman, Jessye Cohen-Filipic, Susan Darlow et al., "Psychiatric and Addictive Symptoms of Young Adult Female Indoor Tanners," *American Journal of Health Promotion* 28, no. 3 (2014): 168–74.

3. Mingfeng Zhang, Abrar A. Qureshi, Alan C. Geller et al., "Use of Tanning Beds and Incidence of Skin Cancer," *Journal of Clinical Oncology* 30, no. 14 (2012): 1588–93.

4. Leah M. Ferrucci, Brenda Cartmel, Annette M. Molinaro et al., "Indoor Tanning and Risk of Early-Onset Basal Cell Carcinoma," *Journal of the American Academy of Dermatology* 67, no. 4 (2012): 552–62.

5. Sherry L. Pagoto, Stephenie C. Lemon, Jessica L. Oleski et al., "Availability of Tanning Beds on US College Campuses," *JAMA Dermatology* 151, no. 1 (2015): 59–63.

6. Sungat K. Grewal, Ann F. Haas, Mark J. Pletcher et al., "Compliance by California Tanning Facilities with the Nation's First Statewide Ban on Use Before the Age of 18 Years," *Journal of the American Academy of Dermatology* 69, no. 6 (2013): 883–89.

7. Derek D. Reed, "Ultra-Violet Indoor Tanning Addiction: A Reinforcer Pathology Interpretation," *Addictive Behaviors* 41 (2015): 247–51.

8. C. R. Harrington, T. C. Beswick, J. Leitenberger et al., "Addictive-Like Behaviours to Ultraviolet Light Among Frequent Indoor Tanners," *Clinical and Experimental Dermatology* 36 (2010): 33–38.

REFERENCES AND RESOURCES

Magazines, Journals, and Newspapers

Banerjee, Smita C., Jennifer L. Hay, Alan C. Geller et al. "Quitting the 'Cancer Tube': A Qualitative Examination of the Process of Indoor Tanning Cessation." *Translational Behavioral Medicine* 4, no. 2 (2014): 209–19.

Ferrucci, Leah M., Brenda Cartmel, Annette M. Molinaro et al. "Indoor Tanning and Risk of Early-Onset Basal Cell Carcinoma." *Journal of the American Academy of Dermatology* 67, no. 4 (2012): 552–62.

Grewal, Sungat K., Ann F. Haas, Mark J. Pletcher et al. "Compliance by California Tanning Facilities with the Nation's First Statewide Ban on Use Before the Age of 18 Years." *Journal of the American Academy of Dermatology* 69, no. 6 (2013): 883–89.

Harrington, C. R., T. C. Beswick, J. Leitenberger et al. "Addictive-Like Behaviours to Ultraviolet Light Among Frequent Tanners." *Clinical and Experimental Dermatology* 36 (2010): 33–38.

Heckman, Carolyn J., Jessye Cohen-Filipic, Susan Darlow et al. "Psychiatric and Addictive Symptoms of Young Adult Female Indoor Tanners." *American Journal of Health Promotion* 28, no. 3 (2014): 168–74.

Heckman, Carolyn J., Teja Munshi, Susan Darlow et al. "The Association of Tanning Behavior with Psychotropic Medication Use Among Young Adult Women." *Psychology, Health & Medicine* 21 (2016): 60–66.

Mosher, Catherine, and Sharon Danoff-Burg. "Addiction to Indoor Tanning: Relation to Anxiety, Depression, and Substance Use." *Archives of Dermatology* 146, no. 4 (2010): 412–17.

Pagoto, Sherry L., Stephenie C. Lemon, Jessica L. Oleski et al. "Availability of Tanning Beds on U.S. College Campuses." *JAMA Dermatology* 151, no. 1 (2015): 59–63.

Reed, Derek D. "Ultra-Violet Indoor Tanning Addiction: A Reinforcer Pathology Interpretation." *Addictive Behaviors* 41 (2015): 247–51.

Seidenberg, Andrew B., Aditya Mahalingam-Dhingra, Martin A. Weinstock et al. "Youth Indoor Tanning and Skin Cancer Prevention." *American Journal of Preventive Medicine* 48, no. 2 (2015): 188–94.

Zhang, Mingfeng, Abar A. Qureshi, Alan C. Geller et al. "Use of Tanning Beds and Incidence of Skin Cancer." *Journal of Clinical Oncology* 30, no. 14 (2012): 1588–93.

Web Sites

American Academy of Dermatology. www.aad.org.
U.S. Food and Drug Administration. www.fda.gov.

Get Enough Sleep

OVERVIEW

Like people of all ages, teens need sleep. According to the National Sleep Foundation, "sleep is food for the brain." While people sleep, "important body functions and brain activity occur." Without sufficient sleep, you compromise your ability to learn, listen, concentrate, and solve problems. You will have trouble focusing on tasks. A brain that is tired will find a way to obtain sleep. It may even fall asleep while driving. It has been estimated that drowsiness causes more than 100,000 car crashes each year.[1]

Most teens require more than nine hours of sleep. But unlike people of other ages, teens naturally tend to stay up later at night. In general, teens have trouble falling asleep before 11 pm. During adolescence, their internal clock, known as circadian rhythm, shifts them in that direction. Some normally stay up even later. Still, they must awaken relatively early to attend school and/or work at their jobs. As a result, teens may easily have a chronic sleep shortage. It is not uncommon for them to yawn and even fall asleep during the school day. According to an article published in 2014 in *Pediatric Nursing*, 87 percent of teens do not obtain adequate amounts of sleep.[2]

WHAT THE EXPERTS SAY

There Appears to Be an Association between Sleep and Academic Performance

In a study published in 2012 in the *Journal of School Health*, researchers from Hong Kong examined the association between sleep patterns, naps, and sleep disorders and the academic performance of students. The cohort consisted of 22,678 students between the ages of 12 and 18 years. They all completed questionnaires on various characteristics, including sleep patterns and academic performance. The researchers learned that during regular school nights only 27.4 percent of the students slept more than eight hours. On the other hand, during non-school nights, 86.4 percent of the students slept more than eight hours. The researchers found an association between late weekend bedtimes and poor academic performance. After-school naps and insufficient sleep also appeared to be associated with poor academic performance. At the same time, delays in awakening on the weekend improved academic performance. The researchers advised students with academic performance problems to "seek medical advice for maintaining a better health-related lifestyle including sufficient rest time."[3]

There Is a Relationship between Adolescent Sleep and School Attendance

In a population-based study published in 2015 in the *Scandinavian Journal of Public Health*, researchers from Norway wanted to learn more about the relationship between adolescent sleep and non-attendance at school. The cohort consisted of 8,347 teens between the ages of 16 and 19 years. Sleep measures included a number of factors such as bedtime, rise time, sleep efficiency, sleep duration, sleep onset latency, waking after sleep onset, insomnia, tiredness, and sleepiness. The researchers found that there was an association between most of these sleep measures and school nonattendance. "Adolescent sleep problems were related to an important functional outcome: school absence." For example, the researchers found adolescents who slept too little were four times as likely to have "substantial school absence." The researchers concluded that students who are identified as having excessive school absences should have their sleep behaviors evaluated.[4]

Insufficient Sleep May Create Safety Concerns

In a study published in 2013 in the *Journal of Adolescent Health*, researchers from Birmingham, Alabama, noted that each year over 8,000 American teens between the ages of 14 and 15 years require medical attention as a result of a pedestrian injury. The researchers wondered if the lack of sleep placed teens at increased risk for these injuries. The cohort consisted of 55 teens between the ages of 14 and 15 years. After one night of four hours of sleep and another night of 8 1/2 hours of sleep, these teens participated in a virtual reality pedestrian environment, which "replicated a two-lane, bidirectional, mid-block street crossing near a local elementary school." Caffeine consumption, which could alter levels of fatigue, was prohibited during those mornings. The teens completed 25 trials while sleep restricted and 25 trials while adequately rested. The results were dramatic. Compared to a night of adequate sleep, following a night of restricted sleep, the teens took more time to begin crossing the street, had less time before contact with vehicles, had more close calls or actual virtual hits, and looked right and left more often. The researchers commented that "inadequate sleep may influence cognitive functioning to the extent that pedestrian safety is jeopardized among adolescents capable of crossing streets safely when rested."[5]

In a study published in 2014 in the *Journal of Clinical Sleep Medicine*, researchers from Virginia and Texas examined the association between the times that teens begin their school day and rates of car crashes. From their earlier research on the topic, the researchers hypothesized that the schools that began their day earlier would have more teens in car crashes. Those teens would need to awaken earlier. The researchers obtained their data on weekday crashes in 16- to 18-year-old teens as well as adults from the Virginia Department of Motor Vehicles. The researchers compared data from Chesterfield County, which starts school 85 minutes earlier, with data from Henrico County, which has a later starting time. As they expected, the researchers found teens who were traveling to schools with the earlier starting times had statistically significant higher rates of crashes. The researchers noted that their findings "adds to the body of research that suggests that early high school start times may be disadvantageous for teen driving safety."[6]

There Is an Association between
Sleep Problems and Excess Weight

In a population-based study published in 2013 in the *Journal of School Health*, researchers from Taiwan investigated the association between sleep quality and weight status, according to body mass index—BMI, among teenagers. The cohort consisted of 2,113 teens between the ages of 15 and 17 years and 5,496 other family members. Sleep quality was divided into three types—difficulty in initiating sleep, difficulty in maintaining sleep, and nonrestorative sleep. The researchers found that 20.9 percent of the teens experienced one of these sleep problems. And, there was an association between difficulty in initiating sleep and higher levels of BMI. The researchers concluded that their findings "suggest that efforts to address childhood overweight and obesity need to take into consideration sleep problems that are highly prevalent among teens."[7]

BARRIERS AND PROBLEMS

Use of Cellular Phones among Teens Is Probably Interfering with Sleep

In an article published in 2013 in *Health Services Insights*, researchers from the University of Rhode Island noted that the use of cellular phones among teens has emerged as an "important factor" that is interfering with both the quality and quantity of teen sleep. Use of phones among teens has grown astronomically; according to these researchers, it is not uncommon for teens to send 100 texts per day. In addition, teens often use phones in bed before falling asleep. As a result, their ability to fall asleep and remain sleeping may be compromised. For example, they may awaken to answer text messages. Moreover, "emerging research points to the prevalence of patterns of problematic phone use among adolescents that are akin to behavioral addiction." Thus, it is very difficult to restrict or "place boundaries" on the phone use of teens. The researchers advised medical providers to ask teens candid questions about their sleep practices. And, if appropriate, medical providers should discuss the importance of establishing boundaries between sleep and phones. "Given the importance of sleep on growing minds and bodies, any efforts to improve adolescent sleep quantity and quality should be considered a worthwhile investment."[8]

Screen Viewing Devices Negatively Impact Sleep

In a study published in 2014 in the *International Journal of Environmental Research and Public Health*, researchers from China investigated the impact that screen viewing devices, such as phones and personal computers, have on sleep duration, sleep quality, and daytime sleepiness among Hong Kong adolescents.

According to these researchers, while the American Academy of Pediatrics recommends that screen viewing time be no more than one to two hours per day, "screen viewing has becomes a crucial activity in the everyday life of adolescents."

The cohort consisted of 762 teens who ranged in age from 12 to 20 years, with a mean age of 15.27 years. Sleeping assessments were made using the Chinese version of the Sleep Quality Index, and the teens reported the exact amount of time that they spent viewing televisions, computers, portable devices, and mobile phones. While the teens noted that they slept an average of 7.74 hours per night, 414 teens or 55.6 percent reported sleeping less than 8 hours per night. At the same time, the teens said that they used screen devices an average of 5 hours 54 minutes per day. The researchers found no association between watching television and any of the sleep variables, and the only sleep variable associated with computer viewing was daytime sleepiness. Similarly, portable devices were only related to sleep duration. On the other hand, mobile phone viewing was correlated with all three sleep variables. Why are these findings so important? According to the researchers, obtaining adequate quality sleep is a crucial component of a successful adolescence. That is why "determining the recommended level of screen viewing among adolescents is a matter of public health."[9]

Video-Game Use before Bedtime Negatively Impacts Sleep

In a study published in 2014 in the *Journal of Adolescence*, researchers from Australia noted that video-gaming is incredibly popular among teens in the United States, with more than three-quarters of all children and teens playing them every week. They wanted to learn more about the association between the use of video games before bedtime and subsequent sleep, working memory (short-term memory), and sustained attention performance. Their cohort consisted of 21 healthy teens (16 males) between the ages of 15 and 20 years. All of the teens were considered "good sleepers." During a one-night stay in the sleep laboratory, a number of different measurements were taken. The researchers learned that, on average, the participants spent four hours gaming in one pre-bedtime session and obtained slightly less than seven hours of sleep. Males spent significantly more time gaming and obtained significantly less sleep. They slept less because they spent so much time gaming, not because they had a problem falling asleep. Because gaming reduced the number of hours slept, it diminished sustained attention in the morning, but not working memory. The researchers noted that their findings "highlight the potential performance deficits associated with evening gaming, especially if repeated on consecutive nights, which may have important consequences in domains such as school achievement and accident risk." To mitigate these problems, "video games should be used in moderation and not too close to the sleep period."[10]

When Someone Sleeps Appears to Make a Difference

In a study published in 2011 in *SLEEP*, researchers from Australia wanted to learn more about the association between early and late bedtimes and wake up time and weight status on preteens and teens in Australia. The cohort consisted of 2,200 preteens and teens between the ages of 9 and 16 years. The preteens and teens were divided into one of four groups: early bed/early rise, early bed/late rise, late bed/early rise, and late bed/late rise. The groups were then evaluated for several factors, including weight status. Despite the fact that they obtained essentially the same amounts of sleep, the preteens and teens who went to bed later and slept later in the morning were 1 1/2 times more likely to become obese than those who went to bed earlier and awakened earlier. Those who went to bed later and slept later in the morning were less physically active and had far more screen time. They were "1.8 times more likely to be insufficiently active, and 2.9 times more likely to have excessive screen time." The researchers said that they find it "somewhat concerning" that the obviously healthier pattern is not "characteristically observed during adolescence." The researchers concluded that their findings "indicate the importance of bed time, as opposed to sleep duration, may have been relatively overlooked to date."[11]

NOTES

1. National Sleep Foundation, http://sleepfoundation.org.

2. Shirley A. Wiggins and Jackie L. Freeman, "Understanding Sleep During Adolescence," *Pediatric Nursing* 40, no. 2 (2014): 91–98.

3. K-K. Mak, S-L Lee, S-Y Ho et al., "Sleep and Academic Performance in Hong Kong Adolescents," *Journal of School Health* 82, no. 11 (2012): 522–27.

4. Mari Hysing, Siren Haugland, Kjell Morten Stormark et al., "Sleep and School Attendance in Adolescence: Results from a Large Population-Based Study," *Scandinavian Journal of Public Health* 43, no. 1 (2015): 2–9.

5. Aaron L. Davis, Kristin T. Avis, and David C. Schwebel, "The Effects of Acute Sleep Restriction on Adolescents' Pedestrian Safety in a Virtual Environment," *Journal of Adolescent Health* 53 (2013): 785–90.

6. Robert Daniel Vorona, Mariana Szklo-Coxe, Rajan Lamichhane et al., "Adolescent Crash Rates and School Start Times in Two Central Virginia Counties, 2009–2011: A Follow-Up Study to a Southeastern Virginia Study, 2007–2008," *Journal of Clinical Sleep Medicine* 10, no. 11 (2014): 1169–1177E.

7. Duan-Rung Chen, Khoa D. Truong, and Meng-Ju Tsai, "Prevalence of Poor Sleep Quality and Its Relationship with Body Mass Index Among Teenagers: Evidence from Taiwan," *Journal of School Health* 83, no. 8 (2013): 582–88.

8. Sue K. Adams, Jennifer F. Daly, and Desireé N. Williford, "Adolescent Sleep and Cellular Phone Use: Recent Trends and Implications for Research," *Health Services Insights* 6 (2013): 99–103.

9. Yim Wah Mak, Cynthia Sau Ting Wu, Donna Wing Shun Hui et al., "Association Between Screen Viewing Duration and Sleep Duration, Sleep Quality, and Excessive Daytime Sleepiness Among Adolescents in Hong Kong," *International Journal of Environmental Research and Public Health* 11, no. 11 (2014): 11201–19.

10. Jasper Wolfe, Kellyann Kar, Ashleigh Perry et al., "Single Night Video-Game Use Leads to Sleep Loss and Attention Deficits in Older Adolescents," *Journal of Adolescence* 37 (2014): 1003–9.

11. Tim S. Olds, Carol A. Maher, and Lisa Matricciani, "Sleep Duration or Bedtime? Exploring the Relationship Between Sleep Habits and Weight Status and Activity Patterns," *SLEEP* 34, no. 10 (2011): 1299–307.

REFERENCES AND RESOURCES

Magazines, Journals, and Newspaper

Adachi-Mejia, Anna M., Patricia M. Edwards, Diane Gilbert-Diamond et al. "TXT Me I'm Only Sleeping: Adolescents with Mobile Phones in their Bedroom." *Family & Community Health* 37, no. 4 (2014): 252–57.

Adams, Sue K., Jennifer F. Daly, and Desireé N. Williford. "Adolescent Sleep and Cellular Phone Use: Recent Trends and Implications for Research." *Health Services Insights* 6 (2013): 99–103.

Chang, Anne-Marie, Daniel Aeschbach, Jeanne F. Duffy, and Charles A. Czeisler. "Evening Use of Light-Emitting eReaders Negatively Affects Sleep, Circadian Timing, and Next-Morning Alertness." *Proceedings of the National Academy of Sciences of the USA* 112, no. 4 (2015): 1232–37.

Chen, Duan-Rung, Khoa D. Truong, and Meng-Ju Tsai. "Prevalence of Poor Sleep Quality and Its Relationship with Body Mass Index Among Teenagers: Evidence from Taiwan." *Journal of School Health* 83, no. 8 (2013): 582–88.

Davis, Aaron L., Kristin T. Avis, and David C. Schwebel. "The Effects of Acute Sleep Restriction on Adolescents' Pedestrian Safety in a Virtual Environment." *Journal of Adolescent Health* 53 (2013): 785–90.

Hysing, Mari, Siren Haugland, Kjell Morten Stormark et al. "Sleep and School Attendance in Adolescence: Results from a Large Population-Based Study." *Scandinavian Journal of Public Health* 43, no. 1 (2015): 2–9.

Mak, K-K., S-L Lee, S-Y Ho et al. "Sleep and Academic Performance in Hong Kong Adolescents." *Journal of School Health* 82, no. 11 (2012): 522–27.

Mak, Yim Wah, Cynthia Sau Ting Wu, Donna Wing Shun Hui et al. "Association Between Screen Viewing Duration and Sleep Duration, Sleep Quality, and Excessive Daytime Sleepiness Among Adolescents in Hong Kong." *International Journal of Environmental Research and Public Health* 11, no. 11 (2014): 11201–19.

Olds, Tim S., Carol A. Maher, and Lisa Matricciani. "Sleep Duration or Bedtime? Exploring the Relationship Between Sleep Habits and Weight Status and Activity Patterns." *SLEEP* 34, no. 10 (2011): 1299–307.

Vorona, Robert Daniel, Mariana Szklo-Coxe, Rajan Lamichhane et al. "Adolescent Crash Rates and School Start Times in Two Central Virginia Counties, 2009–2011: A Follow-Up Study to a Southeastern Virginia Study, 2007–2008." *Journal of Clinical Sleep Medicine* 10, no. 11 (2014): 1169–1177E.

Wiggins, Shirley A., and Jackie L. Freeman. "Understanding Sleep During Adolescence." *Pediatric Nursing* 40, no. 2 (2014): 91–98.

Wolfe, Jasper, Kellyann Kar, Ashleigh Perry et al. "Single Night Video-Game Use Leads to Sleep Loss and Attention Deficits in Older Adolescents." *Journal of Adolescence* 37 (2014): 1003–9.

Web Site

National Sleep Foundation. http://sleepfoundation.org.

Improve Health Literacy Skills

OVERVIEW

It is important that everyone is able to obtain, process, and understand basic health information. This information may then be used to make appropriate and necessary health decisions. Ideally, teens and young adults have at least one parent or other family member to assist with health literacy. But, sometimes, teens and young adults must travel this route by themselves or with the assistance of a nonadult friend. While maintaining a healthy lifestyle may not be easy for many teens and young adults, those who have better health literacy skills may find the process a little easier.

Health literacy requires some degree of mathematical skills. These are needed to calculate such figures as cholesterol and blood sugar levels, measure medications, and understand nutrition labels. Mathematical skills also help with calculating premiums and determining amounts of copays and deductibles. On the other hand, analytical skills may be used to select a health plan or compare prescription drug coverage.[1]

People with limited health literacy skills have an increased risk of making health care mistakes. To make better health care decisions, it is important to take steps to improve one's health literacy.

WHAT THE EXPERTS SAY

Curriculums May Be Designed to Improve Health Literacy

In an article published in 2016 in the journal *Health Education & Behavior*, researchers from Boston and Somerville, Massachusetts, wanted to learn more about how a biology curriculum that focused on infectious diseases improved health literacy. The curriculum was implemented between 2010 and 2013 in elective Biology II classes in three public high schools in Massachusetts, one public high school in Ohio, and a private school in Virginia. The 273 student participants were compared to an age-matched nonparticipant peer group of 125 students from the same schools. The participants in each of the school settings demonstrated increases in conceptual content knowledge and an improved ability to apply scientific principles to health claim evaluation and risk assessment. In addition, the school participants had greater knowledge about infectious diseases, and they shared their information with their social networks. As a result of their findings, the researchers suggested that high school biology classes were a "viable setting" to foster health literacy skills to diverse populations, and these classes "should be used more extensively."[2]

It Is Important to Use Credible Online Health Sources

In a study published in 2012 in the *Journal of School Health*, researchers from Harlingen, Texas, and Ann Arbor, Michigan, wrote that there has been little research on the association between credible online health information sources and adolescent health literacy. As a result, the researchers decided to explore health literacy among predominantly Hispanic teens and to determine if they are exposed to credible online health resources. The researchers administered an online survey to a cross-sectional random sample of high school students, with a mean age of 16 years, in southern Texas. In general, the vast majority of the students searched online for health information. Of the 261 students who completed the survey, 56 percent had heard of MedlinePlus®, a health information Web site developed and maintained by the National Library of Medicine, and 52 percent had adequate levels of health literacy. When compared to the students who had not heard of MedlinePlus®, the students who had heard of this Web site reported higher levels of perceived skills and confidence in looking for health information and more adequate levels of health literacy. Thus, their exposure to credible sources of online health information improved their levels of health literacy. The researchers commented that their results "supported the importance of introducing adolescents to credible online health information resources."[3]

Low Health Literacy Is Associated with Poorer Health Outcomes

In a systematic review published in 2011 in the journal *Annals of Internal Medicine*, researchers based in Durham, North Carolina, examined research articles on the association between low health literacy and health outcomes. After identifying close to 4,000 studies published from 2003 to May 2010, the researchers selected 96 studies in 111 articles, which they rated as having good or fair quality. The researchers found that low health literacy was consistently associated with more hospitalization, greater use of emergency care, lower use of mammography screening, lower use of influenza vaccine, poorer compliance with medications, less ability to understand labels and messages, and, among the elderly, poorer health status and higher mortality. The researchers concluded that "low health literacy is associated with poorer health outcomes and poorer use of health care services."[4]

Teens from Less Advantaged Environments
May Improve Their Health Literacy

In a study published in 2015 in the *Journal of the Medical Library Association*, researchers from Bethesda, Maryland, and Charleston, South Carolina, evaluated a small program designed to improve health literacy, leadership skills, and interest in health careers in high school students living in a low-income, primarily minority community. Students enrolled in the program at the beginning of 11th or 12th grade. The cohort consisted of 11 students who had participated in the program; there were nine females and two males, all

African American. During the program, the students learned about reliable, authoritative health information Web sites. The students used information from these Web sites to create and conduct school and community outreach activities, such as mentoring their peers and exhibiting at local health fairs. All of the students participated in semistructured interviews. The researchers determined that the program had a positive impact on the students' health information competency, leadership skills, academic orientation, and interest in health careers. They concluded that "health information can provide a powerful context for enabling disadvantaged students' community engagement and academic success."[5]

BARRIERS AND PROBLEMS

Everyone Does Not Have Sufficient Health Literacy. Health Materials Need to Be Designed to Direct Readers to the Most Important Information

In a study published in 2013 in the *Journal of Health Communication*, researchers from Texas and Arizona wanted to learn more about how people with different levels of health literacy visualize health related information. The researchers recruited 25 university administrative staff members, whom they assumed would have adequate health literacy skills, and 25 adults enrolled in an adult literacy program, whom they assumed would have limited health literacy skills. During the trial, each subject participated in a health literacy assessment that involved answering questions about an ice cream nutrition label while viewing the label. Two of the questions involved finding information and four required numerical calculations. The researchers found that the subjects with less health literacy spent more time looking at information that was not relevant to the question asked. In fact, those with lower levels of health literacy looked at one spot, even if it was irrelevant, for longer amounts of time than those with high levels of health literacy. As a result of their findings the researchers concluded that health information for patients "should be designed to help them better distinguish important from unimportant information."[6]

Teens with Low Levels of Health Literacy Appear to Have Fewer Healthful Nutritional Behaviors

In a cross-sectional study published in 2010 in the *Journal of Clinical Nursing*, researchers from Taiwan examined the association between health literacy and health status and health-promoting behaviors. The cohort consisted of 1,601 senior/ vocational high school students from six counties in Taiwan. There were slightly more males than females, and the mean age was 17 years. Data were obtained on the following health-promoting behaviors: nutrition, exercise, stress management, interpersonal relations, health responsibility, and self-actualization. The researchers found an association between low health literacy and poorer health status and fewer nutritional-health-promoting behaviors. The researchers concluded that "health literacy is vital for promoting health in adolescence, especially in the domains of nutrition and interpersonal relations."[7]

Nurses Tend to Overestimate the Health Literacy of Their Patients

In a trial published in 2013 in the *Journal of Health Communication*, researchers from Chicago noted that it is very important for nurses to be aware of their patients' level of health literacy. It is "integral to patient care, safety, education, and counseling." The researchers wanted to learn if inpatient nurses were properly assessing levels of health literacy. The cohort consisted of 65 patients and 30 nurses from two inpatient cardiac units; the study was conducted over a six-month period of time. The patients were primarily female African Americans who had heart failure as their diagnosis. The researchers found that the nurses incorrectly identified patients with low health literacy. Overestimates outnumbered underestimates by six to one. The researchers commented that "the overestimation of a patient's health literacy by nursing personnel may contribute to the widespread problem of poor health outcomes and hospital readmission rates." Apparently, there is a need for providing nurses with more training in health literacy. Unfortunately, "while some nursing schools now include HL [health literacy] education in their curriculum, most nurses do not receive this education."[8]

NOTES

1. U.S. Department of Health and Human Services, http://health.gov.

2. Jacque Berri, Susan Koch-Weser, Russell Faux, and Karina Meiri, "Addressing Health Literacy Challenges with a Cutting-Edge Infectious Disease Curriculum for the High School Biology Classroom." *Health Education & Behavior* 43 (2016): 43–53.

3. Suad F. Ghaddar, Melissa A. Valerio, Carolyn M. Garcia, and Lucy Hansen, "Adolescent Health Literacy: The Importance of Credible Sources for Online Health Information," *Journal of School Health* 82 (2012): 28–36.

4. Nancy D. Berkman, Stacey L. Sheridan, Katrina E. Donahue et al., "Low Health Literacy and Health Outcomes: An Updated Systematic Review." *Annals of Internal Medicine* 155 (2011): 97–107.

5. Alla Keselman, Einas A. Ahmed, Deborah C. Williamson et al., "Harnessing Health Information to Foster Disadvantaged Teens' Community Engagement, Leadership Skills, and Career Plans: A Qualitative Evaluation of the Teen Health Leadership Program," *Journal of the Medical Library Association* 103, no. 2 (2015): 82–86.

6. Michael Mackert, Sara E. Champlin, Keryn E. Pasch, and Barry D. Weiss, "Understanding Health Literacy Measurement Through Eye Tracking," *Journal of Health Communication* 18 (2013): 185–96.

7. Li-Chun Chang, "Health Literacy, Self-Reported Status and Health Promoting Behaviours for Adolescents in Taiwan," *Journal of Clinical Nursing* 20 (2010): 190–96.

8. Carolyn Dickens, Bruce L. Lambert, Terese Cromwell, and Mariann R. Piano, "Nurse Overestimation of Patients' Health Literacy," *Journal of Health Communication* 18, Supplement (2013): 62–69.

REFERENCES AND RESOURCES

Magazines, Journals, and Newspapers

Berkman, Nancy D., Stacey L. Sheridan, Katrina E. Donahue et al. "Low Health Literacy and Health Outcomes: An Updated Systematic Review." *Annals of Internal Medicine* 155 (2011): 97–107.

Chang, Li-Chun. "Health Literacy, Self-Reported Status and Health Promoting Behaviours for Adolescents in Taiwan." *Journal of Clinical Nursing* 20 (2010): 190–96.

Dickens, Carolyn, Bruce L. Lambert, Terese Cromwell, and Mariann R. Piano. "Nurse Overestimation of Patients' Health Literacy." *Journal of Health Communication* 18, Supplement 1 (2013): 62–69.

Ghaddar, Suad F., Melissa A. Valerio, Carolyn M. Garcia, and Lucy Hansen. "Adolescent Health Literacy: The Importance of Credible Sources for Online Health Information." *Journal of School Health* 82, no. 1 (2012): 28–36.

Jacque, Berri, Susan Koch-Weser, Russell Faux, and Karina Meiri. "Addressing Health Literacy Challenges with a Cutting-Edge Infectious Disease Curriculum for the High School Biology Classroom." *Health Education & Behavior* 43 (2016): 43–53.

Keselman, Alla, Einas A. Ahmed, Deborah C. Williamson et al. "Harnessing Health Information to Foster Disadvantaged Teens' Community Engagement, Leadership Skills, and Career Plans: A Qualitative Evaluation of the Teen Health Leadership Program." *Journal of the Medical Library Association* 103, no. 2 (2015): 82–86.

Mackert, Michael, Sara E. Champlin, Keryn E. Pasch, and Barry D. Weiss. "Understanding Health Literacy Measurement Through Eye Tracking." *Journal of Health Communication* 18 (2013): 185–96.

Morrison, Andrea, Ruben Chanmugathas, Marilyn M. Schapira et al. "Caregiver Low Health Literacy and Non-Urgent Use of the Pediatric Emergency Department for Febrile Illness." *Academic Pediatrics* 14, no. 5 (2014): 505–9.

Stewart, Diana W., Claire E. Adams, Miguel A. Cano et al. "Associations Between Health Literacy and Established Predictors of Smoking Cessation." *American Journal of Public Health* 103, no. 7 (2013): e43–e49.

Ye, Xiao-Hua, Yi Yang, Yan-Hui Gao et al. "Status and Determinants of Health Literacy Among Adolescents in Guangdong, China." *Asian Pacific Journal of Cancer Prevention* 15, no. 20 (2014): 8735–40.

Web Site

U.S. Department of Health and Human Services. http://health.gov.

Learn More About Internet Addiction

OVERVIEW

It must be obvious to just about anyone that large numbers of teens spend a good amount of time on the Internet. Most teens manage to balance time on the Internet with a host of other academic, athletic, and social interests. However, for some teens, time on the Internet turns into a serious behavior disorder that is more than a desire to be on the Internet too many hours of the day. Like other addictive behaviors, teen addiction to the Internet is characterized by a progressive loss of control over the ability to avoid, limit, or regulate the time spent on the Internet.

Thus far, experts have been unable to determine a specific cause for teen Internet addiction. It is generally thought that teens who suffer from disorders such as depression, anxiety, low self-esteem, poor self-image, and attention deficit hyperactivity disorder are at increased risk for Internet addiction. For these teens, spending time on the Internet releases endorphins, or brain chemicals that trigger feelings of pleasure. It is nearly impossible for them to limit their time on the Internet, even as their grades in school, outside activities, and friendships suffer from their hours online. It is not uncommon for them to distort or actually lie about their time on the Internet. Teens who are addicted to the Internet may also suffer a number of physical symptoms, including vision problems, insomnia, carpal tunnel syndrome, poor nutrition and/or personal hygiene, headaches, and back and neck pain.[1]

WHAT THE EXPERTS SAY

Some Researchers Consider Internet Addiction to Be a Major Health Problem among Teens

In a cross-sectional study published in 2014 in the *Journal of the Pakistan Medical Association*, researchers from Turkey wanted to learn more about the frequency of Internet addiction among secondary and high school students in a rural area of Turkey where most people lived by farming and animal husbandry. The cohort consisted of 1,157 students—55 percent males and 45 percent females between the ages of 11 and 19 years. All the participants completed questionnaires. According to the Internet Addiction Scale, 7.9 percent of the students were addicted to the Internet. Students who described themselves as having a Type A personality and students who started using the Internet at younger ages had higher rates of Internet addiction. The researchers also found that students who used the Internet every day or at least 14 hours per week were at increased risk for addiction. Since they spend so much time sitting at the computer, they are at increased risk for being overweight or even obese. The incidence of Internet addiction was much higher in the obese students. Addiction was less prevalent in those who used the Internet for homework and research than those who used it for entertainment and social relationships. Internet addiction was also associated with loneliness. The researchers concluded that "Internet addiction was found to be a major health problem in middle and high school students."[2]

Teens Who Are Addicted to the Internet Have an Increased Risk for Being Overweight

In a cross-sectional study published in 2014 in the journal *Cyberpsychology, Behavior, and Social Networking*, researchers from Turkey investigated the association between Internet addiction and eating attitudes and body mass index (BMI). The cohort consisted of 1,938 students between the ages of 14 and 18 years who completed a questionnaire. Slightly over half the students were female. The researchers found that 12.4 percent of the teens had an Internet addiction. And, having a computer with an Internet connection was associated with an increased BMI. Students who surfed the Internet, watched videos, talked in chat rooms and via instant messaging, and played online games were significantly associated with increased BMI. But, students who used the Internet for academic activities had lowered BMI. Other Internet activities, such as checking email and shopping, were not associated with BMI.[3]

Internet Addiction May Exacerbate Depression and Hostility in Teens and Improvements in Internet Addiction May Be Useful in Lowering Levels of Depression, Hostility, and Social Anxiety

In a prospective study published in 2014 in the journal *Comprehensive Psychiatry*, researchers from Taiwan wanted to learn if an addiction to the Internet would exacerbate symptoms of depression, hostility, and social anxiety. The researchers recruited 2,293 students in grade 7 and assessed their Internet addiction, depression, hostility, and social anxiety. One year later, the same assessment was repeated. The teens who evolved from not addicted during the first assessment to addicted in the second assessment had increases in depression, especially among girls, and hostility. The teens who evolved from addicted in the first assessment to not addicted in the second assessment showed lower levels of depression, hostility, and social anxiety. The researchers noted that their study "revealed the negative mental health consequences of Internet addiction." But, it also showed that students who were in "remission" from Internet addiction exhibited "beneficial mental health effects." They recommended the implementation of prevention and intervention programs as early as possible to teens addicted to the Internet.[4]

Parental Involvement Appears to Reduce the Incidence of Internet Addiction and Related Problems

In a study published in 2015 in *Comprehensive Psychiatry*, researchers from Taiwan wanted to learn more about the association between parental mediation and involvement and Internet addiction, cyberbullying, substance use, and depression in teens. The cohort consisted of over 1,800 junior high school students who completed questionnaires in 2013. One-seventh of the students were found to have an Internet addiction; the addiction was more likely to occur in male students than female students. And, students with poor school performance had an increased risk for Internet addiction. The researchers found that the students who perceived lower levels of parental attachment were more likely to experience Internet addiction, cyberbullying, smoking, and depression. On the other hand, students who reported higher levels of parental restrictions were less likely to experience Internet addiction or engage in cyberbullying. Adolescent Internet addiction was found to be associated with cyberbullying, victimization/perpetration, smoking, consumption of alcohol, and depression. The researchers noted that "measures such as promoting family functions and parental mediation of Internet use by children were needed to prevent Internet addiction and online risks."[5]

University Students Who Are Addicted to the Internet Tend to Be Shy and Aggressive

In a study published in 2013 in the journal *Computers in Human Behavior*, researchers from Turkey investigated the association between problematic Internet use and shyness, narcissism, loneliness, aggression, and self-perception in 424 male and female Turkish university students. The students ranged in age from 17 to 23 years. The researchers found positive associations between problematic Internet use and shyness and aggression. No statistically significant correlation was seen between problematic Internet use and narcissism, loneliness, or self-perception. The researchers concluded that their findings "will assist practitioners and researchers in identifying risk groups, taking preventive measures and adopting policies aimed at those risk groups."[6]

Parent-Adolescent Interaction May Well Play a Role in Fostering or Preventing Internet Addiction

In a study published in 2014 in the journal *BMC Psychiatry*, researchers from Shanghai wanted to learn more about the association between family-based factors and adolescent Internet addiction. From October to November 2007, 5,122 junior and senior students, with a mean age of 15.9 years, from 16 high schools, completed questionnaires. The researchers found that strong parental disapproval of the Internet was associated with Internet addiction. Bad mother-adolescent relationships were more strongly associated with Internet addiction than bad father-adolescent relationships. The researchers maintained that their study "showed the importance of improving parent-adolescent communication." It appeared that "parental supervision and parent-adolescent harmonious interaction" played a key role in the prevention of adolescent Internet addiction.[7]

BARRIERS AND PROBLEMS

Problematic Internet Use by Parents May Well Be Associated with Problematic Internet Use by Teens, Especially When the Teens Are Stressed

In a study published in 2015 in the *Journal of Adolescent Health*, researchers from Australia and Hong Kong investigated the association between parental problematic Internet use and problematic Internet use among their teenage children, who were 13 to 17 years old. Although the researchers began with over 1,000 parent and teen dyads, 263 teens and 62 parents were classified as moderate to severe problematic users of the Internet. About 14 percent of the teens were classified as having moderate to severe levels of stress. The researchers found a significant association between parental and teen problematic Internet use. The parents of the teens who had moderate to severe problematic Internet use were more than three times as likely to be classified with moderate to severe problematic Internet use. However, this relationship only held true for the teens who did not experience high levels of stress. The relationship became insignificant among teens who experienced high levels of stress. The researchers noted that their findings "have a direct implication on the clinical treatment, management, and prevention of PIU [problematic Internet use] among young people, particularly in East Asian countries where adolescent PIU is prevalent, and where parental influence on adolescents is a cultural characteristic."[8]

It Appears to Be Useful to Distinguish between Generalized Internet Addiction and Specific Internet Addiction

In a study published in 2015 in the journal *Asia-Pacific Psychiatry*, researchers from Germany, China, and Taiwan wanted to determine if it was important to distinguish between generalized and specific Internet addiction. They explained that generalized Internet addiction refers to the problematic use of the Internet "covering a broad range of Internet-related activities." That contrasted with specific Internet addiction, which is the problematic use of particular online activities, such as excessive video gaming or devoting excessive time to social networks. The cross-cultural cohort consisted of 636 participants from China, Taiwan, Sweden, and Germany. In questionnaires, the researchers assessed generalized Internet addiction as well as addictive behaviors in online video gaming, online shopping, online social networks, and online pornography. They found that the participants had "distinct forms of specific Internet addiction." There was only one exception. The researchers determined that there was a correlation between online social network addiction and generalized Internet addiction. This was most often seen in Germany. The researchers concluded that "specific and generalized Internet addiction can be distinguished."[9]

NOTES

1. Net Addiction, netaddiction.com, and Psych Central, psychcentral.com.

2. Tugce Koyuncu, Alaettin Unsal, Didem Arslantas, "Assessment of Internet Addiction and Loneliness in Secondary and High School Students," *Journal of the Pakistan Medical Association* 64, no. 9 (2014): 998–1002.

3. Faith Canan, Osman Yildirim, Tuba Yildirim Ustunel et al., "The Relationship Between Internet Addiction and Body Mass Index in Turkish Adolescents," *Cyberpsychology, Behavior, and Social Networking* 17, no. 1 (2014): 40–45.

4. Chih-Hung Ko, Tai-Ling Liu, Peng-Wei Wang et al., "The Exacerbation of Depression, Hostility, and Social Anxiety in the Course of Internet Addiction Among Adolescents: A Prospective Study," *Comprehensive Psychiatry* 55 (2014): 1377–84.

5. Fong-Ching Chang, Chiung-Hui Chiu, Nae-Fang Miao et al., "The Relationship Between Parental Mediation and Internet Addiction Among Adolescents, and the Association with Cyberbullying and Depression," *Comprehensive Psychiatry* 57 (2015): 21–28.

6. Hatice Odaci and Çiğdem Berber Çelik, "What Are Problematic Internet Users? An Investigation of the Correlations Between Problematic Internet Use and Shyness, Loneliness, Narcissism, Aggression and Self-Perception," *Computers in Human Behavior* 29 (2013): 2382–87.

7. Jian Xu, Li-xiao Shen, Chong-huai Yan et al., "Parent-Adolescent Interaction and Risk of Adolescent Internet Addiction: A Population-Based Study in Shanghai," *BMC Psychiatry* 14 (2014): 112+.

8. Lawrence T. Lam and Emmy M. Y. Wong, "Stress Moderates the Relationship Between Problematic Internet Use by Parents and Problematic Internet Use by Adolescents," *Journal of Adolescent Health* 56 (2015): 300–306.

9. Christian Montag, Katharina Bey, Peng Sha et al., "Is It Meaningful to Distinguish Between Generalized and Specific Internet Addiction? Evidence from a Cross-Cultural Study from Germany, Sweden, Taiwan and China," *Asia-Pacific Psychiatry* 7 (2015): 20–26.

REFERENCES AND RESOURCES

Magazines, Journals, and Newspapers

Canan, Faith, Osman Yildirim, Tuba Yildirim Ustunel et al. "The Relationship Between Internet Addiction and Body Mass Index in Turkish Adolescents." *Cyberpsychology, Behavior, and Social Networking* 17, no. 1 (2014): 40–45.

Carli, V., T. Durkee, D. Wasserman et al. "The Association Between Pathological Internet Use and Comorbid Psychopathology: A Systematic Review." *Psychopathology* 46 (2013): 1–13.

Chang, Fong-Ching, Chiung-Hui Chiu, Nae-Fang Miao et al. "The Relationship Between Parental Mediation and Internet Addiction Among Adolescents, and the Association with Cyberbullying and Depression." *Comprehensive Psychiatry* 57 (2015): 21–28.

Király, Orsolya, Mark D. Griffiths, Róbert Urbán et al. "Problematic Internet Use and Problematic Online Gaming Are Not the Same: Findings from a Large Nationally Representative Adolescent Sample." *Cyberpsychology, Behavior, and Social Networking* 17, no. 12 (2014): 749–54.

Ko, Chih-Hung, Tai-Ling Liu, Peng-Wei Wang et al. "The Exacerbation of Depression, Hostility, and Social Anxiety in the Course of Internet Addiction Among Adolescents: A Prospective Study." *Comprehensive Psychiatry* 55 (2014): 1377–84.

Koyuncu, Tugce, Alaettin Unsal, and Didem Arslantas. "Assessment of Internet Addiction and Loneliness in Secondary and High School Students." *Journal of the Pakistan Medical Association* 64, no. 9 (2014): 998–1002.

Lam, Lawrence T., and Emmy M. Y. Wong. "Stress Moderates the Relationship Between Problematic Internet Use by Parents and Problematic Internet Use by Adolescents." *Journal of Adolescent Health* 56 (2015): 300–306.

Montag, Christian, Katharina Bey, Peng Sha et al. "Is It Meaningful to Distinguish Between Generalized and Specific Internet Addiction? Evidence from a Cross-Cultural Study from Germany, Sweden, Taiwan and China." *Asia-Pacific Psychiatry* 7 (2015): 20–26.

Odaci, Hatice, and Çiğdem Berber Çelik. "Who Are Problematic Internet Users? An Investigation of the Correlations Between Problematic Internet Use and Shyness, Loneliness, Narcissism, Aggression, and Self-Perception." *Computers in Human Behavior* 29 (2013): 2382–87.

Park, Subin, Kang-E M. Hong, Eun J. Park et al. "The Association Between Problematic Internet Use and Depression, Suicidal Ideation and Bipolar Disorder Symptoms in Korean Adolescents." *Australian & New Zealand Journal of Psychiatry* 47, no. 2 (2013): 153–59.

Şenormanci, O., G. Şenormanci, O. Güçlü, and R. Konkan. "Attachment and Family Functioning in Patients with Internet Addiction." *General Hospital Psychiatry* 36 (2014): 203–7.

Szczegielniak, Anna, Karol Palka, and Krzysztof Krysta. "Problems Associated with the Use of Social Networks—A Pilot Study." *Psychiatria Danubina* 25, Supplement 2 (2013): 212–15.

Xu, Jian, Li-xiao Shen, Chong-huai Yan et al. "Parent-Adolescent Interaction and Risk of Adolescent Internet Addiction: A Population-Based Study in Shanghai." *BMC Psychiatry* 14 (2014): 112+.

Yao, Bin, Wei Han, Lingxia Zeng, and Xiong Guo. "Freshman Year Mental Health Symptoms and Level of Adaptation as Predictors of Internet Addiction: A Retrospective Nested Case-Control Study of Male Chinese College Students." *Psychiatry Research* 210 (2013): 541–47.

Web Sites

Net Addiction. netaddiction.com.
Psych Central. psychcentral.com.

Limit Exposure to Electromagnetic Fields

OVERVIEW

Electric and magnetic fields are areas of energy that surround electrical devices. Electric fields are created by differences in voltage; the higher the voltage, the stronger the field. Electric fields are produced by the local build-up of electric charges in the atmosphere. Magnetic fields are formed when electric current flows; the greater the current, the stronger the magnetic field.

Electric fields are at their strongest when they are close to a charge or a charged conductor. Their strength diminishes with distance. In addition, walls, buildings, and trees may serve as barriers to electric fields. When power lines are buried in the ground, their electric fields are barely detectable. Magnetic fields are strongest when they are close to their area of origin, and they weaken with distance. But unlike electric fields, magnetic fields are not blocked by structures.

Though invisible to the human eye, electromagnetic fields, which combine electric and magnetic fields, are everywhere in the environment. In addition to the natural sources of electromagnetic fields, there are sources that have been designed by humans. For example, every power socket emits low frequency electromagnetic fields. Other sources include power lines, electrical wiring, microwave ovens, computers, and cell phones.

Researchers are strongly divided on the issue of whether or not electromagnetic fields pose a significant health risk to humans. To highlight this lack of consensus, this chapter is set up differently than others in the book. The first section discusses studies suggesting that electromagnetic fields are harmful, while the second section highlights studies suggesting that electromagnetic fields are not harmful. Although the jury is still out on this matter, avoiding excess exposure to electromagnetic fields may still be a good habit to follow.

STUDIES THAT SUGGEST
ELECTROMAGNETIC FIELDS ARE HARMFUL

Chronic Exposure to Electromagnetic Fields May Trigger Changes in Serum Lipid Levels

In a cross-sectional study published in 2016 in the journal *Environmental Science and Pollution Research International*, researchers from China wanted to learn if the chronic exposure to electromagnetic fields altered serum lipid levels. The study was carried out at electric power plants in the Zhejiang province in China. The researchers recruited 1,073 people, including 863 males and 210 females, between the ages of 22 and 60 years. All the participants were divided into one of two groups—high occupational exposure to electromagnetic fields and low occupational exposure to electromagnetic fields. Eight hundred and seventy-five participants completed the study. The researchers found a significant positive association between occupational exposure to electromagnetic fields and LDL ("bad cholesterol") levels. Those with high electromagnetic field exposure, longer employment duration, and more cell phone use had significantly higher total cholesterol levels, LDL levels, and levels of triglycerides. These higher levels placed the subjects at increased risk for cardiovascular disease. The researchers commented that their findings demonstrated that chronic exposure to electromagnetic fields "was associated with the change in serum lipids levels."[1]

Exposure to the Electromagnetic Fields of Cell Phones May Trigger Spontaneous Abortions in Pregnant Women

In a study published in 2015 in the *Journal of Environmental Health Science & Engineering*, researchers from Iran wanted to determine the association between the use of cell phones by pregnant women and the spontaneous abortion of a growing fetus. The cohort consisted of 292 women who had unexplained spontaneous abortions before 14 weeks of gestation and 308 women who were pregnant for 14 weeks. All the women were between the ages of 18 and 35 years. Data were collected on both groups of women, who were recruited from 10 hospitals in Tehran. Information on cell phone use was also obtained. The researchers found an association between the use of cell phones and spontaneous abortions. "Although the mechanisms underlying the effects of EMF [electromagnetic fields] on the risk of spontaneous abortions are not well understood, early embryos are known to be sensitive to environmental exposures."[2]

Following the Construction of a New High-Voltage Power Line, Residents Report Symptoms

In a study published in 2015 in the journal *Environmental Research*, researchers from the Netherlands and New Zealand tested residents before and after the construction of a nearby high-voltage power line. Both residents living close to the power line and those living a little further away participated in the two tests that occurred before the power line and the two tests that took place after construction of the power line. The researchers found that the residents living closer to the power line and who had higher incomes were more likely to agree to participate in the study. At baseline, symptom reports of residents living closer to the power line did not differ significantly from residents living further away. Participants were asked about 16 different nonspecific somatic symptoms such as headaches, dizziness, and low back pain. Health complaints tended to begin during construction of the power line. After the power line was opened, those living closest reported symptoms. "This increase in reported symptoms occurred largely parallel to the increase in the belief that these symptoms are caused by a power line."[3]

Electromagnetic Fields from Wireless Devices
May Impair Memory in Teens

In a prospective study published in 2015 in the journal *Environment International*, researchers from Switzerland wanted to determine if the electromagnetic fields from wireless devices had any effect on the memory of adolescents. The cohort consisted of 439 teens, between the ages of 12 and 17 years, from 24 schools in rural and urban areas in central Switzerland. The baseline study took place between June 2012 and February 2013. Students completed questionnaires and performed a computerized memory test. Parents also completed questionnaires. The study was repeated one year later with 425 of the same students and the same study managers. The researchers gained even more information from a subgroup of 95 teens. For three days, these teens carried an exposimeter, a portable measuring device, and kept diaries on a time-activity diary application installed in smartphones. The researchers determined that the exposure to the electromagnetic fields appeared to have an effect on memory. "A change in memory performance over one year was negatively associated with cumulative duration of wireless phone use and more strongly with RF-EMF [radiofrequency electromagnetic fields] dose."[4]

STUDIES THAT SUGGEST
ELECTROMAGNETIC FIELDS ARE NOT HARMFUL

Short-Term Exposure to Mobile Phone Electromagnetic Fields
Does Not Appear to Affect Human Cognitive Performance

In a study published in 2012 in the journal *Bioelectromagnetics*, researchers from Austria wanted to learn more about the association between short-term exposure to mobile phone electromagnetic fields and human cognitive performance. The researchers conducted a meta-analysis of the topic that included 17 studies with 749 subjects. The researchers were unable to locate any credible evidence that mobile phones had any short-term impact on human cognitive performance. The cognitive abilities were neither impaired nor improved by the phones' electromagnetic fields. The researchers concluded that their findings "suggested that a substantial short-term impact of high frequency electromagnetic fields emitted by mobile phones can essentially be ruled out."[5]

When People Consider Their Medical Problems to Be
Caused by Electromagnetic Fields, There May Also
Be a Psychological Component

In a qualitative study published in 2016 in *Bioelectromagnetics*, a researcher from France wanted to learn more about people who report having physical symptoms from exposure to electromagnetic fields. The cohort consisted of 11 men and

29 women, with a mean age of 51 years. Detailed interviews were conducted primarily in the participants' homes. The four most common electromagnetic field exposure problems experienced by the participants were sleep disturbances, headaches, pain in various locations, and abnormal fatigue. The researchers found that the subjects typically blamed electromagnetic fields after they were unable to obtain a medical solution to their problem. It was then that they decided that electromagnetic fields are noxious and responsible for their symptoms. "Subjects, thus, became able to link their symptoms to EMF exposure in a distinctly adversarial manner." The researcher concluded that in at least some of these cases there was a psychological component to the symptoms. So, their medical concerns were probably less a function of contact with electromagnetic fields and more related to "psychological mechanisms."[6]

The Media Attention on Electromagnetic Fields Appears to Trigger Symptoms in Some People

In a study published in 2013 in the *Journal of Psychosomatic Research*, researchers from the United Kingdom and Germany examined the role that media might play in the development of symptoms related to exposure to electromagnetic fields. The cohort consisted of 147 subjects who were randomly assigned to watch a television report about the adverse health effects of WiFi (n=76) or a control film (n=71), which was the same length but addressed the security of mobile phone transmission. After watching the films, the subjects received a sham exposure to a WiFi signal for 15 minutes. The testing took place between January and June 2012 in London. Eighty-two subjects (54 percent) reported symptoms that they maintained were the result of their exposure to WiFi. In addition, the experimental film increased worries about electromagnetic fields among subjects with higher levels of pre-existing anxiety, a greater tendency for somatosensory amplification, and among those who considered themselves to have a higher sensitivity to electromagnetic fields. "Media reports about the adverse effects of supposedly hazardous substances can increase the likelihood of experiencing symptoms following a sham exposure and developing an apparent sensitivity to it." And, these effects have the potential to continue for longer periods of time. Had the researchers not debriefed the subjects on what had actually occurred, "it is possible that this belief would have made future symptomatic reactions to electromagnetic stimuli more likely."[7]

NOTES

1. Z. Wang, L. Wang, S. Zheng et al.. "Effects of Electromagnetic Fields on Serum Lipids in Workers of a Power Plant," *Environmental Science and Pollution Research International* 23 (2016): 2495–504.

2. F. S. Mahmoudabadi, S. Ziaei, M. Firoozabadi, and A. Kazemnejad, "Use of Mobile Phone During Pregnancy and the Risk of Spontaneous Abortion," *Journal of Environmental Health Science & Engineering* 13 (2015): 34+.

3. Jarry T. Porsius, Liesbeth Claassen, Tjabe Smid et al., "Symptom Reporting After the Introduction of a New High-Voltage Power Line: A Prospective Field Study," *Environmental Research* 138 (2014): 112–17.

4. Anna Schoeni, Katharina Roser, and Martin Röösli, "Memory Performance, Wireless Communication and Exposure to Radiofrequency Electromagnetic Fields: A Prospective Cohort Study in Adolescents," *Environment International* 85 (2015): 343–51.

5. Alfred Barth, Ivo Ponocny, Timo Gnambs, and Robert Winkler, "No Effects of Short-Term Exposure to Mobile Phone Electromagnetic Fields on Human Cognitive Performance: A Meta-Analysis," *Bioelectromagnetics* 33, no. 2 (2012): 159–65.

6. Maël Dieudonné, "Does Electromagnetic Hypersensitivity Originate from Nocebo Responses? Indications from a Qualitative Study," *Bioelectromagnetics* 37, no. 1 (2016): 14–24.

7. Michael Witthöft and G. James Rubin, "Are Media Warnings About the Adverse Health Effects of Modern Life Self-Fulfilling? An Experimental Study on Idiopathic Environmental Intolerance Attributed to Electromagnetic Fields (IEI-EMF)," *Journal of Psychosomatic Research* 74 (2013): 206–12.

REFERENCES AND RESOURCES

Magazines, Journals, and Newspapers

Barth, Alfred, Ivo Ponocny, Timo Gnambs, and Robert Winkler. "No Effects of Short-Term Exposure to Mobile Phone Electromagnetic Fields on Human Cognitive Performance: A Meta-Analysis." *Bioelectromagnetics* 33, no. 2 (2012): 159–65.

Dieudonné, Maël. "Does Electromagnetic Hypersensitivity Originate from Nocebo Responses? Indications From a Qualitative Study." *Bioelectromagnetics* 37, no. 1 (2016): 14–24.

Goedhart, Geertje, Martine Vrijheid, Joe Wiart et al. "Using Software-Modified Smartphones to Validate Self-Reported Mobile Phone Use in Young People: A Pilot Study." *Bioelectromagnetics* 36 (2015): 538–43.

Kato, I., A. Young, J. Liu et al. "Electric Blanket Use and Risk of Thyroid Cancer in the Women's Health Initiative Observational Cohort." *Women & Health* 55, no. 7 (2015): 829–41.

Mahmoudabadi, F. S., S. Ziaei, M. Firoozabadi, and A. Kazemnejad. "Use of Mobile Phone During Pregnancy and the Risk of Spontaneous Abortion." *Journal of Environmental Health Science & Engineering* 13 (2015): 34+

Porsius, Jarry T., Liesbeth Claassen, Tjabe Smid et al. "Symptom Reporting After the Introduction of a New High-Voltage Power Line: A Prospective Field Study." *Environmental Research* 138 (2015): 112–17.

Qi, G., X. Zuo, L. Zhou et al. "Effects of Extremely Low-Frequency Electromagnetic Fields (ELF-EMF) Exposure on B6C3F1 Mice." *Environmental Health and Preventive Medicine* 20, no. 4 (2015): 287–93.

Schoeni, Anna, Katharina Roser, and Martin Röösli. "Memory Performance, Wireless Communication and Exposure to Radiofrequency Electromagnetic Fields: A Prospective Cohort Study in Adolescents." *Environment International* 85 (2015): 343–51.

Wang, Z., L. Wang, S. Zheng et al. "Effects of Electromagnetic Fields on Serum Lipids in Workers of a Power Plant." *Environmental Science and Pollution Research International* 23 (2016): 2495–504.

Witthöft, Michael, and G. James Rubin. "Are Media Warnings About the Adverse Health Effects of Modern Life Self-Fulfilling? An Experimental Study on Idiopathic

Environmental Intolerance Attributed to Electromagnetic Fields (IEI-EMF)." *Journal of Psychosomatic Research* 74 (2013): 206–12.

Web Sites

MedlinePlus. www.nim.nih.gov/medlineplus.
World Health Organization. www.who.int/.

Limit Screen Time

OVERVIEW

Although it may be impossible to imagine, there was a time when there were no screens. Before the invention of the television, people listened to radio. However, by the mid-1900s, many people had televisions in their homes. Generally, those televisions were placed in the living or family room. That was the single screen for the entire family.

Of course, televisions still exist. But, there are also a host of other screens. From computers to phones, each day teens spend hours looking at screens. In fact, large numbers of adults are now expressing concern over the amount of time that teens spend looking at screens.

According to the National Center for Health Statistics, in 2012, during the previous 30 days, 98.5 percent of teens ages 12 to 15 years reported watching television and 91.1 percent reported using the computer every day outside of school. Almost one-third of the teens (29.5 percent) watched television for two hours a day. A stunning 6.9 percent watched television for five hours or more per day, and 5.1 percent used a computer for five hours or more per day. Spending more than two hours per day of screen time has been theorized to be associated with a number of problems in teens. These are believed to include elevated blood pressure, elevated serum cholesterol, and excess weight. An expert panel from the National Heart, Lung, and Blood Institute and the American Academy of Pediatrics recommends no more than two hours per day of screen time.[1]

WHAT THE EXPERTS SAY

Screen Time Appears to Be Associated with Amounts of Body Fat

In a study published in 2010 in the *American Journal of Epidemiology*, researchers based in Canada wanted to learn more about the association between screen time during secondary school and the amount of body fat in the students. The cohort consisted of 744 Canadian adolescents who were 12 to 13 years old when the study began. Fourteen percent of them were overweight. Over 57 months, the participants completed self-reported questionnaires on television viewing and computer use. The majority of the participants had between 25 and 30 hours of screen time per week. However, almost 30 percent of the cohort had screen times that increased, decreased, or remained high. The researchers found that "physically inactive boys who increased or maintained high screen time and physically active girls who increased screen time gained the most body fat." And, they concluded that there is an "urgent need for population-level strategies aimed at reducing screen time."[2]

Increased Screen Time Is Associated with Higher Body Mass Index (BMI)

In a study published in 2013 in the journal *Pediatrics*, researchers from Boston examined the association between screen use and body mass index in 91 teens between the ages of 13 and 15 years. Over a one-week period of time, the participants completed a weekday and Saturday 24-hour diary in which they recorded the amount of screen time they devoted to television, computers, and video games. In addition, the participants carried handheld computers and responded to four to seven questionnaires per day about their various primary, secondary, and tertiary activities. The researchers found that the participants spent the most time watching television, and television watching was most often designated as where they were directing their primary attention. Moreover, there was an association between paying primary attention to television and a higher BMI. The researchers concluded that their findings "support the notion that attention to TV is a key element of the increased obesity risk associated with TV viewing." The researchers wondered if the teens were influenced by "TV commercials . . . [with] preferences for energy-dense, nutritionally questionable foods and/or eating while distracted by TV."[3]

There Appears to Be an Association between Screen Time and Depression and Anxiety

In a study published in 2015 in the journal *Preventive Medicine*, researchers from Canada wanted to learn more about the relationship between screen time and depression and anxiety. The cohort consisted of 2,482 English-speaking students in grades 7 to 12. Data were collected from 2006 to 2010 as part of a larger study. The researchers found that the time spent in sedentary screen-based activities was significantly associated with the severity of depression and anxiety. The longer the screen time, the more profound the cases of depression and anxiety. "Screen time may represent a risk factor for, or a marker of these psychiatric disorders among youth." The researchers advised healthcare providers to ask about screen time when assessing children and teens who want treatment for depression and anxiety. When the researchers looked further into the types of screen-based activities, they found that computer use and video game playing were significantly associated with depressive symptoms, but only video gaming was significantly associated with anxiety.[4]

Greater Screen Time Is Associated with More Reports of Somatic Symptoms

In a study published in 2014 in *Preventive Medicine*, researchers from Iceland, Sweden, New York City, and West Virginia investigated the relationship between screen time in 10- to 12-year-old preteens and their reports of somatic symptoms, or symptoms for which no physical cause could be determined. Data were obtained from the population-based 2011 Youth in Iceland school survey, which included 10,829 students. Among the many questions, students were asked about screen time and the incidence of the symptoms of dizziness, tremors, headaches, stomachaches, and multiple symptoms. Interestingly, the reported prevalence of symptoms increased with the amount of hours spent on the screen. Both the males and females who spent more screen time had more symptoms. "This held for all individual screen activities as well as the cumulative measure of daily minutes spent on screen-based media and prevalence of one or more somatic symptoms." And, the students who spent four hours or more per day on screen-based activities had the highest rates of all forms of somatic symptoms.[5]

BARRIERS AND PROBLEMS

Many Teens Are Not Limiting Their Screen Time

In a study published in 2015 in the journal *BMC Public Health*, researchers from Australia wanted to assess the actual amount of time Australian children and adolescents spend on all types of screens. Their cohort consisted of 1,373 males and 1,247 females between the ages of 8 to 16 years. They were all students at 25 Australian government and nongovernment primary and secondary schools. The researchers found that 45 percent of the 8-year-old students and 80 percent of the 16-year-old students had more than two hours of screen time each day. The most popular screen activities were watching television and videos. The researchers concluded that it may no longer be possible to limit screen time to no more than two hours per day. According to the researchers, "screen based media are central in the everyday lives of children and adolescents."[6]

Screens and Televisions in the Bedroom Reduce Sleep Duration and Delay Bedtimes

In a longitudinal study published in 2013 in *BMC Public Health*, researchers from Finland noted that screens and televisions are an ever-growing presence in the bedrooms of children. The researchers wanted to learn more about the effects these screens and televisions have on the sleep habits of children aged 10 and 11 years in the fourth and fifth grades. The cohort consisted of 353 children from 27 schools; they answered baseline questionnaires in 2006 and follow-up questionnaires in 2008. The researchers found an association between screen use and television viewing and significantly shorter sleep duration and later bedtimes. "The more children used a computer or watched a TV, the greater was the decrease in sleep duration and the delay in bedtime." The researchers concluded that "parents, teachers and health care providers should be aware that television viewing and computer use may have an adverse impact on sleep, which in turn may lead to daytime tiredness, attention and behavioral problems as well as increased health risk in the long run."[7]

In a study published in 2015 in *Pediatrics*, researchers from Berkeley, California; Boston; and Berlin examined the association between different sized screens in the bedroom and sleep duration and restfulness. The cohort consisted of 2,048 fourth and seventh graders who participated in the Massachusetts Childhood Obesity Research Demonstration Study in 2012 and 2013. The researchers determined that 54 percent of the children slept near a small screen and 75 percent slept in a room with a television. More seventh graders (65 percent) slept with a small screen than fourth graders (46 percent). When compared to the children who slept without a nearby screen, children who slept near a small screen had 20.6 fewer minutes of sleep. In addition, the children who slept near a small screen were more likely to think that they had insufficient rest or sleep. When compared to children who slept in a room without a television, children who slept in a room with a television had 18 fewer minutes of sleep. According to the researchers, their findings "caution against children's unfettered access to screen-based media in their rooms."[8]

Transitioning to a New School May
Reduce Physical Activity and Increase Screen Time

In an innovative study published in 2015 in the *International Journal of Behavioral Nutrition and Physical Activity*, researchers from Australia investigated the effect of the transition from primary to secondary school on physical activity and sedentary activity, such as screen time. Fifteen schools in Victoria, Australia, were included in the trial. In nine schools, students who completed year six transitioned to a new school for year seven; in six schools, students remained in the same school environment from year six to year seven. Data were collected from the students when they were in their sixth year and again when they were in their seventh year. The researchers found that the students who transitioned to a new school had lower rates of daily moderate to vigorous physical activity and increases in average daily sedentary behavior, such as screen time. On the other hand, screen time for those students who remained in the same school environment actually declined. The researchers commented that "changing school environments results in greater change in types of behaviour, showing this influential life stage is a critical target for the reduction of unhealthy behaviours."[9]

NOTES

1. National Center for Health Statistics, www.cdc.gov/nchs.

2. Tracie A. Barnett, Jennifer O'Loughlin, Catherine M. Sabiston et al., "Teens and Screens: The Influence of Screen Time on Adiposity in Adolescents," *American Journal of Epidemiology* 172, no. 3 (2010): 255–62.

3. David S. Bickham, Emily A. Blood, Courtney E. Walls et al., "Characteristics of Screen Media Use Associated with Higher BMI in Young Adolescents," *Pediatrics* 131, no. 5 (2013): 935–41.

4. Danijela Maras, Martine F. Flament, Marisa Murray et al., "Screen Time Is Associated with Depression and Anxiety in Canadian Youth," *Preventive Medicine* 73 (2015): 133–38.

5. Richard E. Taehtinen, Inga Dora Sigfusdottir, Asgeir R. Hegason, and Alfgeir L. Kristjansson, "Electronic Screen Use and Selected Somatic Symptoms in 10–12 Year Old Children," *Preventive Medicine* 67 (2014): 128–33.

6. Stephen Houghton, Simon C. Hunter, Michael Rosenberg et al., "Virtually Impossible: Limiting Australian Children and Adolescents' Daily Screen Based Media Use," BMC *Public Health* 15, no. 5 (2015).

7. Teija Nuutinen, Carola Ray, and Eva Roos, "Do Computer Use, TV Viewing, and the Presence of the Media in the Bedroom Predict School-Aged Children's Sleep Habits in a Longitudinal Study?" BMC *Public Health* 13 (2013): 684+.

8. J. Falbe, K. K. Davison, R. L. Franckle et al., "Sleep Duration, Restfulness, and Screens in the Sleep Environment," *Pediatrics* 135, no. 2 (2015): e367–e375.

9. J. Marks, L. M. Barnett, C. Strugnell, and S. Allender, "Changing from Primary to Secondary School Highlights Opportunities for School Environment Interventions Aiming to Increase Physical Activity and Reduce Sedentary Behaviour: A Longitudinal Cohort Study," *International Journal of Behavioral Nutrition and Physical Activity* 12 (2015): 59.

REFERENCES AND RESOURCES

Magazines, Journals, and Newspapers

Barnett, Tracie A., Jennifer O'Loughlin, Catherine M. Sabiston et al. "Teens and Screens: The Influence of Screen Time on Adiposity in Adolescents." *American Journal of Epidemiology* 172, no. 3 (2010): 255–62.

Bickham, David S., Emily Blood, Courtney E. Walls et al. "Characteristics of Screen Media Use Associated with Higher BMI in Young Adolescents." *Pediatrics* 131, no. 5 (2013): 935–41.

Falbe, J., K. K. Davison, R. L. Franckle et al. "Sleep Duration, Restfulness, and Screens in the Sleep Environment." *Pediatrics* 135, no. 2 (2015): e367–e375.

Feng, Qi, Qing-le Zhang, Yue Du et al. "Associations of Physical Activity, Screen Time with Depression, Anxiety and Sleep Quality Among Chinese College Freshmen." *PLoS ONE* 9, no. 6 (2014): e100914+.

Houghton, Stephen, Simon C. Hunter, Michael Rosenberg et al. "Virtually Impossible: Limiting Australian Children and Adolescents' Daily Screen Based Media Use." *BMC Public Health* 15, no. 5 (2015).

Kremer, Peter, Christina Eishaug, Eva Leslie et al. "Physical Activity, Leisure-Time Screen Use and Depression Among Children and Young Adolescents." *Journal of Science and Medicine in Sport* 17, no. 2 (2014): 183–87.

Maras, Danijela, Martine F. Flament, Marisa Murray et al. "Screen Time Is Associated with Depression and Anxiety in Canadian Youth." *Preventive Medicine* 73 (2015): 133–38.

Marks, J., L. M. Barnett, C. Strugnell, and S. Allender. "Changing from Primary to Secondary School Highlights Opportunities for School Environment Interventions Aiming to Increase Physical Activity and Reduce Sedentary Behaviour: A Longitudinal Cohort Study." *International Journal of Behavioral Nutrition and Physical Activity* 12 (2015): 59.

Melkevik, Ole, Torbjørn Torsheim, Ronald J. Iannotti, and Bente Wold. "Is Spending Time in Screen-Based Sedentary Behaviors Associated with Less Physical Activity: A Cross National Investigation." *International Journal of Behavioral Nutrition and Physical Activity* 7 (2010): 46+.

Nuutinen, Teija, Carola Ray, and Eva Roos. "Do Computer Use, TV Viewing, and the Presence of the Media in the Bedroom Predict School-Aged Children's Sleep Habits in a Longitudinal Study?" *BMC Public Health* 13 (2013): 684+.

Taehtinen, Richard E., Inga Dora Sigfusdottir, Asgeir R. Helgason, and Alfgeir L. Kristjansson. "Electronic Screen Use and Selected Somatic Symptoms in 10–12 Year Old Children." *Preventive Medicine* 67 (2014): 128–33.

Web Site

National Center for Health Statistics. www.cdc.gov/nchs.

Reduce Stress

OVERVIEW

In today's very hectic, fast-paced, and often economically challenged world just about all teens deal with some degree of stress. School days start early and are frequently jam-packed with responsibilities. There may also be specific issues with teachers and peers; there may be problems mastering a specific subject or several subjects. After-school hours may include participation in a sports team and/or a part-time job. When a teen finally returns home, there may be hours of homework and at least a few household chores.

And the home front may be a source of even more stress. Parents may be trying to juggle two very hectic schedules, while also finding the time for everyday

household tasks. Parents may be fighting over issues, separating, or even divorc-
ing. Teens may be traveling back and forth between their parents' separate homes.
There may be significant others in the picture, and they may have their own
children. So, the family dynamics may have their own stressors.

Moreover, teens may be dealing with even worse situations. The family may
face severe economic insecurity resulting in a lost home, shelter living, or home-
lessness. Sometimes, teens may be forced to deal with the untimely death of a
parent. Clearly, teens may become overloaded with stress. That is why it is important to learn ways to reduce stress.

WHAT THE EXPERTS SAY

Physical Exercise Reduces Stress

In a study published in 2013 in the *American Journal of Health Promotion*,
researchers from Minneapolis, Minnesota, wanted to learn more about the association between vigorous physical exercise and perceived stress, mental health,
and socializing among 14,706 four-year college students. The data, which were
obtained from the Harvard School of Public Health Study of College Health
Behaviors, were collected from 94 schools in 2004. The researchers determined
that the students who met vigorous physical activity recommendations were less
likely to report perceived stress and poor mental health. The researchers commented that "interventions to improve mental well-being of college students
should also consider promoting physical activity."[1]

Music Appears to Be Useful in Reducing Stress

In a study published in 2015 in the journal *Psychoneuroendocrinology*, researchers from Germany examined the association between listening to music in everyday life and stress reduction. The initial cohort consisted of 55 healthy university
students, with 35 females and 20 males. They ranged in age from 18 to 31 years,
with a mean age of 23.2 years. The participants were studied during a five-day
regular term week at the beginning of a semester and during a five-day examination week at the end of a semester. Four times per day, the participants rated their
music listening behavior and their perceived stress levels. A subgroup of 25 students provided saliva samples on two consecutive days during both weeks. The
researchers learned that listening to music decreased subjective stress levels and
lowered cortisol concentrations, which suggested reductions in stress. According
to the researchers, their findings indicated that "music listening can be considered a means of stress reduction in daily life, especially if it is listened to for the
reason of relaxation."[2]

In a randomized study published in 2014 in the *International Journal of Clinical
Pediatric Dentistry*, researchers from India wondered if music would be useful in
reducing the stress levels of anxious pediatric dental patients about to undergo

tooth extraction. The cohort consisted of 60 children between the ages of 6 and 12 years. Thirty children were placed in a group that listened to music; the other 30 children did not listen to any music. Did music provide a sufficient level of distraction to reduce anxiety? The researchers determined that the children who listened to music had reduced levels of anxiety. For example, the pulse rate in the control group was greater than in the music group. And, the systolic blood pressure was lower in the music group than the control group. The researchers commented that the "audio distraction [music] did decrease the anxiety in pediatric patients to a significant extent." In addition, "patients had an overwhelming response to music presentations and wanted to hear them in their subsequent visits."[3]

Stress Reduction Interventions May
Alter Stress Levels in College Students

In a study published in 2014 in the journal *Health Promotion Practice*, researchers from Oklahoma State University wanted to determine what stress reduction interventions would alter stress levels in male and female college students. They examined various aspects of stress such as overall perceived stress, test anxiety, and personal burnout. The cohort consisted of 531 students (293 males and 238 females) taking college courses that focused on cognitive-behavioral stress management, cardiovascular fitness, or generalized physical activity. They also formed a control group. By the end of the semester, the students in the stress management and physical activity groups had significantly lower levels of perceived stress, text anxiety, and personal burnout. The students in the fitness group had significantly lower levels of perceived stress and personal burnout, but there were no differences in scores for text anxiety. The researchers commented that "a combination of stress reduction strategies may be the most effective means of reducing stress indices in male and female college students."[4]

Qigong, a Traditional Chinese Exercise,
Appears to Be Useful for Stress Reduction

In a study published in 2013 in the journal *Complementary Therapies in Clinical Practice*, researchers from Brunei and Singapore wanted to learn if qigong, a traditional Chinese mind-body exercise, would be useful for reducing stress, anxiety, and depression. The initial cohort consisted of 34, mostly female, first-year nursing and midwifery students from Brunei, who were believed to be at increased risk for high levels of stress. The intervention group of 18 students practiced qigong for an hour twice weekly and the control group of 16 students refrained from practicing any qigong. Unfortunately, five students from the qigong group and seven students from the control groups dropped out of the study. Still, the students completed self-administered questionnaires, and there were important findings. After 10 weeks, the students in the intervention group had significant reductions in stress, anxiety, and depression. The researchers concluded that a 10-week program of qigong "may be a cost effective means to manage stress and improve mood status and immune function among nursing and midwifery students."[5]

Biofeedback Appears to Be Useful for Stress and Other Problems

In a study published in 2015 in the journal *Nursing Research and Practice*, researchers from California and Thailand investigated the use of biofeedback to reduce stress, anxiety, and depression in Thai graduate students in public health nursing. Sixty students, who ranged in age from 21 to 52 years, were randomly assigned to either a four-week biofeedback intervention group or a control group with no intervention. The participants in the intervention group were told to use their portable biofeedback devices three times per day and to record their practice times in a log. By the end of the intervention, the intervention students experienced significantly reduced levels of stress, anxiety, and depression. The students in the control group had increases in the medical problems. The researchers noted that learning stress reduction techniques should be very important for these students. "As future leaders in the public health nursing arena, it is important for graduate students in public health nursing programs to learn strategies and interventions to help them manage their lives and cope with life stressors."[6]

BARRIERS AND PROBLEMS

Teens May Have a Medical Problem, Such as Type 1 Diabetes, That Adds Stress to Their Lives

In a study published in 2016 in the *Journal of Pediatric Health Care*, researchers from Philadelphia and Orange, Connecticut, wanted to learn more about the stressors associated with having type 1 diabetes in early adolescence. Type 1 diabetes is actually a somewhat common childhood disorder. Each year, about 15,000 new cases are diagnosed in the United States. Type 1 diabetes necessitates a fairly rigorous self-management routine. "Diabetes self-management is complex and demanding, requiring frequent blood glucose monitoring, carbohydrate counting, administration of insulin, and treatment of events of hypo- and hyperglycemia." Data were obtained from 205 students between the ages of 11 and 14 years; 58 percent were female. The participants were asked to identify their top three stressors, and they responded to open-ended questions. Eighty-two percent of the students reported that school was the top stressor. That was followed by social life (49 percent) and diabetes (48 percent). So, almost half the students considered their chronic illness to be a top stressor in their lives. The researchers also identified three diabetic-specific stressors—"just having diabetes, dealing with emotions, and managing diabetes."[7]

Certain Foods May Increase the Risk of Perceived Stress

In a trial published in 2014 in the *Central European Journal of Public Health*, researchers from the United Kingdom and Saudi Arabia examined the association between nutritional behavior and stress and depressive symptoms. The trial included 3,706 undergraduate students at seven universities in the United Kingdom. The self-administered questionnaire included 12 questions on food frequency. The researchers found that the consumption of unhealthy foods, such as sweets and cookies, was significantly associated with perceived stress and depressive symptoms in females. Conversely, the consumption of healthier foods, such as salad, fresh fruits, and cooked vegetables, was significantly negatively associated with perceived stress and depressive symptoms for males and females. The researchers commented that "interventions to reduce depressive symptoms and stress among students could also result in the consumption of healthier foods."[8]

For Many Teens, School Is a Source of a Great Deal of Stress

In a study published in 2011 in the *European Journal of Public Health*, researchers from several different European countries investigated the association between adolescent perceived stress and adiposity. As part of this study, the researchers examined 10 different stress dimensions. The cohort consisted of 1,121 teens (484 males and 637 females) between the ages of 12.5 and 17.5 years from six European cities. The researchers found that although female teens reported more levels of stress than the male teens, they had similar stress profiles. Males and females both reported that their highest levels of stress came from school related events or situations. According to the researchers, "it is important that school communities and managers are aware of this and that they are involved in developing strategies to turn down the experience of stress in adolescents and to ameliorate their coping capacities."[9]

NOTES

1. Nicole A. VanKim and Toben F. Nelson, "Vigorous Physical Activity, Mental Health, Perceived Stress, and Socializing Among College Students," *American Journal of Health Promotion* 28, no. 1 (2013): 7–15.

2. A. Linnemann, B. Ditzen, J. Strahler et al., "Music Listening as a Means of Stress Reduction in Daily Life," *Psychoneuroendocrinology* 60 (2015): 82–90.

3. Divya Singh, Firoza Samadi, JN Jaiswal, and Abhay Mani Tripathi, "Stress Reduction through Audio Distraction in Anxious Pediatric Dental Patients: An Adjunctive Clinical Study," *International Journal of Clinical Pediatric Dentistry* 7, no. 3 (2014): 149–52.

4. Timothy Baghurst and Betty C. Kelley, "An Examination of Stress in College Students Over the Course of a Semester," *Health Promotion Practice* 15, no. 3 (2014): 438–47.

5. Ee Suen Chan, David Koh, Yan Choo Teo et al., "Biochemical and Psychometric Evaluation of Self-Healing Qigong as a Stress Reduction Tool Among First Year Nursing and Midwifery Students," *Complementary Therapies in Clinical Practice* 19 (2013): 179–83.

6. Paul Ratanasiripong, Orawan Kaewboonchoo, Nop Ratanasiripong et al., "Biofeedback Intervention for Stress, Anxiety, and Depression Among Graduate Students in Public Health Nursing," *Nursing Research and Practice* (2015) Article ID 160746.

7. A. M. Chao, K. E. Minges, C. Park et al., "General Life and Diabetes-Related Stressors in Early Adolescents with Type 1 Diabetes," *Journal of Pediatric Health Care* 30 (2016): 133–42.

8. Walid El Ansari, Hamed Adetunji, and Reza Oskrochi, "Food and Mental Health: Relationship Between Food and Perceived Stress and Depressive Symptoms Among University Students in the United Kingdom," *Central European Journal of Public Health* 22, no. 2 (2014): 90–97.

9. Tineke De Vriendt, Els Clays, Lea Maes et al., "European Adolescents' Level of Perceived Stress and Its Relationship with Body Adiposity—The HELENA Study," *European Journal of Public Health* 22, no. 4 (2011): 519–24.

REFERENCES AND RESOURCES

Magazines Journals, and Newspapers

Baghurst, Timothy, and Betty C. Kelley. "An Examination of Stress in College Students Over the Course of a Semester." *Health Promotion Practice* 15, no. 3 (2014): 438–47.

Chan, Ee Suen, David Koh, Yan Choo Teo et al. "Biochemical and Psychometric Evaluation of Self-Healing Qigong as a Stress Reduction Tool Among First Year Nursing and Midwifery Students." *Complementary Therapies in Clinical Practice* 19 (2013): 179–83.

Chao, A. M., K. E Minges, C. Park et al. "General Life and Diabetes-Related Stressors in Early Adolescents with Type 1 Diabetes." *Journal of Pediatric Health Care* 30 (2016): 133–42.

De Vriendt, Tineke, Els Clays, Lea Maes et al. "European Adolescents' Level of Perceived Stress and Its Relationship with Body Adiposity—The HELENA Study." *European Journal of Public Health* 22, no. 4 (2011): 519–24.

El Ansari, Walid, Hamed Adetunji, and Reza Oskrochi. "Food and Mental Health: Relationship Between Food and Perceived Stress and Depressive Symptoms Among University Students in the United Kingdom." *Central European Journal of Public Health* 22, no. 2 (2014): 90–97.

Linnemann, A., B. Ditzen, J. Strahler et al. "Music Listening as a Means of Stress Reduction in Daily Life." *Psychoneuroendocrinology* 60 (2015): 82–90.

Ratanasiripong, Paul, Orawan Kaewboonchoo, Nop Ratanasiripong et al. "Biofeedback Intervention for Stress, Anxiety, and Depression Among Graduate Students in Public Health Nursing." *Nursing Research and Practice* (2015), Article ID 160746.

Regehr, Cheryl, Dylan Glancy, and Annabel Pitts. "Interventions to Reduce Stress in University Students: A Review and Meta-Analysis." *Journal of Affective Disorders* 148 (2013): 1–11.

Simon, Arun K., T. V. Bhumika, and N. Sreekumaran Nair. "Does Atraumatic Restorative Treatment Reduce Dental Anxiety in Children? A Systematic Review and Meta-Analysis." *European Journal of Dentistry* 9, no. 2 (2015): 304–9.

Singh, Divya, Firoza Samadi, JN Jaiswal, and Abhay Mani Tripathi. "Stress Reduction through Audio Distraction in Anxious Pediatiric Dental Patients: An Adjunctive Clinical Study." *International Journal of Clinical Pediatric Dentistry* 7, no. 3 (2014): 149–52.

VanKim, Nicole A., and Toben F. Nelson. "Vigorous Physical Activity, Mental Health, Perceived Stress, and Socializing Among College Students." *American Journal of Health Promotion* 28, no. 1 (2013): 7–15.

Web Site

American Academy of Child & Adolescent Psychiatry. www.aacap.org.

Use Sunscreen

OVERVIEW

Just about everyone should be aware that the sun may damage the skin. Sun exposure has been associated with the premature development of skin wrinkles as well as several types of skin cancer. For decades, dermatologists, the physicians who specialize in skin problems, have been advising people of all ages to wear sunscreen or products that contain a number of different ingredients that help prevent the sun's ultraviolet (UV) radiation from harming the skin. Both types of ultraviolet radiation, UVA and UVB, may damage the skin and cause premature aging and skin cancer.

Sunscreen labels list their SPF or sun protector factor, a measure of their ability to protect the skin from UVB damage. Thus, if it takes 20 minutes for unprotected skin to start turning red, using a sunscreen with a SPF of 15 should multiply that amount of time by 15 or to about five hours. It is best to use a sunscreen with a SPF of at least 15. Many recommend higher numbers. Some sunscreens, known as broad-spectrum sunscreens, protect the skin from both UVA and UVB rays. Yet, while exact figures vary, according to the Skin Protection Foundation, less than one-third of the youth in America practice effective sun protection.[1]

WHAT THE EXPERTS SAY

Some Programs Have Been Successful in Improving the Use of Sunscreen

In a study published in 2015 in the journal *Preventive Medicine*, researchers from Australia wanted to learn more about the ability of a single-session online intervention to improve sun-protective behaviors among Australian adults. The cohort consisted of 532 Australian adults with a mean age of 39.3 years. The men and women were randomly placed in an intervention group of 265 or a control group of 267. The researchers noted that the online intervention focused on "fostering positive attitudes, perceptions of normative support, and control perceptions for sun protection." The participants reported more positive attitudes toward sun protection and the use of products that provide protection from the sun's rays in the subsequent month. However, "it is unknown whether sunscreen protective measures were used effectively (e.g. whether sunscreen was reapplied)."[2]

A Smartphone Mobile Application Informs People That They Need to Reapply Sunscreen

In a study published in 2015 in *JAMA Dermatology*, researchers from Colorado and New Mexico evaluated the ability of a smartphone application to provide real-time sun protection advice, such as informing a person that he/she should reapply sunscreen. The trial, which was conducted in 2012, included a sample of 604 adults who owned Android smartphones. The treatment group included 305. Two hundred and thirty-two people downloaded the application, but only 125 actually used it. The researchers learned that users of the smartphone mobile application reported that they spent less time in the sun and employed more sun protective behaviors, such as the use of sunscreen and wearing protective clothing. The researchers noted that "use of the mobile app was lower than expected but associated with increased sun protection."[3]

An Appealing Appearance-Based Video May Foster More Sunscreen Use Than a Health-Based Video

In a study published in 2015 in the *Dermatology Online Journal*, researchers from California and Colorado wanted to determine if viewing videos could improve the use of sunscreen among 50 California high school students. In 2012, the students were randomized to view one of two different five-minute educational videos that promoted the use of sunscreen. The students rated the usefulness of the appearance-based video significantly higher than the health-based video. The appearance-based video emphasized that the regular use of sunscreen could help to prevent premature aging, sagging skin, uneven skin tone, and the development of wrinkles. On the other hand, the educational-based video discussed how exposure to ultraviolet light and insufficient sun protection increased the risk of skin cancer. This video showed images of skin cancer, and noted that not wearing sunscreen could lead to melanoma. Six weeks after viewing the videos, satisfaction surveys were administered. In terms of usefulness, educational content, and message appeal, the teens rated the appearance-based video higher than the health-based video. The researchers commented that "focusing on the short-term risk of UV light on physical appearance may have increased the salience of sun protection and consequently the perceived value of such behavior." Moreover, "this may be especially pertinent among adolescent patients who have lower perceived risk of experiencing disease, such as skin cancer."[4]

Televised Advertising Campaigns May Increase Sun Protection Behaviors, Including the Use of Sunscreen

In a study published in 2015 in the *American Journal of Preventive Medicine*, researchers from Australia noted that an advertising campaign known as SunSmart has been encouraging people to use sun protection for decades. The researchers investigated these advertisements broadcast during the summers between 1987 and 2011. They wanted to determine if these advertisements were increasing the use of sun protective behaviors such as using sunscreen. Cross-sectional weekly telephone surveys of Melbourne residents were conducted over the summers from 1987–1988 to 2010–2011, and analyzed in 2012–2014. Twenty-one percent of the respondents were 14 to 24 years old. The researchers asked the participants about their sun-related attitudes and sun protection and sunburn on the weekend prior to the interviews. They were also questioned about their exposure to television advertising during the four weeks before the interviews. The researchers found that viewing of the advertisements was associated with increased sun protective behaviors, including the use of sunscreen. "After more than two decades of public education on skin cancer, the amount of exposure to SunSmart TV advertising continues to be strongly associated with improved compliance in sun-related attitudes and behaviors across time periods and age groups."[5]

BARRIERS AND PROBLEMS

Age and Gender Appear to Influence the Use of Sunscreen

In a multicenter, cross-sectional study published in 2015 in the *American Journal of Clinical Dermatology*, researchers from Australia evaluated age and gender differences and the use of sunscreen. The researchers were primarily interested in learning more about sunscreen knowledge, attitudes, and behaviors.

The cohort consisted of 416 participants who were over the age of 18 years. Forty-two percent were male. The researchers learned that 94 percent of the participants between the ages of 18 and 30 years experienced at least one sunburn during the previous year. Only 15 percent of the participants used the recommended amount (40 ml) of sunscreen. Women were twice as likely as men to use sunscreen, and they knew more about sunscreen and sun protection than the men. The women were also more likely to reapply the sunscreen. While both men and women had high rates of sunscreen use during warmer weather, there were significantly lower rates of use during cooler months. So, it was not surprising that men had twice the incidence of skin cancer. And, among both men and women, the incidence of skin cancer increased with age. Younger participants were more likely to spend time sunbathing, but less likely to use sunscreen. The researchers commented that "there are knowledge, attitude, and behavior deficiencies within each demographic group that need to be specifically targeted through educational and public health efforts in order to improve general sun protection measures and decrease the incidence of skin cancers."[6]

Parents of Children Who May Be at Increased Risk for Skin Cancer Are Not Using a Sufficient Amount of Sunscreen

In a study published in 2015 in *Cancer Epidemiology, Biomarkers & Prevention*, researchers from Los Angeles and Philadelphia wrote that first-degree relatives of melanoma survivors have a "substantially higher" lifetime risk for melanoma, the most serious type of skin cancer. As a result, parents of these children must be even more vigilant with their use of sunscreen. The researchers wanted to learn if these parents were actually using sufficient sunscreen. A survey was administered by mail, telephone, or online to 324 Latino and non-Latino survivors of melanoma and 324 of their children, who had an average age of 9 years. Eighty-four percent of the cohort were non-Latino white and 70 percent were females. The researchers learned that these children had high rates of exposure to the sun, and their rates of sunburn were equal to or higher than estimates from average-risk populations. The Latino children were less likely to wear sunscreen and hats and more likely to wear sunglasses. As the children grew older they were less likely to use sun protection, and they had an increased risk for sunburns. The researchers underscored the need for melanoma survivors to be aware that their children are at increased risk. Then, survivors could "consider discussing this issue with a health care provider." The researchers noted that these discussions were infrequent occurrences in their sample. "Interventions to improve sun protection and reduce sun exposure and sunburns in high-risk children are needed."[7]

Not All Sun Protection Interventions Are Effective

In a study published in 2015 in the journal *Health Education Research*, researchers from the University of Southern California evaluated the effectiveness of a multiyear pilot sun safety education program conducted from 2006 to 2012 among Hispanic and Latino early adolescents in sunny Los Angeles. The researchers recruited 777 students from 19 schools with high Hispanic and Latino enrollment. Trained college students conducted the program, which consisted of three one-hour lessons over a three-week period of time, during regular school hours. From the pre- and post-testing, it was evident that the students learned a good deal about the need for protecting the skin from the sun with sunscreen. But, that knowledge did not, necessarily, translate into changes in behavior. "Due to rapidly increasing rates of melanoma in Hispanics, the largest and one of the fastest growing ethnic groups in the United States, increased sun safety education targeted to Hispanic children and adolescents is needed."[8]

Some College Students Are
Exposing Themselves to Too Much Sun

In a pilot study published in 2012 in the *Journal of American College Health*, researchers from Wayne, New Jersey, and New York City noted that melanoma is the second most common cancer diagnosed among people between the ages of 15 and 29 years. That is why these researchers wanted to learn more about the behaviors, barriers, and beliefs relevant to sun exposure and protective behaviors. The initial cohort consisted of 153 undergraduate students at a large state university in western New York. One hundred and thirty-nine of the participants completed an online survey. According to the students, in the summer they spent more than three hours per day outside. But, only 17.3 percent reported using some type of sunblock. Meanwhile, 60 percent reported recent indoor tanning, and 41 percent reported having more than 10 lifetime sunburns. Most often, the students indicated that they forgot to use sunscreen. A smaller number noted that they did not burn, so there was no need for sunscreen. The researchers commented that "demographics coupled with inconsistent and low levels of sunblock use, high annual prevalence of indoor tanning, and multiple lifetime sunburns indicate that this sample is at high risk for skin cancer."[9]

NOTES

1. Skin Cancer Foundation, www.skincancer.org.
2. K. M. White, C. Starfelt, R. M. Young et al., "A Randomised Controlled Trial of an Online Theory-Based Intervention to Improve Adult Australians' Sun-Protection Behaviours," *Preventive Medicine* 72 (2015): 19–22.
3. D. B. Buller, M. Berwick, K. Lantz et al., "Smartphone Mobile Application Delivering Personalized, Real-Time Sun Protection Advice: A Randomized Clinical Trial," *JAMA Dermatology* 151, no. 5 (2015): 497–504.
4. W. Tuong and A. W. Armstrong, "Participant Satisfaction with Appearance-Based Versus Health-Based Educational Videos Promoting Sunscreen Use: A Randomized Controlled Trial," *Dermatology Online Journal* 21, no. 2 (February 2015).
5. Suzanne J. Dobbinson, Angela Volkov, and Melanie A. Wakefield, "Continued Impact of SunSmart Advertising on Youth and Adults' Behaviors," *American Journal of Preventive Medicine* 49, no. 1 (2015): 20–28.
6. Andrew Lee, Kieran Benjamin Garbutcheon-Singh, Shreya Dixit et al., "The Influence of Age and Gender in Knowledge, Behaviors, and Attitudes Towards Sun Protection: A Cross-Sectional Survey of Australian Outpatient Clinic Attendees," *American Journal of Clinical Dermatology* 16 (2015): 47–54.
7. B. A. Glenn, T. Lin, L. C. Chang et al., "Sun Protection Practices and Sun Exposure Among Children with a Parental History of Melanoma," *Cancer Epidemiology, Biomarkers & Prevention* 24, no. 1 (2015): 169–77.

8. K. A. Miller, B. M. Langholz, T. Ly et al., "SunSmart: Evaluation of a Pilot School-Based Sun Protection Intervention in Hispanic Early Adolescents," *Health Education Research* 30, no. 3 (2015): 371–79.

9. Corey Hannah Basch, Grace Clarke Hillyer, Charles E. Basch, and Alfred Neugut, "Improving Understanding About Tanning Behaviors in College Students: A Pilot Study," *Journal of American College Health* 60, no. 3 (2012): 250–56.

REFERENCES AND RESOURCES

Magazines, Journals, and Newspapers

Basch, Corey Hannah, Danna Ethan, Grace Clarke Hillyer, and Alyssa Berdick. "Skin Cancer Prevention Coverage in Popular US Women's Health and Fitness Magazines: An Analysis of Advertisements and Articles." *Global Journal of Health Science* 6, no. 4 (2014): 42–48.

Basch, Corey Hannah, Grace Clarke Hillyer, Charles E. Basch, and Alfred I. Neugut. "Improving Understanding About Tanning Behaviors in College Students: A Pilot Study." *Journal of American College Health* 60, no. 3 (2012): 250–56.

Buller, D. B., M. Berwick, K. Lantz et al. "Smartphone Mobile Application Delivering Personalized, Real-Time Sun Protection Advice: A Randomized Clinical Trial." *JAMA Dermatology* 151, no. 5 (2015): 497–504.

Dobbinson, Suzanne J., Angela Volkov, and Melanie A. Wakefield. "Continued Impact of SunSmart Advertising on Youth and Adults' Behaviors." *American Journal of Preventive Behaviors* 49, no. 1 (2015): 20–28.

Glenn, B. A., T. Lin, L. C. Chang et al. "Sun Protection Practices and Sun Exposure Among Children with a Parental History of Melanoma." *Cancer Epidemiology, Biomarkers & Prevention* 24, no. 1 (2015): 169–77.

Gould, M., M. D. Farrar, R. Kift et al. "Sunlight Exposure and Photoprotection Behaviour of White Caucasian Adolescents in the UK." *Journal of the European Academy of Dermatology and Venereology* 29, no. 4 (2015): 732–37.

Lee, Andrew, Kieran Benjamin Garbutcheon-Singh, Shreya Dixit et al. "The Influence of Age and Gender in Knowledge, Behaviors and Attitudes Towards Sun Protection: A Cross-Sectional Survey of Australian Outpatient Clinic Attendees." *American Journal of Clinical Dermatology* 16 (2015): 47–54.

Miller, K. A., B. M. Langholz, T. Ly et al. "SunSmart: Evaluation of a Pilot School-Based Sun Protection Intervention in Hispanic Early Adolescents." *Health Education Research* 30, no. 3 (2015): 371–79.

Tuong, W., and A. W. Armstrong. "Participant Satisfaction with Appearance-Based Versus Health-Based Educational Videos Promoting Sunscreen Use: A Randomized Controlled Trial." *Dermatology Online Journal* 21, no. 2 (February 2015).

White, K. M., C. Starfelt, R. M. Young et al. "A Randomised Controlled Trial of an Online Theory-Based Intervention to Improve Adult Australians' Sun-Protection Behaviours." *Preventive Medicine* 72 (2015): 19–22.

Web Site

Skin Cancer Foundation. www.skincancer.org.

Glossary

Aerodigestive: the combined organs and tissues of the respiratory tract and the upper part of the digestive tract

Algorithm: a procedure or formula for solving a problem

Allostatic load: wear and tear on the body

Alloxan: an oxidized product of uric acid that destroys islet cells of the pancreas, thereby causing diabetes

Androgenetic alopecia: the absence of hair from skin areas in which it is normally present. It is the most common type of hair loss; it is due to male hormones.

Angina: a type of chest pain caused by reduced blood flow to the heart muscle

Anterior cruciate ligament: a ligament in the knee

Anthropometric: human body measurements

Antiandrogenic: a substance that blocks the actions of androgens, the hormones responsible for male characteristics

Anti-atherogenic activity: helps to prevent the formation of plaque

Antiproliferative: inhibit the growth of cells as in inhibiting the growth of cancer cells

Antipyretic: has properties that reduce fever

Apoptosis: cell death

Atherogenesis: formation of fatty lesions on arterial walls

Atherosclerosis: also known as hardening of the arteries, atherosclerosis is the build-up of fat, cholesterol, and other substances in the walls of arteries and the formation of hard structures called plaque

Atopic dermatitis: a chronic skin disorder in which there are scaly and itchy rashes

Atrial fibrillation: an erratic heart rhythm originating in the atrium

Autism spectrum disorder: a brain disorder characterized by deficits in social interaction, verbal and nonverbal communication, and restricted and repetitive behaviors

Benign prostatic hyperplasia: enlargement of the prostate gland

Binge eating disorder: recurrent episodes of compulsive overeating

Body mass index (BMI):   a body measurement based on a person's height and weight

Bone mineral density: a measurement of bone density reflecting the strength of the bones

Calculus: hardened dental plaque

Carcinogenic: cancer causing

Cerebral infarction: blockage of the flow of blood in the brain

Cheilitis: painful inflammation and cracking of the mouth

Chondroitin: a molecule occurring naturally in the body that is a major component of cartilage

Citraturia: levels of citric acid in the urine

Copra oil: oil made from dried coconut flesh

Coronary angiography: a medical test that uses dyes and special x-rays to evaluate the coronary arteries

Coumaphos: a highly toxic insecticide

Crackles: pathological breath sounds heard in the lungs of people with respiratory illness, such as pneumonia, or heart failure

C-reactive protein: a protein produced by the liver that rises when there is inflammation in the body

Cytotoxic: toxic to living cells

Disclosing agent: preparations that contain a coloring agent which is used to identify bacterial plaque in the mouth

Distal radial fracture: fracture of the radial bone near the wrist

Dyslexia: a developmental reading disorder in which the brain has a specific information processing problem

Dyslipidemia: an abnormal amount of lipids in the blood

Dysmenorrhea: painful menstruation

Dyspepsia: indigestion

Ellagic Acid: a phytochemical found in some plant foods such as strawberries and raspberries. It is believed to have anti-cancer properties.

Enterocolitis: inflammation of the colon and small intestine

Erythema: a skin condition characterized by redness

Erythrocytes: red blood cells

Esophagogastroduodenoscopy: a diagnostic endoscopic procedure used to see the upper portion of the gastrointestinal tract

Essential fatty acids: fatty acids that the body requires to function, but the body is unable to produce them, so they must be ingested

Euthymic: a relatively normal mood in people: not depressed but not highly elevated

Fasting plasma glucose: also known as the fasting blood sugar test, this test measures blood sugar levels when the patient is fasting

Gingivitis: inflammation of the gums

Granuloma: small nodule

Hemodynamic: movement of blood

Hepatotoxicity: liver injury usually caused by drugs

Hypercholesterolemia: elevated levels of serum cholesterol

Hyperlipidemia: elevated levels of lipids in the blood

Hypertension: elevated blood pressure

Hypoxia: deprived of adequate oxygen supply

Idiopathic: arising spontaneously from an obscure or unknown cause

Inguinal hernia: the protrusion of intestine into the groin area

Insulin resistance: an impaired ability of cells to respond to insulin

Interproximally: areas between adjoining teeth

Irritable bowel syndrome: a disorder in which there are recurrent episodes of abdominal distension and bloating, abdominal pain, and altered bowel habits with constipation and/or diarrhea, and an urgency to defecate

Isoenergetic: equal

Isoflavones: phytochemicals or compounds produced by plants that may have an effect on the body

Laparotomy: surgical incision into the abdominal cavity

Legumes: a family of plants that bear edible seeds in pods

Lipemia: abnormally high concentrations of lipids in the blood

Lipids: a broad group of naturally occurring molecules that include fat, waxes, sterols, and fat-soluble vitamins

Liposomes: microscopic artificial sacs composed of fatty substances that contain a water droplet mixture and an active ingredient. It is often used in experimental research

Locavore: a person who prefers to eat local food

Lycopene: a carotenoid that gives fruits and vegetables a red color

Mastalgia: breast pain

Metabolic syndrome: also known as insulin resistance, with this disorder there is extra weight around the waist, high blood pressure, and elevated levels of cholesterol

Metastasis: the spreading of cancer from its initial site to other parts of the body

Mucositis: breaking down of mucous membranes leading to ulceration and infection

Neoplasm: a new and abnormal growth, especially characteristic of cancer

Nephrectomy: the surgical removal of all or part of a kidney

Nocebo: in medicine, an inert substance or form of therapy that creates harmful effects in a patient

Nociception: pain from the stimulus of nerve cells

Nocturia: getting up during the night to urinate

Obesogenic: supportive of obesity, promoting obesity

Oleuropein: a phenolic compound found in olive oil

Osteoarthritis: a degenerative joint disease characterized by damage to the cartilage that cushions the joints

Osteocalcin: a marker of bone formation

Osteopenia: bone mineral density that is lower than normal but not low enough to be classified as osteoporosis

Osteoporosis: a condition in which the bones lose too much mineralization. The weakened bones are at increased risk for breakage

Ozone: a gas composed of three oxygen atoms

Parenteral: introduction of nutrition, medicine, or other substances into the body via a route other than the mouth

Periodontal disease: inflammation of the gums and the loss of attachment of the periodontal ligament

Photoaging: damage to the skin from UV radiation

Phytic acid: a dietary fiber component found in most grains and legumes that has been shown to have antioxidant and anticancer properties

Plant polyphenols: naturally occurring plant compounds that offer protection from a number of different illnesses

Postprandial lipemia: elevated lipid levels after the consumption of a meal

Post-traumatic stress disorder: a mental health condition triggered by exposure to traumatic events

Preterm delivery: delivery of a baby before 37 weeks of gestation

Proapoptotic: programmed cell death

Pruritus: itching

Psoriasis: a common skin condition that causes redness and irritation. People with psoriasis often have thick, red skin with flaky silver-white patches called scales

Psychotropic medication: medication affecting the mind, emotions, and behavior

Radical prostatectomy: removal of the prostate gland and surrounding tissue

Reepithelilialization: restoring the soundness from injury of external surfaces of the body

Rheumatoid arthritis: in this disorder, the immune system attacks the joints, making them swollen, stiff, and painful

Sarcopenia: the degenerative loss of skeletal muscle mass and strength associated with aging

Silver sulphadiazine: a topical antibacterial cream used for burns

Sjogren's syndrome: an autoimmune disorder in which the body attacks glands in the body that produce moisture, such as the salivary and tear glands

Social anxiety disorder: a condition in which a person fears being evaluated by others and avoids social situations

Static balance: the ability to maintain one's balance when not moving

Strangury: frequent, painful urination of small amounts of urine

Tear film osmolarity: the salt content of the eye, which tends to be higher in people with dry eyes

Teratology: the study of malformations

Triglycerides: a type of fat in the blood that provides energy to the body

Ulcerative colitis: a type of inflammatory bowel disease that affects the lining of the large intestine and rectum

Urolithiasis: process of forming stones in the kidneys, bladder, or urethra

Viremia: viruses entering the bloodstream

Visceral adiposity: excess weight in the abdominal area

Working memory: short-term or recent memory

Index

Academic Pediatrics, 18

Accident Analysis & Prevention, 162–163, 166

Acta Paediatrica, 39

Active commuting: barriers and problems, 99–100; cardiovascular health, 97; employers and, 99–100; habit formation and, 98; HDL cholesterol and, 99; increasing numbers of people who, 99; infrastructure changes that increase, 98; metabolic health and, 99; psychological well-being and, 97–98; study of, Australia, 99; study of, California, 98; study of, Finland, 98; study of, Portugal, 99; study of, U.K., 97–100

Acute respiratory tract infections (ARTI), 106–107

Addictive Behaviors, 233

Adolescent Medicine: State of the Art Reviews, 149

Advances in Nutrition, 33

AIDS Patient Care and STDs, 207

Alabama, studies, 146, 167, 244

Alameda County Medical Center, 207

Alcohol abuse, 18, 55, 146, 166, 235–236

Alcoholism: Clinical & Experimental Research, 55

American Academy of Neurology, 163

American Academy of Orthopaedic Surgeons, 154

American Academy of Pediatrics, 245, 265

American Heart Association, 80

American Journal of Clinical Nutrition, 79, 117

American Journal of Dentistry, 121

American Journal of Emergency Medicine, 168–169

American Journal of Epidemiology, 39, 87, 265

American Journal of Health Promotion, 189, 238

American Journal of Managed Care, 213–214

American Journal of Orthodontics and Dentofacial Orthopedics, 122

American Journal of Preventive Medicine, 97, 234, 238

American Speech-Language-Hearing Association, 132

Angle Orthodontist, 120

Anorexia, 2, 116

Antibiotics: adults and, 104–105; beneficial bacteria and, 105; body mass index (BMI), 105–106; celiac disease and, 105; children and, 104–105; early-life body mass, 106; farm animals and, 104–105; gender and, 105–106; infants and, 105–106, 107; obesity and, 104–105; overuse of, 104, 106–107; reduction in use, 104; reduction in use, barriers and problems, 106–107; respiratory infections and, 103–104, 106–107; side effects, 104; study of, Maryland, 104; study of, New York, 104, 106; study of, New Zealand, 105–106; study of, Pennsylvania, 107; study of, Taiwan, 106; study of, Thailand, 106; subtherapeutic antibiotic therapy, 140–105; teens and, 104–105; therapy, 104; unnecessary use of, 103–107; what the experts say about, 104–106

Antimicrobial Agents and Chemotherapy, 106

Appetite, 9, 11, 23, 28–29, 45, 56, 72, 203

Applied Physiology, Nutrition, and Metabolism, 17, 51

Archives of Pediatrics & Adolescent Medicine, 155, 184

Archives of Public Health, 183

Arizona, studies, 23, 151

Asia Pacific Journal of Clinical Nutrition, 7, 25, 61–62

Asia-Pacific Psychiatry, 257

Atheroschlerosis, 34, 38

Attention deficit/hyperactivity disorder (ADHD), 39–40

Attentional bias modification, 43

Auburn University, 140–141

Australia, studies, 6, 11, 29, 56, 62, 89–90, 99, 126, 129, 184, 189–191, 246–247

Australian Bureau of Statistics, 99

Australian Census of Population and Housing, 99

Avon Longitudinal Study of Parents and Children, 106

Bangor University, Wales, 24

Bariatric surgery, 49

Belgium, studies, 45

Bicycling: diabetes, 97; hypertension, 97; what the experts say about, 97–99

Biology of Reproduction, 229

Bipolar disorder, 180–181

Birth Defects Research, 234

Blaser, Martin, 105

Blood glucose levels, 1

BMC Endocrine Disorders, 117

BMC Gastroenterology, 105

BMC Medicine, 154

BMC Muscular Disorders, 115

BMC Pediatrics, 8, 179

BMX Psychiatry, 256

BMC Public Health, 14, 51, 186, 235

BMJ, 50, 78, 129

Body Image, 196

Body image: depression and, 195; Facebook and, 197–198; female models and, 196; gender and, 195–197; ideal body types and, 196; maintaining a healthy, 194–198; maintaining a healthy, barriers and problems, 196–198; obesity and, 195; physical activity and, 195; post-baby bodies of celebrities and, 197; preoccupation of, 194; race and, 195–196; school-based interventions, 196; study of, Brazil, 194; study of, Illinois, 197; study of, Korea, 197; study of, Texas, 195; study of, Vietnam, 195; teasing and, 197; what the experts say about, 195–196

Body mass index (BMI): ideal, 1; study of, Texas, 49; unhealthy dieting and, 2–36

Bone density: abdominal fat and, 111–118; anorexia nervosa and, 116; building and maintaining strong bones, 114; calcium and, 115–116; diet and, 114–115; exercise and, 115; gender and, 115; low-dose oral contraceptives and, 117; maintaining good, 114–118; maintaining good, barriers and problems, 116–118; physical activity and, 116; resistance training and, 115; study of, Brazil, 115, 117; study of, China, 116; study of, Finland, 115–117; study of, Greece, 116; study of, Michigan, 117; study of, Tennessee, 115–116; teens and, 116; Vitamin D and, 114–115, 117, 129–130; Vitamin K and, 115; what the experts say about, 115–116

Brain Sciences, 54

Brazil, studies, 46, 60–61, 115, 117, 138, 194

Breakfast: academic achievement and, 8; access to food and, 8; barriers and problems, 8–9; behavioral problems and, 7; bone mineral density and, 7–8; bullying/cyberbullying and, 9; frequent eaters of, 6; gender and, 7; obesity and eating, 6; protein-rich, 7; psychosocial health and, 8; satiety and, 7; school, 8; skipping, x, 6–9; study of, Australia, 6; study of, Canada, 9; study of, Japan, 7; study of, Norway, 7; study of, South Africa, 8; teens and, 6–7; what the experts say about, 6–8

British Household Panel Survey, 98

British Journal of General Practice, xiv

British Journal of Nutrition, 6, 28, 116

British Journal of Sports Medicine, 156, 160

Brown University, 194

Buddhist meditation, 200

Bulimia nervosa, 2

Bulletin of the World Health Organization, 40–41

Bullying, 183–187; advantages, 186; barriers and problems, 185–187; definition of, 183–184; negative body image and, 185–186; parenting style and, 185; school-based programs, 184, 187; school environment and, 184; skipping breakfast and, 9; socioeconomic status and, 186–187; study of, Australia, 184; study of, Czech Republic, 185; study of, Finland, 184; study of, Netherlands, 184–186; study of, Slovakia, 185; teachers and, 184, 186–187; what the experts say about, 184–185

Burger King, 48

Cadernos de Saúde Pública (Reports in Public Health), 46

Caffeine and energy drinks, 244; academic achievement and, 55; adolescent intake of, 54–57; alcohol dependence and, 55–56; anxiety and, 56; cognitive function and, 56–57; definition of, 53–54; depression and, 56; gender and, 54, 56; limit intake of, 53–58; limit intake of, barriers and problems, 56–57; mood and, 56; sleep behavior and, 54–55;

sleep depth and, 54–55; stress and, 56; study of, Australia, 56; study of, California, 56; study of, Colorado, 54; study of, Maryland, 55; study of, Switzerland, 54; study of, U.K., 56–57; teens and, 54–57; what the experts say about, 54–56; withdrawal effects, 55

California, studies, 56, 77, 98, 110, 134, 163, 214, 233, 240

California Health Interview Survey (2007), 214

CAMELIA project, 61

Canada, studies, 9, 17, 51, 73, 88–89, 133–134, 156, 162–163, 179, 192, 265–266

Canadian Diabetes Association 2013 Clinical Practice Guidelines, 88

Canadian Food Inspection Agency, 74

Canadian Hospitals Injury Reporting and Prevention Program, 161

Canadian Journal of Public Health, 54

Cancer Causes & Control, 128

Cancer Epidemiology, Biomarkers & Prevention, 212

Cardiovascular health: active commuting, 97; exercise and physical activity, 87–88; sugar and, 76, 79

Celiac disease, 69, 105

Centers for Disease Control and Prevention (CDC), 65, 67, 143, 159; Youth Risk Behavior Surveillance—United States, 2013, 33

Cheers for Ears, 132

Child Abuse & Neglect, 151, 179, 185

Child and Adolescent Mental Health, 190

Childhood Obesity, 46

Children's Hospital of Philadelphia, 166

Children's of Alabama, 160

China, studies, 66, 116, 128, 179, 229, 238, 261–262,

Chlamydia Screening Implementation, 205

Cholesterol levels, 1

Chronic Diseases and Injuries in Canada, 161

Circulation, 1, 50

Clinical and Experimental Dermatology, 241

Clinical Psychological Science, 192

Coaching Boys into Men (CBIM), 149
Cognitive Behaviour Therapy, 190
Collegium Antropologicum, x
Colorado, studies, 54,
Columbia University Medical Center, 38
Community Dentistry and Oral
    Epidemiology, 120
Community supported agriculture (CSA)
    groups, 22–24
Compendium of Continuing Education in
    Dentistry, 121
Comprehensive Psychiatry, 255–256
Computers in Human Behavior, 256
Conidi, Frank, 163
Connecticut, studies, 180
Contraception: emergency, 227–231
Contraception, 229–231
Cook, Ken, 28
Cornish Academies Project, 56
Critical Reviews in Food Science and
    Nutrition, 33
Current Drug Abuse Reviews, 51–52
Current Opinion in Clinical Nutrition and
    Metabolic Care, 81
Cyberbullying, 256; definition of, 183;
    skipping breakfast and, 9
Cyberprogram 2.0, 189
Cyberpsychology, Behavior, and Social
    Networking, 146, 255
Czech Republic, studies, 185

Danish National Patient Register,
    211–212
Dating relationships: college-based
    courses on, 217; community-based in-
    teractive theater programs modeling,
    217; cultivating healthy, 216–220; de-
    pression, 218; Facebook and, 218–219;
    gender and, 216–217; healthy, barriers
    and problems, 218–220; healthy, spe-
    cific characteristics of, 216–217; mod-
    eling healthy, 216; race and, 216–217;
    same-sex relationships, 218; sisters and,
    218; study of, Florida, 217; study of,
    Maryland, 216–217; study of, Texas,
    217; study of, Utah, 217; teens, 216–
    217; violence and abuse, 219–220; what
    the experts say about, 216–218

Denmark, studies, 89; 28–29, 211–212
Dental care: anxiety, 123; barriers and
    problems, 122–124; children and, 121;
    difficult economic times and, 120–121;
    disclosing agents, 122; flossing, xiv, 124;
    fluoride and, 121; nutritional deficien-
    cies and, 120; orthodontic appliances,
    122–123; oscillating-rotating power
    brushes, 121; periodontal disease, 123;
    plaque control, compliance with, 122–
    123; practice excellent home, 119–124;
    race and, 123–124; sonic brushes, 121;
    study of, Germany, 121–122; study of,
    Iceland, 120; study of, Indiana, 123;
    study of, Ohio, 121–122; study of,
    Poland, 123; study of, U.K., 122; study
    of, Virginia, 120; teens and, 121; text
    messages to orthodontic patients, 120;
    toothpaste, 122; well-being and, 120;
    what the experts say about, 120–122
Depression: body image, 195; caffeine
    and, 56; dating relationships and, 218;
    dieting and, 3; exercise and, 85–86;
    family meals and, 16; gender and,
    59–60; Internet addiction and, 255;
    mindfulness and, 200; processed
    foods and, 59–60; resilience and, 181;
    safer sex and, 225; screen time and,
    266–267; trans fats and, 40; unhealthy
    diets and, 3
Deutsches Ärzteblatt International, 161
Dexa scan, 7
Diabetes: bicycling and, 97; exercise and
    physical activity, 88–89; fast food and,
    50; organically grown food and, 30;
    stress and, 273; sugar and, 76–77; Type
    1, 273; Type 2, 50, 76–77, 88–89, 127;
    Vitamin D and, 127, walking and, 97
Dieting: barriers and problems to, 3–4;
    depression and, 3; fad, x; study of,
    Minnesota, 2–3; teens and, 2; triggers,
    3–4; unhealthy, avoiding, 1–20; what
    the experts say regarding, 2–3
Disordered eating, 194, 201; family meals
    and, 2–3, 18–19; peers behaviors and,
    4, 6
Driving: barriers and problems, 145–147;
    college students, 145; distracted,

143–146; drinking and, 146, 166–167; fatalities, 144; Google Glass and, 145; seatbelts, 166–169; study of, Alabama, 146; study of, Kenya, 144; study of, Spain, 145; study of, Turkey, 145; study of, U.K., 145–146; study of, U.S., 144; texting while, 143–147; texting while, laws regarding, 143; visual-manual phone tasks and, 144; what the experts say about, 144–145
Drug use, 18, 166

Early Intervention in Psychiatry, 201
Eastern Ontario 2011 Youth Risk Behavior Survey, 9
Eating Behaviors, 3, 43, 195, 201
Edinboro University, 229
Edmonton Minor Soccer Association, 156
El Joven Noble, 152
Electromagnetic fields: chronic exposure to, 260–261; limiting exposure to, 260–263; memory loss in teens, 262; mobile phones, 262; psychosomatic medical problems, 262–263; serum lipid levels and exposure to, 260–261; spontaneous abortions, 261; study of, China, 260–261; studies suggesting the harmful effects of, 260–262; studies suggesting the safety of, 262–263
Electronic cigarettes (e-cigarettes), 233–236; alcohol use and, 235; barriers and problems, 235–236; college students and, 236; definition of, 233; environmental impact of, 235; gender and, 236; nicotine in, 234–235; pregnancy and, 234–235; study of, California, 233; study of, New York, 235; study of, Texas, 234, 236; study of, U.K., 235; teens and, 234, 235–236; tobacco use and, 234; what the experts say about, 233–235; young adults and, 233–234
Emergency contraception, 227–231; barriers and problems, 229–231; benefits of, 228–229; college students and, 229–230; education about, 29–230; efficacy rates of, 230; exposure to, 229; gender and, 231; IUDs, 228, 230; obesity and, 230; Plan B, 228; Plan B One-Step,

228; problems purchasing, 230–231; reasons for using, 228; study of, China, 229; study of, India, 230; ulipristal acetate (Ella), 228; what the experts say about, 228–229
England, studies, 34
Environmental Research, 29
Environmental Science and Pollution Research International, 260
Environmental Working Group, 28; Clean Fifteen, 31; Dirty Dozen, 31
European Child & Adolescent Psychiatry, 128
European Hydration Institute, 11
European Journal of Dentistry, 122
European Journal of Clinical Nutrition, 66, 126
European Journal of Nutrition, 33, 49
European Journal of Pediatrics, 185
European Journal of Psychotramatology, 180
European Journal of Public Health, 166–167
Exercise and physical activity, xiii, 85–100; age-appropriate, 86; anxiety, 85; barriers and problem, 88–89; bicycling, 97–100; cancer and, 87; cardiovascular health and, 87–88; depression, 85–86; gender and, 86; group sports, 91–95; harmful, 89; heart failure and, 88; immune system and, 85; incentive programs, xiv; intake of water and, 12; making time for frequent, 85–89; mortality and, 87; race and, 87–88; regular, 85; running strenuously, 89; stress and, 86–87; stroke and, 88; study of, Canada, 88–89; study of, Denmark, 89; study of, Lebanon, 86–87; study of, Minnesota, 87; study of, Mississippi, 87; study of, Missouri, 89; study of, Netherlands, 85; study of, Switzerland, 86–87, 89; study of, U.K., 88; Type 2 diabetes and, 88–89; usefulness of different, 89; walking, 97–100; what the experts say regarding, 16–17, 86–88
Explore, 200

Facebook: body image and, 197–198; dating relationships and 218–219
Family Dinner Project, 16–17

Family meals, 2–3, 16–20; after-school activities, 20; barriers and problems, 19–20; BMI and, 17–18; depression and, 16; disordered weight control behaviors and, 17–19; frequency of, 17–20; improvements in nutritional health and, 17; mental health benefits of, 17; obesity and, 17–18; overall healthy eating and, 18; race and, 18; self-esteem and, 17; sports, 20; substance abuse and, 16, 18; study of, Canada, 17; study of, U.K., 17; study of, U.S., 2, 16–19; teen pregnancy and, 16; work schedules and, 20

Farmers' markets, 24-25

Fast food: addiction, 51–52; availability of, 51; coronary heart disease and, 50 ; definition of, 48; drive-up windows, 48; gender and, 48; limiting intake of, 48–52; limiting intake of, barriers and problems to, 51–52; metabolic syndrome and, 49–50; preference for, 51; race and, 48; study of, Canada, 51; study of, Iran, 49; study of, Scotland, 51; study of, Singapore, 50; study of, UK, 50; study of, U.S., 50; taxing, 50; Type 2 diabetes and, 50; weight gain and, 49–50; what the experts say about, 49–50

Fatality Analysis Reporting System, 169

Federal Motor Carrier Safety Administration, 143

Federal Railroad Administration, 143

Feet: flip-flops, 140–141; fungus, 138–139; gender, 138, 140; high heels, 140; in-shoe pressure, 138–139; infections, 139; odors, 139; pain, 138; running on grass, 138–139; shock-absorbing insoles, 139; shoe selection, 140–141; study of, Brazil, 138; study of, Italy, 139; taking care of, 137–141; taking care of, barriers and problems, 140–141; warts, 138; what the experts say about, 138–139

Finland, studies, 33–34, 78, 98, 115–117, 184

Fleming, Alexander, 103

Florida, studies, 217

Food and healthy eating, 1–81; avoiding unhealthy diets and weight-loss methods, 1–4; breakfast, skipping, 6–9; caffeine and energy drinks, limit the intake of, 53–58; family meals, 16–20; fast food intake, limiting, 48–52; food labels, reading, 69–74; fruits and vegetables, eating the recommended amount of, 32–36; incorporating healthier snacks into your diet, 43–46; locally produced foods, 21–25; organically grown foods, 27–31; processed food, limiting, 59–63; sodium and salt intake, 64–68; sugar, reduce intake of, 76–81; trans fats, eliminating or greatly reducing from diet, 38–41; water, drinking sufficient, 11–14

Food & Nutrition Research, 7

Food deserts, 25

Food intolerance, 69

Food labels, 40; Cleveland, Ohio, 41; college students and, 71; definition of, 69–70; gender and, 70–72; healthy eating and, 70–71; incorrect information on, 73–74; incorrect reading of, 72–73; reading, 69–74; reading, barriers and problems, 72–74; requirements, Canada, 41; requirements, U.S., 41; study of, Canada, 73; study of, India, 73; study of, Korea, 70–71; study of, Minnesota, 71; study of, New Zealand, 73; study of, Switzerland, 71; weight loss and, 70; what the experts say about, 70–73

France, studies, 12–13, 68

Fruits and vegetables, eating the recommended amount of, 32–36; barriers and problems, 35–36; benefits of, 33–35; cancer and, 33–34; coronary heart disease and, 35; expenses related to, 35; lifespan and, 33–34; strokes and, 34–35; study of, England, 34; study of, Finland, 33–34; study of, Norway, 33; study of, Sweden, 33–34; teens and, 36; what the experts say about, 33–35

Gender: antibiotics and, 105–106; body image and, 195–197; BMI and, 115;

breakfast and, 7; caffeine and energy drinks, 54, 56; dating relationships and, 216–217; depression and, 59–60; electronic cigarettes and, 59–60; emergency contraception and, 231; exercise and physical activity and 86; fast food and, 48; feet and, 138, 140; food labels and, 70–72; sexually transmitted diseases and, 206; social connections and friendships with peers, 175; sports and, 93–95; sunscreen use and, 278–279; tanning beds and, 238; trans fats and, 40; violence and, 149–150;
Genetically-modified organisms (GMOs), 27–28
George Mason University, 192
Georgia, studies, 79
Germany, studies, 121–122, 190
Girls on the Go!, 189
Google Glass, 145
Greece, studies, 116
Guangzhou Asian Games, 2010, 157

Habits: dietary, Croatian adolescents, x; establishing healthy, ix, xiii–xv, 28–29; formation, definition of, xiii; forming and reforming, xiii–xv; incentive programs, x, xiii–xiv; incentive programs, Minnesota, xiv; intervention programs, Utah, xiii–xiv; making a new healthy, xv; triggers, xiii
Happy Being Me, 196
Harvard University, 41; Harvard Prevention Research Center, 44
Health Affairs, 60, 80
Health Behaviour in School–Aged Children, 186
Health Education & Behavior, 249
Health Habits Program (HHP), x
Health literacy skills: adolescent, 250–252; barriers and problems, 251–252; improving, 249–252; low, 250–252; materials for, 251; nurses and, 252; nutritional behaviors and, 251–252; over-estimating, 252; study of, Massachusetts, 249; study of, Michigan, 249–250; study of, Ohio, 249; study of, Taiwan, 251–252; study of, Texas, 249;

study of, Virginia, 249; using credible online health sources, 249–250; what the experts say about, 249–251
Health Promotion Journal of Australia, 99
Health Services Insights, 245
Hearing: children, 132–133; headphones and, 132; impairment, 131; interventions to prevent loss of, 133–134; loss, 131–132; loss, noise-induced, 132, 135–136; personal listening device behavior, 132–133; protecting, 131–136; protecting, barriers and problems, 134–136; study of, Australia, 129–130; study of, California, 134; study of, Canada, 133–134; study of, Minnesota, 134; study of, South Africa, 132; study of, U.K., 135; study of, Wisconsin, 133–134; teens, 134–135; undergraduate music students, 135–136; what the experts say, 132–133
HORMONES, 116
Human Factors, 145
Human Movement, 140
Human papillomavirus (HPV): cancer and, 210–211, 213; definition of, 210–211; genital warts and, 211–212; school-based educational programs, 212; sexual behavior and, 211; study of, Denmark, 211–212; study of, Italy, 212; study of, North Carolina, 212; study of, Ohio, 212; transmission of, 210; vaccination, 109, 210–211; vaccination, barriers and problems, 212–214; vaccination, insurance coverage of, 213–214; vaccination, rates of, 212–213; vaccination, safety of, 212; vaccination, timely administration of, 213; what the experts say about, 211–212
Human Vaccine & Immunotherapeutics, 212
Hypertension, 66

Iceland, studies, 120
Illinois, studies, 151, 163, 168, 197
India, studies, 73;
Indian Journal of Community Medicine, 230
Indian Journal of Endocrinology and Metabolism, 6

Indian Journal of Medical Research, 228
Indiana, studies, 123
International Journal of Audiology, 135
International Journal of Behavioral Medicine, 86, 88
International Journal of Eating Disorders, 2, 196
International Journal of Environmental Research and Public Health, 245
International Journal of Obesity, 105–106
International Journal of Preventive Medicine, 45
International Journal of STD & AIDS, 208
Internet addiction, 254–256; aggression and, 255–256; barriers and problems, 257–258; depression and, 255; parent-adolescent interaction and, 256–257; parental involvement and, 256; parents and, 257; reasons for, 254; shyness and, 256; study of, Taiwan, 255; study of, Turkey, 254, 256; teens and, 254–257; university students, 256; weight problems and, 255; what the experts say about, 254–257
Internet Addiction Scale, 254
Iran, studies, 45, 49
Iranian Journal of Public Health, 168
Iraq, studies, 150
Israel, studies, 180, 190
Israel Journal of Psychiatry and Related Sciences, 180
Italy, studies, 11, 122, 139;

JAMA Dermatology, 239
JAMA International Medicine, 79
JAMA Pediatrics, 3, 234
Japan, studies, 7
Joslin Diabetes Center, 19
Journal of Abnormal Child Psychology, 192
Journal of Adolescence, 55, 190
Journal of Adolescent Health, 2, 4, 18, 85, 109–110, 151–152, 189, 191, 244, 257
Journal of Advanced Prosthetics, 157
Journal of Affective Disorders, 180
Journal of Clinical Oncology, 238
Journal of Clinical Sleep Medicine, 244
Journal of Alternative and Complementary Medicine, 200

Journal of American College Health, 201, 236
Journal of Antimicrobial Chemotherapy, 104
Journal of Athletic Training, 139
Journal of Behavioral Nutrition and Physical Activity, 99
Journal of Bone and Mineral Research, 115–116
Journal of Clinical and Diagnostic Research, 49
Journal of Clinical Nutrition, 127
Journal of Clinical Nursing, 251–252
Journal of Community Health, 169
Journal of Community Health Nursing, 217
Journal of Dentistry, 78
Journal of Educational Psychology, 184
Journal of Epidemiology & Community Health, 17, 34
Journal of Family and Community Medicine, 150
Journal of Family Psychology, 217
Journal of Health Economics, xiii
Journal of Health Communication, 251
Journal of Health Psychology, 140
Journal of Human Nutrition and Dietetics, 62
Journal of Interpersonal Violence, 149, 186
Journal of Lesbian Studies, 181
Journal of Neurology, 164
Journal of Nutrition, 13, 39
Journal of Nutrition Education, 19
Journal of Nutrition Education and Behavior, 22
Journal of Occupational Health, 86–87
Journal of Oral Research and Review, 122
Journal of Orthopaedic and Sports Physical Therapy, 139
Journal of Paediatrics and Child Health, 126
Journal of Pediatric and Adolescent Gynecology, 59–60
Journal of Pediatric Surgery, 160
Journal of Primary Care & Community Health, 163
Journal of Primary Prevention, 216
Journal of Psychiatric Research, 195
Journal of Psychopharmacology, 56
Journal of Public Health Dentistry, 123

Journal of Safety Research, 144, 167

Journal of School Health, 44, 46, 150, 243–244, 249–250

Journal of School Nursing, 8

Journal of School Violence, 185

Journal of Sports Sciences, 138

Journal of the Academy of Nutrition and Dietetics, 71–72

Journal of the American Academy of Dermatology, 239, 240

Journal of the American College of Cardiology, 89

Journal of the American Dietetic Association, 19, 23

Journal of the American Podiatric Medical Association, 140–141

Journal of the Medical Library Association, 250

Journal of the Pakistan Medical Association, 254

Journal of the Pediatric Infectious Diseases Society, 107

Journal of the Science of Food, 25

Journal of the Science of Food and Agriculture, 29–30

Journal of Trauma and Acute Care Surgery, 144

Journal of Urology, 168

Kabat-Zinn, Jon, 200

Kansas, studies, 151

Kentucky Fried Chicken, 48

Kenya, studies, 144;

Knee Surgery, Sports Traumatology, Arthroscopy, 160

KNHANES, 70

Korea, studies, 39–40, 59–60, 70–71, 157, 181, 197

Korean Journal of Family Medicine, 70

Koru training, 201–202

Kurdistan, studies, 168

Language, Speech, and Hearing Services in School, 134

The Laryngoscope, 133

Lebanon, studies, 86–87

Lebanon War, 180

Local Harvest, 22

Locally produced foods, 21–25; barriers and problems, 24–25; children who grow their own produce, 23; community-supported agriculture programs, 23–24; farmers' markets and, 24; food deserts and, 25; food safety issues, 25; income and, 23; interventions, 23–24; nutrition and, 24–25; study of, Arizona, 23; study of, North Carolina, 23–24; transportation, 25; what the experts say about, 23–24; workplace flexibility and, 24

Maryland, studies, 55, 104, 216–217

Massachusetts, studies, 60, 79, 238, 249, 266

Massachusetts General Hospital, ix

Massachusetts Medical School, 200

Mayo Clinic, 39

McDonald's, 48

Meat and meat products, consuming, x

Medical care and avoiding medical issues, 103–141; antibiotics, unnecessary use of, 103–107; bone density, maintaining good, 114–118; dental care, practice excellent home, 119–124; feet, taking care of, 137–141; hearing, protecting, 131–136; vaccinations for teens, 109–113; Vitamin D deficiency, preventing, 125–130

Medical Problems of Performing Artists, 135

Medicine & Science in Sports & Exercise, 87

MedLine Plus, 250

Mental, emotional, and social health, 173–203; body image, maintaining a healthy, 194–198; bullying, 183–187; mindfulness, 199–203; resilience, building, 178–182; self-esteem, improving, 188–192; social connections and friendships with peers, building, 173–176

Mexico, studies, 12

Michigan, studies, 117, 137–138, 249–250

Michigan Podiatric Medical Association, 137–138

Mindfulness, 199–203; anxiety and, 200–201; at-risk teens and, 202–203; barriers and problems, 202–203 ; benefits of, 200; bipolar disease, 201; depression and, 200; disordered eating and, 201; emotional well-being and, 200; Koru training, 201–202; psychiatric disorders and, 200–201; race and, 202–203; study of, North Carolina, 200–202; study of, Ohio, 201; study of, Pennsylvania, 200–202; study of, Texas, 202; study of, U.K., 200; theory, 190–191; weight loss and, 203; what the experts say about, 200–202

Mindfulness, 202

Minnesota, studies, 2–3, 46, 71, 87, 134, 162–163, 191

Mississippi, studies, 87

Missouri, studies, 89

Morbidity and Mortality Weekly Report, 33

National Ambulatory Care Survey, 106–107

National Cancer Institute, 87

National Center for Health Statistics, 48, 265

National Health and Nutrition Examination Surveys, 1, 65

National Heart, Lung, and Blood Institute, 265

National Highway Safety Administration, 143

National Highway Traffic Safety Administration, 144, 169

National Hospital Ambulatory Care Survey, 107

National Institutes of Deafness and Other Communication Disorders, 131

National Institutes of Health, 19

National Longitudinal Survey of Children, 192

National Sleep Foundation, 242

National Survey of Children's Exposure to Violence II, 151

National Traffic Highway Safety Administration, 166

National Trauma Data Bank (NTDB), 168

National Youth Tobacco Surveys, 234

Nature, 104–105

Netherlands, studies, 29–30, 40, 85, 128, 184–186

New Hampshire, studies, 151

New Statesman, 103

New York, studies, 104, 106, 149, 168–169, 235

New York Presbyterian Hospital, 38

New York University, 106; Langone Medical Center, 105

New Zealand, studies, 29, 62, 73, 78, 105–106, 179,

Nicotine & Tobacco Research, 235

Noise & Health, 132

North Carolina, studies, 23–24, 46, 60, 200–202, 212

North Carolina Child Health Assessment and Monitoring Program, 22–23

Norway, studies, 7, 33

Nurses' Health Study, 79

Nursing and Midwifery Studies, ix

Nutrición Hospitalaria, x, 12, 194

Nutrients, 66, 73

Nutrition Facts label, 70

Nutrition Labeling and Education Act of 1990, 70

Nutrition, Metabolism & Cardiovascular Diseases, 38

NutriTrack database, 62

Obesity: antibiotics and, 104–105; body image and, 195; breakfast and, 6; emergency contraception and, 230; family meals and, 17–18; organically grown foods and, 30; salt and, 66; seatbelt use and, 168–169; snacking and, 44–45; sports and, 93; sugar and, 76; Vitamin D and, 126–127

Obesity Surgery, 49

Occupational & Environmental Medicine, 133

Ohio, studies, 121–122, 201, 212

Oral Health & Preventive Dentistry, 123

Organically grown foods, 27–31; antioxidants in, 28; barriers and problems, 30–31; cadmium in, 28; definition of, 27–28; diabetes and, 30; government standards regarding, 28; healthy eating habits and, 28–29; obesity and, 30;

overall health improvements and, 29–30; overall health and, 30; pesticides in, 28–30; reasons for eating, 29–30; study of, Australia, 29; study of, Denmark, 28–29; study of, Netherlands, 29–30; study of, New Zealand, 29; study of, U.K., 28; what the experts say about, 28–30
Osteoporosis, 115–116
Osteoporosis International, 115

Pakistan Journal of Biological Sciences, 72
Palo Alto Medical Foundation, 148
Parental education, 18
Pediatric Nursing, 243
Pediatrics, 17, 65, 211, 213, 266
Pennsylvania, studies, 80, 107, 200–202
Perceptual and Motor Skills, 89
Pesticides, 27–29
Pew Research Center for the 2010 Spring Change Assessment, 146
Plan B, 228
Plan B One-Step, 228
PLoS ONE, 12, 30, 35, 40, 68, 77–78, 80, 117, 129
Poland, studies, 123
Portugal, studies, 99
Positive Youth Development programs, 179
Post–traumatic stress disorder (PTSD), 180
Preventing Chronic Disease, 23, 44, 67
Preventive Medicine, xiv, 60, 88, 98, 266
Primary Care: Clinics in Office Practice, 211
Proceedings of the Nutrition Society, 24
Processed foods, 38–41; availability of, 62–63; children and, 60; definition of, 59; depression and, 59–60; fast food and, 61–62; limiting, 59–63; limiting, barriers and problems, 61–63; metabolic syndrome in adolescents and, 61; sodium and, 60; study of, Australia, 62; study of, Brazil, 60–61; study of, Korea, 59–62; study of, Massachusetts, 60; study of, New Zealand, 62; study of, North Carolina, 60; study of, Singapore, 60; study of, U.K., 60; taste

and, 62; teens and, 60; weight gain and, 60–61; what the experts say about, 59–60
Project EAT, 2, 4
Psychology & Behavior, 43
Psychology of Sport and Exercise, 195
Psychoneurendocrinology, 271
Public Health Nutrition, 13, 18, 24, 61–62, 71, 73

Quality of Life Research, 181
Quebec Health Insurance Board, 88

Resilience: anxiety and, 181; barriers and problems, 180–182; bipolar disorder and, 180–181; building, 178–182; characteristics of resilient children and teens, 178–179; common characteristics of resilient people, 180; depression and, 181; exposure to violence and, 180; interventions, teacher-delivered, 180; lesbian youth and, 181–182; optimism and, 180; physical activity and, 179–180; positive youth development and, 179; study of, Canada, 179; study of, China, 179; study of, Connecticut, 180; study of, Israel, 180; study of, Korea, 181; study of, New Zealand, 179; what the experts say about, 179–180

Safer sex, practicing, 221–226; barriers and problems to, 224–227; condoms, 222, 224–225; culturally sensitive media messages, 223; depression and, 225; education, 222–223; emotional component, 222–223; lesbians and, 225–226; online focus groups, 223–224; socioeconomic status and, 224–225; STIs and, 224, 226; what the experts say about, 222–224
Safety: protective gear, wearing, 158–164; seatbelts, wearing, 166–169; sports injuries, preventing, 153–157; texting while driving, 143–147; violence, learn ways to prevent, 148–152
Salt: children's preference for, 68; deficiencies, 65; excess, 66; limiting intake,

64–68; limiting intake, barriers and problems, 66–68; obesity and, 66; study of, China, 66; study of, France, 68; study of, U.K., 66; teens and, 64–65; what the experts say about, 65–66

Salud Pública de México (Public Health in Mexico), 14

San Diego Immunization Registry, 110

Scandinavian Journal of Medicine & Science in Sports, 156

Scandinavian Journal of Public Health, 243

School-Wide Positive Behavioral Intervention and Supports (SWPBIS), 184

Scientific American, 41

Scotland, studies, 51;

Screen time, limiting, 265–269; anxiety and, 266–267; barriers and problems to limiting, 267–269; body fat and, 265–267; BMI and, 266; depression and, 266–267; new schools and, 268–269; somatic symptoms and, 267; study of, Canada, 265–266; study of, Massachusetts, 266; teens and, 267; televisions and screens in the bedroom, 267–268; what the experts say about, 265–267

Second Step: Student Success Through Prevention (SS–SSTP), 151

Seatbelts, 166–169; barriers and problems to using, 168–169; factors influencing drivers who use, 167–168; incorrect use of, 169; kidney trauma and, 168; laws enforcing use of, 167; obesity and, 168–169; people who don't wear, 166–167; socioeconomic status and use of, 168; study of, Alabama, 167; study of, Illinois, 168; study of, Kurdistan, 168; study of, New York, 168–169; study of, Spain, 166–167; study of, Texas, 168; traffic injuries and, 167; vehicle collisions and, 168; what the experts say about, 166–168

Self-esteem: barriers and problems to, 191–192; body dissatisfaction and, 191; chronic illness and, 192; cyberprogram 2.0, 189; definition of, 188–189; exposure to violence and, 191; generalized

social anxiety and, 192; Girls on the Go!, 189; group mindfulness programs, 190–191; improving, 188–192; instability, 192; multiple social identities, 190; positive self-images, 190; study of, Australia, 189–191; study of, Canada, 192; study of, Germany, 190; study of, Israel, 190; study of, Minnesota, 191; study of, Spain, 189; study of, Texas, 191; study of, U.K., 190; teens, 190; what the experts say about, 189–191

Sex and dating, 205–231; dating relationships, cultivating healthy, 216–220; emergency contraception, 227–231; HPV vaccinations, 210–214; safer sex, practicing, 221–226; STIs, screening for, 205–208

Sex Roles, 197

Sexually Transmitted Diseases, 205, 207, 211

Sexually Transmitted Infections, 206

Sexually-transmitted infections (STIs): chlamydia, 205, 208; concurrent sexual relationships and, 206; gender and, 206; gonorrhea. 208; HIV, 206–208; medical providers and screening for, 207–208; medication therapy, 207; pharmacists and screening for, 207; screening for, 205–208; screening for, barriers and problems, 207–208; screening for, behavior changes as a result of, 205; screening, out-of-pocket costs, 208; self-collected samples for screening, 206–207; study of, U.S., 206–208; types of, 205; what the experts say about, 205–207

Singapore, studies, 50, 60

Singapore Chinese Health Study, 50

Skipping meals, x, 2

Sleep: academic performance and, 243; barriers and problems, 245–247; behavior and, 54–55; benefits of, 246–247; cellular phones and, 245; caffeine and, 54–55; circadian rhythm, 243; depth, 54–55; electroencephalogram (EEG), 54; getting enough, 242–247; safety concerns from not getting enough, 244; screen viewing decides and, 245–246;

study of, Alabama, 244; study of, Australia, 246–247; study of, Texas, 244; study of, Virginia, 244; video game use and, 246; weight problems and inadequate, 244–245; what the experts say about, 243

SLEEP, 246

Sleep Quality Index, 246

Slovakia, studies, 185

Smoking, 2, 18, 176, 234

Snack foods/snacking, 18; after school programs and, 44–45; container size, 45; costs of, 44–46; definition, 43; healthier, 43–46; healthier, barriers and problems accessing, 45–46; obesity and, 44–45; prompting people to eat healthier, 43–44; reasons for snacking, 43–45; school cafeteria, 45; study of, Belgium, 45; study of, Brazil, 46; study of, Iran, 45; study of, Minnesota, 46; study of, North Carolina, 46; teens and, 45–46; vending machines, 46; what the experts say about, 43–45

Social anxiety disorder, 192

social connections and friendships with peers: barriers and problems to building, 175–176; building, 173–176; gender and, 175; harmful, 175–176; instant messaging and, 175; negative influences, 176; parental support and building, 175; role in adolescent physical activity, 174–175; smoking and, 176; support from, 173–174; what the experts say about, 173–175

Socioeconomic status: bullying and, 186–187; safer sex practices and, 224–225; seatbelt use and, 168

Sodium, 60; blood pressure readings in children and adolescents, 65–66, 66–67; cardiovascular disease and, 65; food labeling of, 67; limiting intake, 64–65; limiting intake, barriers and problems, 66–68; restaurant meals, 67–68; teens and, 64, 66–67; what the experts say about, 65–66

Soft drinks, x, 78–80

South Africa, studies, 8, 132

Southern Community Cohort Study, 87

Southern Medical Journal, 146, 162, 167

Spain, studies, 40, 145, 166–167, 189

Sports: ADHD and, 92–93; after-school, 93–94; children, 92; football programs, 93, 95; drinks, 65; gender and, 93–95; group, participating in, 91–95; group, participating in, barriers and problems, 94–95; group, participating in, benefits of, 92; injuries, 94–95; injuries, lower-limb, 154; injuries, preventing, 153–157; injuries, preventing, problems and barriers, 156–157; knee injuries, 156; neuromuscular warm-ups, 154; obesity and, 93; orofacial injuries, 155–156; overuse injuries, 154; protective gear, 158–164; school-based injury preventive programs, 155, 156–157; soccer, 94; study of, Canada, 156; study of, Korea, 157; study of, Sweden, 156; study of, Turkey, 155; teen, 92, 153–154, 156–157; what the experts say about, 92–94, 154–156, 158160–162; youth development and, 93–94

Stanford Children's Health, 154

Sports, protective gear, 158–164; barriers and problems, 162–164; boxing, 161; concussions and, 163–164; cost of, 162; eye protection, 159; flag football, 160–161; helmets, 159, 161–164, 168; hockey, 162; mouthguards, 155–157; nonmotorized wheeled activities, 161–162; pads, 159, 160; risk-taking and, 162–163; safety education programs, 163; snowboarders and, 160; study of, California, 163; study of, Canada, 162–163; study of, Illinois, 163; study of, Minnesota, 162–163; traumatic brain injury and, 163; water sports, 160; what the experts say about, 160–162

Sports Medicine, 155

Stress: biofeedback and, 273; chronic, 86–87; college students and, 272; diet and, 274; physical activity and. 271–272; qigong and, 272–273; reducing, 270–274; reducing, barriers and problems, 273–274; school, 274; Type 1 diabetes and, 273; what the experts say about, 271–273

Sugar: addiction to, 81; cardiovascular health and, 76, 79; cavities and, 78–79; disaccharides, 76; -free diet, 79–81; insulin resistance, 77; metabolic syndrome, 77; monosaccharides, 76; obesity and, 76; predisposition to like, 80–81; reducing intake of, 76–81; reducing intake of, barriers and problems, 79–81; refined, 76–81; simple, 76; study of, California, 77; study of, Finland, 78; study of, Georgia, 79; study of, Massachusetts, 79; study of, Pennsylvania, 80; study of, New Zealand, 78; study of, Thailand, 78; study of, U.K., 78; -sweetened beverages, 78–79; -sweetened beverages, taxes on, 80; Type 2 diabetes and, 76–77; weight gain and, 78; what the experts say about, 77–79
Sugar Association, 76
St. Mary's Hospital, 103
Stopbullying.gov, 183–184
Sunscreen, 276–280; age and use, 278–279; appearance-based videos promoting use of, 277–278; barriers and problems with using, 278–280; college students and, 280; gender and use, 278–279; ineffective interventions, 279–280; parents and, 279; skin cancer and, 279–280; Smartphone apps, 272; televised advertising campaigns endorsing use of, 278; what the experts say about, 276–278; intervention programs, 276–277; Taekwondo, 157
Sweden, studies, 33–34, 156
Switzerland, studies, 11, 54, 71, 86–87, 89

Taiwan, studies, 106, 251–252, 255
Tanning beds, 238–241; addictive qualities of, 238, 240–241; barriers and problems to avoiding, 239–241; college campuses and, 239–240; gender and, 238; skin cancer and, 238–239; study of, California, 240; study of, China, 238; study of, Massachusetts, 238; underage rules, 240; what the experts say about, 238–239
Teen Driver Source, 166

Teen Medical Academy, 152
Tennessee, studies, 115–116, 151
Texas, studies, 13, 49, 168, 191, 197, 202, 217, 234, 236, 244, 249
Thailand, studies, 78, 106
Traffic Injury Prevention, 145
Trans fats: attention deficit/hyperactivity disorder (ADHD), 39–40; cancer and, 39; cardiovascular system and, 38–39; definition of, 38; depression and, 40; eliminating or greatly reducing, 38–41; eliminating or greatly reducing, barrier and problems, 40–41; gender and, 40; food labeling, 40–41; inventors of, 41; LDL levels and, 38–39; postmenopausal women and, 38–39; study of, Korea, 39–40; study of, Netherlands, 40; study of, Spain, 40; teens and, 39–40; what the experts say about, 38–40
Tufts University Jean Mayer USDA Human Nutrition Research Center on Aging, 38–39
Turkey, studies, 126, 145, 155, 254, 256

Understanding Society, 97
U.K. Department of Health National Diet and Nutrition Survey, 35, 66
U.K. National Diet and Nutrition Survey Rolling Programme, 127
U.K., studies, 17, 28, 50, 56–57, 60, 66, 78, 88, 97–100, 122, 135, 145–146, 190, 200, 235
U.S. Advisory Committee on Immunization Practices (ACIP), 211
U.S. Department of Agriculture, 22
U.S. Department of Health and Human Services, 48
U.S. Department of Transportation, 166
U.S. Food and Drug Administration (FDA), 70
U.S. National Health and Nutrition Examination Survey 2003–2006, 129
University of Alabama at Birmingham, 106
University of Kansas, 240
University of Massachusetts, 196
University of Michigan Health System, 117

University of Minnesota, 18; Fitness Rewards Program, xiv
University of Illinois, Urbana-Champaign, 17
University of Vermont, 22
Urine osmolality, 11–12
US News and World Report, 239
Utah, studies, 217

Vaccinations: barriers and problems, 111–113; childhood, 109; compliance, 109–110; direct messaging to parents about, 109–110; human papillomavirus (HPV), 109, 210–211; influenza, 109; parents and, 111–112; provider recommendations, 111; school-based, 110–112; states and, 112–113; study of, California, 110; teens, 109–113; what the experts say about, 109–111
Vietnam, studies, 195
Violence: adult physical health and childhood, 150; athletic coaches and, 149; childhood exposure to, 150; domestic, 149; family bonding and, 150; gender, 149–150; gun, 148; interventions, 149, 151–152, 180; learn ways to prevent, 148–152; preventing, barriers and problems, 151–152; prevention, teaching, 149, 151–152; race and, 150; school, 150–151; self-esteem and, 1914; study of, Arizona, 151; study of, Kansas, 151; study of, Illinois, 151; study of, Iraq, 150; study of, New Hampshire, 151; study of, New York, 149; study of, Tennessee, 151; study of, Washington, 148–149; what the experts say about, 149–150
Violence and Victims, 191
Virginia, studies, 120, 244, 249
Virginia Commonwealth University, 19
Virginia Department of Motor Vehicles, 244

Visceral adiposity, 117–118
Vitamin D: autism spectrum disorder and, 128; barriers and problems, 128–130; children and, 126, 129–130; coronary artery disease and, 126; deficiency, 125–130; fortification, 128; hypertension and, 126–127; metabolic syndrome and, 127; obesity and, 126–127; purpose of, 125–126; serum concentrations of, 126; sources of, 126; study of, Australia, 126, 129; study of, China, 128; study of, Netherlands, 128; study of, Turkey, 126; sun protection and, 128–129; supplementation, 129–130; teens and, 126, 129–130; Type 2 diabetes and, 127; what the experts say about, 126–128

Walking: diabetes and, 97; hypertension, 97; what the experts say about, 97–99
Washington, studies, 14, 148–149
Water, drinking sufficient, 11–14; barriers and problems, 13–14; cognitive performance and, 11–13; exercise and, 12–13; moods and, 12–13; study of, Australia, 11; study of, France, 12–13; study of, Georgia, 13; study of, Italy, 11; study of, Mexico, 12; study of, Switzerland, 11; study of, Texas, 13; study of, Washington, 14; what the experts say about, 11–13; weight loss and, 14
Water, tap, 13–14
Weight loss: mindfulness and, 203; reading food labels and, 70; walking and, 14
Wendy's, 48
Willett, Walter, 41
Wisconsin, studies, 133–134
World Health Organization (WHO), 32–33, 36, 40, 66

YMCA, 23, 44
Youth in Iceland school survey, 267

About the Authors

MYRNA CHANDLER GOLDSTEIN, MA, has been a freelance writer and independent scholar for more than 25 years. She is the author of *Healthy Oils: Fact versus Fiction*; *Healthy Herbs: Fact versus Fiction*; and *Healthy Foods: Fact versus Fiction*, as well as several other books with Greenwood Press, an imprint of ABC-CLIO.

MARK ALLAN GOLDSTEIN, MD, is founding chief of the Division of Adolescent and Young Adult Medicine at Massachusetts General Hospital and associate professor of pediatrics at Harvard Medical School. He is author or editor of numerous professional and lay publications. His research interests include studying the effects of eating disorders and malnutrition on bone mineralization in adolescents and young adults.